Dyslexia: Its Neuropsychology and Treatment

Dyslexia: Its Neuropsychology and Treatment

Edited by

George Th. Pavlidis
University of Medicine & Dentistry of New Jersey,
Rutgers Medical School, New Jersey

and

Dennis F. Fisher
US Army Human Engineering Laboratory, Maryland

JOHN WILEY & SONS
Chichester · New York · Brisbane · Toronto · Singapore

Library of Congress Cataloging-in-Publication Data:

Main entry under title:

Dyslexia: its neuropsychology and treatment.

    Based on papers from a conference held in Thessaloniki, Greece, June 1983, and co-sponsored by the Orton Dyslexia Society and the International Academy for Research in Learning Disabilities.
    Includes index.
    1. Dyslexia—Congresses.   I. Pavlidis, George Th.   II. Fisher, Dennis F. III.Orton Dyslexia Society.   IV. International Academy for Research in Learning Disabilities. [DNLM: 1. Dyslexia—congresses. WM 475 D9983 1983] RC394.W6D96   1986   616.85′53   85-16780

ISBN 0 471 90875 4

British Library Cataloguing in Publication Data:

Pavlidis, George Th.
    Dyslexia its neuropsychology and treatment.
    1. Dyslexia
    I. Title   II. Fisher, Dennis F.
    616.85′53   RC394.W6

ISBN 0 471 90875 4

Printed and bound in Great Britain.

ΣΤΗ ΜΝΗΜΗ ΤΟΥ ΠΑΤΕΡΑ ΜΟΥ

To the memory of my father

G. Th. P.

To the memory of a brilliant scientist, trusted friend, and an excellent human, to Norman Geschwind.

and

To all children who unknowingly contributed to the knowledge in this book and yet may never be able to read the words it contains.

G. Th. P. & D. F. F.

List of Contributors

ATHEY, I.

Dean, Graduate School of Education, Rutgers, The State University, New Brunswick, NJ 08903, USA

BABBITT, B. C.

Coordinator project Re-ED, University of California, Los Angeles, CA, USA.

BADDELEY, A.

Past President, Experimental Psychology Society, Director, MRC Applied Psychology Unit, 15 Chaucer Road, Cambridge CB2 2EF, England

BAKKER, D. J.

1st Vice President, International Academy for Research on Learning Disabilities; Professor of Psychology, Free University Paedological Institute, Department of Developmental & Educational Neuropsychology, Koningslaan 22, Amsterdam (2), Netherlands

BRYAN, T.

Professor of Education, College of Education, University of Illinois at Chicago, Box 4348, Chicago, IL 60680, USA

CRUICKSHANK, W. M.

Executive Director, International Academy for Research in Learning Disabilities; Professor Emeritus, University of Michigan, Ann Arbor, MI, USA

DUANE, D. D.

Past President, The Orton Dyslexia Society; Associate Professor of Neurology, Mayo Medical School; Consultant, Department of Neurology, Mayo Clinic and May Foundation; Rochester, MN 55905, USA

FISHER, D. F.

Behavioral Research Directorate, US Army Human Engineering Laboratory, MD, USA

GALABURDA, A. M.

Director, The Neurological Unit and Charles A. Dana Research Institute, Beth Israel Hospital, Department *of Neurology, Harvard Medical School, Boston, MA 02115, USA*

GESCHWIND, N.*
James Jackson, Putnam Professor of Neurology, Harvard Medical School; Director, Neurological Unit, Beth Israel Hospital 330 Brookline Avenue, Boston, MA 02215, USA; Professor of Psychology, Massachusetts Institute of Technology

GOLDGAR, D. E.
Boys Town National Institute, Omaha, NE, USA

HOLLANDER, H. E.
Chief Psychologist, Community Mental Health Center, UMDNJ-Rutgers Medical School, NJ 08854, USA

JOHNSON, D. J.
Director, Learning Disabilities Program, Northwestern University, 2299 Sheridan Road, Evanston, IL, 60201, USA

KEOGH, B. K.
Professor of Education, Moore Hall, University of California, Los Angeles, CA 90024, USA

KIMBERLING, W. J.
Boys Town National Institute, Omaha, NE, USA

KINSBOURNE, M.
Eunice Kennedy Schriver Center, 200 Trapelo Road, Waltham, MA 02254, USA

LEONG, C. K.
Professor of Education, Institute of Child Guidance and Development, University of Saskatchewan, Saskatoon, Saskatchewan S7N 0WO, Canada

LICHT, R.
Free University, Paedological Institute, Koningslaan 22, Amsterdam (2), Netherlands

LUBS, H. A.
University of Miami, Miami, FL, USA

MATĚJČEK, Z.
Postgraduate Medical Institute, Nam. Kub. Revoluce 24, 100 00 Praha 10, Czechoslovakia

MILES, T. R.
Head, Department of Psychology, University College of North Wales, Department of Psychology, Bangor, Gwynedd LL57 2DG, Wales, United Kingdom

PAVLIDIS, G. TH.
2nd Vice President, International Academy for Research in Learning Disabilities; Director, Eye movement and Dyslexia project Department of Pediatrics, UMDNJ-Rutgers Medical School, Piscataway, NJ 08854 USA; Research Professor of Psychology, F. D. University

* Deceased

PENNINGTON, B. F.   *Professor of Genetics, University of Colorado, Health Sciences Center, Denver, CO, USA*

RAWSON, M. B.   *Editor-in Chief for The Orton Dyslexia Society, Box 31, Route 12, Frederick, MD 21701; Formerly Associate Professor of Sociology, Hood College, MD, USA*

RAYNER, K.   *Professor of Psychology, Department of Psychology, University of Massachusetts, Amherst, MA, USA*

SMITH, S. D.   *Boys Town National Institute, Omaha, NE, USA*

STURMA, J.   *Child Psychiatric Clinic, Dolni Pocernice, Praha, Czechoslovakia*

TORGESEN, J. K.   *Professor of Psychology, Psychology Department, Florida State University, Tallahassee, FL 32306, USA*

WILSON, B.   *Rivermead Rehabilitation Centre, Abington Road, Oxford OX1 4XD, England*

WOLF, N.   *Psychology Department, Florida State University, Tallahassee, FL 32306, USA*

Contents

EXPERIMENTAL FINDINGS

TREATMENT

Foreword

Dyslexia, a term which appeared in the literature for the first time about 1886. It is a term which, since that time, is replete with widely differing definitions and misunderstood by many practitioners. The second edition of *Webster's Unabridged Dictionary* omits the word entirely, although the publication of that volume appeared many years after 1886. The problem, however, is compounded because professional usage of the word goes beyond the dictionary definition (when that can be found). The term derives from 'logos' meaning 'the word' in ancient Greek. Some translators also define it to mean 'speech', but this usage does not appear frequently in modern professional literature. The meaning leans also on the French language and perhaps more so on so-called new Latin.

The Greek logos, while coming close to the English use of the word in modern scientific papers, doesn't convey the meaning exactly. In St John's Gospel there occurs a phrase and sentence: 'In the beginning was the *word*, and the word was God.' In this instance word, or logos, referred to a specific dogma handed down from a spiritual source for the people to follow. That is a far cry from the contemporary definition of dyslexia which, when located ultimately, merely refers to an 'inability to read', the opposite of ability to read words. This simplistic statement is undoubtedly in large measure the cause for the variety of over-simplified usages which appear, particularly in the writings of educators and psychologists, although not one of the professions involved can claim universal accuracy in its use of the term. An authority in the field of reading has recently stated in a new book that 'children with any form of reading impairment are known as dyslexic'.

This concept of dyslexia, while accurate in some instances, is almost totally wrong in its implication that all forms of reading *in children* fall within this definition. There are adults with accurately defined dyslexia as there are adolescents. This is not a problem restricted to the childhood years, and statements to the contrary by those who should know better are misleading and do the field a disservice.

It is interesting, perhaps by coincidence, that the papers included in this volume developed from two independent conferences held in June of 1983 in

Halkidiki in the northern part of Greece. The first was a smaller conference attended by approximately thirty of the world's leadership in this area of human development, and the second was the much larger and 2nd World Congress on Dyslexia, that was co-sponsored professionally by The Orton Dyslexia Society and the International Academy for Research in Learning Disabilities.

It is also interesting to this writer that the issue of the definition of dyslexia never came up in the discussions during the conference as a basis for disagreement or argument. Neuroanatomists, pediatricians, neuropsychologists, neuroeducators, and others representing other disciplines related to dyslexia, spoke from a common consensus and understanding, namely, all learning is neurologically based and dyslexia is a form of learning disability related to reading, the recognition of words, and the interpretation of what is seen visually or heard auditorily which is the result of a neurophysiological dysfunction. Argument regarding this statement was not heard during the first week of the invitational conference, nor indeed during the second week when more than a hundred additional participants joined the original group for a more open forum. To the specialist who knows this problem and who is devoting his or her professional life to a further understanding of its etiological and therapeutic complexities, the concept of neurophysiological dysfunction is a commonly accepted point of view. To those who come upon the term as *dilettanti* during whose college or university training there was little or no emphasis on gross human anatomy, neuroanatomy, or neurophysiology it is easy to understand the often-held misconceptions that dyslexia is but another form of reading dysfunction which will respond to the usual remedial reading approaches of the typical school or clinic reading program. Nothing could be further from the truth. Dyslexia, in whatever form it takes—mild, moderate, or severe—is one of the most complicated central nervous system problems there is. Until today it demands thoughtful, interdisciplinary diagnostic efforts. The absence of diagnosis, leads to insurmountable hurdles to successful life adjustment of the individual.

In 1963 another term appeared in the clinical literature, namely, *learning disabilities*. This term, for which there are recorded more than forty synonyms (one of which is dyslexia) swept the professional world as the be-all and end-all of the perplexing children whom neither professional educators nor parents know how to serve adequately. Some grave errors were made in the early years following the appearance of this term. The International Reading Association claimed ownership of the term, as did the American Speech and Hearing Association. The School Psychology Division of the American Psychological Association, and the American Occupational Therapy Association, among other professional groups, each and all claimed the child with learning disabilities to be its responsibility. Physicians from pediatrics and neurology were among the last to become actively interested in this child, and since usually they had had no orientation to these problems during either their pre-medical or their post-medical training, they were usually unable to be of much service to the clients referred to them. This remains true unfortunately as we write.

More recently 'learning disabilities' has become a much more generic term. It is generally defined as a problem in a child which is illustrated by academic, social, or emotional disabilities, which in turn are the result of perceptual processing deficits (neurological), which in turn finally are the result of a defined (or assumed) neurophysiological dysfunction, the etiology of which is prenatal, perinatal, or postnatal. Although this statement has not been accepted word for word, the concepts are generally those incorporated in the recently adopted definition of the Canadian Association for Children with Learning Disabilities. The same concepts are embodied in the statement, yet unanimously accepted, of the (USA) Joint Committee on the Definition of Learning Disabilities.

Within this generic statement of learning disabilities are identified a number of clinical subsets (on which, it must be pointed out, there is not complete professional agreement). Within this broad grouping of children, adolescents, and adults would be found those with dyslexia and aphasia. Included also is a high percentage (89.9 per cent) of a large group of athetoid and spastic-type cerebral palsy children under sixteen years of age. About one-third of certain subtypes of children with epilepsy show the same psychopathological characteristics as those with learning disabilities, and in varying percentages other clinical populations, for example hyperactive emotionally disturbed children and youth, exogenous mentally retarded children (both educable and trainable), and probably socially maladjusted–delinquent youth. A high incidence of survivors of Reye's disease has been reported as having been learning disabled prior to the onset of the virus, and most recently autism, particularly in some animal forms, has been related to learning disabilities.

It is not my intention through over-simplification to lump many clinical neurological problems together as a single clinical entity. We are stating that a relatively long list of clinical problems, each known to have or to be suspected of having a neurological base, have much in common with accurately defined dyslexia. Nor are we saying that each of the clinical entities mentioned in the preceding paragraphs is synonymous with dyslexia. We are stating that dyslexia forms a neurological problem closely associated with other known neurological dysfunctions, and as such must be considered from this point of view both diagnostically and therapeutically. This point of view is reflected in numerous of the papers included in this volume.

The sad element in this total situation is that preprofessional students in their training rarely receive any understanding of the position of dyslexia in relation to other forms of learning disabilities. Commonalities in terms of psychopathology are rarely pointed out, i.e. attention disturbances, figure–ground pathology, auditory and/or visual perceptual processing deficits, dissociation, perseveration, and a myriad of other commonly recognized neuropsychological and neurophysiological characteristics which invade good academic achievement, social adjustment, and emotional development. Until dyslexia is viewed from this organic point of view, therapeutic regimens will be inappropriately conceptualized, university preparation of new professionals will limit their ability to function adequately, and clients with dyslexia will not receive appropriate efforts to bring them to the maximum of their capacities.

WILLIAM M. CRUICKSHANK, PH.D.
Executive Director,
International Academy for Research in Learning Disabilities,
Ann Arbor, Michigan

Introduction

The interdisciplinary nature of inquiry into the problems of dyslexia has provided a rich source of hypothesis testing and frustration. Why is it that with so many minds working in so many directions that a 'cure' for reading problems has not been found? From the many papers and books that have been published on dyslexia we are a little clearer in our knowledge of what does and what does not work to alleviate the difficulties that the dyslexics have with reading, spelling, arithmetic and with the speedy execution of sequential tasks. This volume aims at providing experimental data and theories that contribute to a better understanding of the causes, effects, diagnosis, and treatment of dyslexia.

The individual dyslexic, of course, is subjected to a number of injustices in school, society, and the work place. Dyslexia is a difficult topic to research because not all dyslexics present the same symptomatology, a fact that often leads to confusion and controversy. A large portion of this volume is dedicated to describing the characteristics, consequences, and subtypes of dyslexia. The perspectives of psychological, educational, neurological, and sociological concerns reported in this volume are in no way meant to be comprehensive, but they are rather directed at giving the reader a sense of the tremendous complexity of the problem that has both interfered with and enhanced our understanding for well over one-hundred years.

SAMPLING AND DEFINING:
METHODOLOGICAL ISSUES

Looking at the person next to you will reveal little about their ability to process language. In Chapter 1 Rawson points out many of the contributors to poor language function. Her model is particularly useful in pointing out characteristics of the disability from interactions of the receptive and expressive components of visible and auditory language. The second chapter in this section features Keogh and Babbitt's concerns for valid comparisons of various reading disabled samples. Their marker system provides a useful means of maximizing similarities within and between groups as well as between reading and mathematic disabilities. Chapter 3 is meant as a cautionary note for researcher, by Fisher and Athey. Too frequently too few controls are designed into the research protocol, or even worse, descriptive statements are made of characteristics of dyslexics without noting the characteristics of normal readers. Part of that requirement is the inclusion of control groups matched for reading and age levels to dyslexics.

Neurological issues

In the first chapter in this section, Galaburda describes some of the more current findings regarding cortical involvement. Here the philosophy of the animal model for examining developing hemispheric specialization is described along with some exciting notions of cell migration and the testosterone connection. That same connection is further described by Geschwind where left-handedness, cerebral dominance, autoimmune disorders, and testosterone levels are correlated with familial incidence. Duane, in the last chapter of this section, describes the contributions of technology to our understanding of cortical anatomy and function. Three of these, computed tomography, nuclear magnetic resonance, and brain electrical activity mapping (BEAM) provide new resources in characterizing the disorder prior to mortality. He is quick to relate limitations however, but is optimistic about future advances.

EMPIRICAL FINDINGS

In his analysis of the contribution of language awareness to reading proficiency, Leong points out that the reading acquisition process is a complex interaction of psycholinguistic (syntactic, semantic) and cognitive awareness. It is therefore possible for each level of processing to break down at any of innumerable loci. Each characteristic of the break down is then traceable to poor systemization, hypothesis generation, surface and/or deep structural confusion among others. The second chapter by Rayner examines some of the perceptual aspects of dyslexia by exploring the possibility that disabled readers simply do not have as great a functional perceptual span as normal readers and therefore cannot process as much information during a single fixation. While both language deficit and visual–spatial deficit dyslexics have somewhat different eye-movement patterns from normal readers, data presented could not confirm these patterns as the cause of the disability or that the smaller span is accountable for the large differences in reading. The third chapter in this section by Pavlidis examines in more detail the three major hypotheses of the relationship between erratic eye movements and dyslexia: These postulate that eye movements: (a) reflect ongoing problems during processing of text; (b) cause dyslexia; and (c) erratic eye movements and dyslexia do not have to be causally related, but rather they stem from common or parallel brain malfunctions.

The fourth chapter in this section by Bakker and Licht makes an account of the differences in processing capability in younger as compared to older readers. A somewhat acknowledged means of describing those differences has been between a concentration early on with visual–perceptual aspects of the text with practice leading to automaticity, and concentrating on the meaning (semantic/syntactic). While the evidence for such a shift has been well documented these authors account for it on the basis of shifting importance of processing from the right to the left hemisphere. When, why, and how may not be as obvious but dyslexics may find it more difficult to make the transition from right to left hemisphere. Miles is concerned with the acknowledgement of the dyslexic into adulthood. He presents data showing that bright adult dyslexics are much slower than younger normal readers in performing reading and non-reading tasks.

In contrast to the more historical perspective that dyslexia is a unitary disability, the notion of subtypes represents an exciting and compelling means of better understanding the problems of dyslexics. Two chapters, the first by Kinsbourne and the second by Smith and her associates, describe some of the important descriptive techniques and hence, insights into remediation that are coming to light. Whether neurological, genetic or statistically isolable each of the subtypes is found to be unique in aspects of poor performance in certain domains but a great amount of overlap also exists between the various subtypes.

Dealing with a disability involves more than remediation of the specifics of that disability as Bryan points out. There are factors of personality that are equally disturbed in terms of self-concept and propensity to learn. An important though frequently overlooked problem is attribution: Who's fault is it 'that I can't do things like the others!' 'I could but . . .', and trying not to fail again leads to a fatalistic attitude. Some dyslexics succeed, some get along in nonliterature occupations but many remain sensitive to failure. The retarded reader from a low socioeconomic background who is the focus of Hollander's chapter experiences problems with delinquency. For some the frustrations seem to get too high and the work too difficult. For others, peer approval or striking out against an unfair society leads to incarceration and further confirmation of failure. Will reading remediation in itself reduce recidivism?

PEDAGOGICAL CONCERNS

In the first chapter of this section, Johnson describes a remediation program for adults developed at Northwestern University which has as its strength the diagnosis of multi-faceted components of the disability. Here the individual is of concern and remediation is targeted to the weaknesses. Making the individual aware of different processing capabilities is as functional to vocational success as it is in attacking reading difficulties. Enhanced self-image is frequently an unexpected reward.

Matějček and Sturma describe some of the models of reading remediation being used in Czechoslovakia. The government is now actively involved in servicing the needs of reading disabled students and screening procedures are in effect throughout the country. Where facilities are not available, the children are taken in residence and given intensive care until ready to return to their community. These educators were pioneers in their country and their account of the developing awareness is intriguing. In the third chapter of this section, Wilson and Baddeley describe a single case remediation plan for an acquired dyslexic. While the method is tedious it is worth the effort especially to set up what might seem to be a propensity to learn. The rigors of the technique are described as are the rewards in what seems like a statement of joy to learn and retain information. A brief overview into the new field of computer-aided instruction is provided by Torgeson and Wolf in the last chapter of this section. They review a number of programs and present their strengths and weaknesses. While they feel the future is bright for such technology much work from classroom data collection to software development must be done.

ORIGINS: A GREEK EXPERIENCE

The complexities inherent in a topic like dyslexia demand ideas from around the world. Such was the case in June of 1983, at Halkidiki, Greece, where just a few steps from the birthplace of Aristotle, many leading researchers and educators met to learn more about dyslexia in two independent meetings. A small *Interdisciplinary Consortium on Dyslexia* was organized by Dennis F. Fisher and was sponsored by the US Army Human Engineering Laboratory.*

The *2nd World Congress on Dyslexia* was a larger meeting that offered the opportunity to experts from eastern and western nations to share their knowledge and experiences. It was organized by George Th. Pavlidis and was sponsored by the International Academy for Research in Learning Disabilities and The Orton Dyslexia Society. It is our hope that future international conferences will continue to better our understanding of dyslexia, to lead to its early diagnosis, and to its effective treatment.

GEORGE TH. PAVLIDIS
DENNIS F. FISHER

* Dr Fisher expresses special appreciation to its director, Dr John Weiss, for his continued support of both basic and applied research.

General—Methodological Issues

CHAPTER 1

Developmental Stages and Patterns of Growth of Dyslexic Persons

MARGARET BYRD RAWSON
Foxes Spy, 7924 Rocky Springs Rd, Frederick, MD 21701, USA

It is too obvious to need stating, but too important to neglect, that each human coming into the world brings a quite unique set of genes into his or her life; but nature has already been, and continuingly will be, influenced by nurture. It is equally obvious that there are characteristics that this person shares, both initially and developmentally, with all other human beings. Here we have his evolutionary inheritance: the limits of bodily form and function, the apparently inherent urge to grow and learn, initial plasticity and adaptiveness, what we sometimes call a social nature, and many other components of this complexity.

There are ways, too, in which he is like some, but not all, other persons: characteristics that categorize him as a member of each of a large number of groups or classes: sex, size, shape, color, and particular mental and physical attributes. As you look about you, you observe that everyone *has* such attributes and, with ease or difficulty, you can find persons who match one or many of the traits you are aware of in yourself or others, supposing that such a match matters to you or to them! In this connection, a book to own and pore over is Spier's (1980) delightful anthropology in pictures: *PEOPLE*. It is frequently convenient, useful, necessary, and even desirable, to see, or sort, or work with, people in groups, where their common characteristics serve a purpose and their differences do not greatly matter.

On the other hand, the essence of personhood lies in those very differences, the pattern of positions that each person takes on the many dimensions of life in nature and nurture, the dynamics of movement on each dimension, and the interactional effects of each upon the others. Our subject is, for instance, older today, perhaps healthier, maybe a more confused student of Arabic, wearing new spectacles, knowing from yesterday's session with the psychologist that 'dyslexia' names the problem he is all-too-familiar with, and yet, from today's hour with the language therapist, that there is real hope of a successful way out. We need not press the familiar point of individual uniqueness beyond reminding ourselves that while we may deal with persons in groups, it is as individuals that they respond, and learn, and grow. This truth is crucial; we neglect to pay attention to it at everyone's cost—our clients', our own, and society's.

Now let us backtrack and consider as our matrix the patterns of development of specifically dyslexic persons of all ages, for this is one of the generally identifiable groups in our world population. Everywhere, across language and cultural boundaries, there seem to be some basic similarities in those we may tag 'dyslexic', or with some equivalent label. The people I am thinking of here have in common a variety of difficulties in mastering the skills their culture expects of them in the use of their mother tongue. This includes the spoken language that each culture on this earth has, and its written or printed form if the culture be a literate one. I have been interested in many languages and cultures and have learned from them—from the Czech to the Chinese, from the Dutch to the Yugoslav, and others. However, English, mostly North American English, is the only language of which I can legitimately speak in depth.

When an American or English child is born, he comes into anything but a homogeneous language community. He may be born with the proverbial 'silver spoon in his mouth', 'the inheritor of a silver tongue' spoken by a family that uses English with ease, precision, grace, and effectiveness. He may be of upper, middle, professional, or working class; with two parents or one; with or without siblings to imitate and stimulate. Perhaps he will find himself in a family and a community where standard English (however defined) has to take its chance with predominant Spanish, Chinese, Gullah, or other speech by which he may be surrounded, or with a marked dialect giving some strong regional flavor to his understanding and speech. Even within such groups there are important differences in the amount and quality of communication, and in the child's place in his family and community.

No matter what the language, some constitutional, many-dimensional differences are obvious from the beginning. Many differences, formerly not easily observed in infancy, have been coming to light in recent years. Some are detectable and measurable in the very young infant, such as response at as early as two to four weeks of age to perceivable differences in speech sounds like the voiced and unvoiced consonants /p/ and /b/. Later, but still before the use of the first utterances that adults define as words, understanding of some speech is apparent, and not a few vocalizations are used with intent to communicate, perhaps even symbolically, Here, one might say, are roots of language development in the individual, even before what I like to call 'the Vygotsky Milestone', (see Vygotsky, 1934)—the stage at which 'thought [evident from behaviour] becomes verbal, and speech [whose elements have

VERBAL LANGUAGE

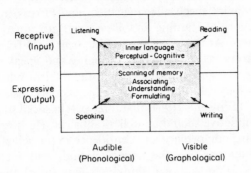

Figure 1. Analysis of verbal language, from Rawson (1975). Reproduced by permission of York Press, Inc.

been practiced] becomes rational'. At these earliest stages the individual's linguistic fingerprints appear, if only we can read them. Someday we may be able to predict with greater confidence who is likely to become 'eulexic' and who 'dyslexic' (using the Greek prefixes *eu-* and *dys-* to distinguish, respectively, those who are *good* or *poor* at acquiring the skills of *lexis—language.*) Then perhaps we can know better how we may enhance the former and help the latter, with concurrent regard for weaknesses, strengths and needs in nonlinguistic as well as language characteristics.

In the time and manner of the young child's achievement of the Vygotsky Milestone, differences between extremes of future eulexia and dyslexia become apparent. These show up in the several sensory modalities: kinesthetic (a relationship too often neglected), auditory, and visual, and in 'getting it all together' in inner language or verbal thinking, looking perhaps especially at left-cerebral hemisphere activity, as in Figure 1, reprinted from an earlier paper (Rawson, 1975) but still opposite.

So far, most of us have reached the anecdotal rather than even the statistical stage of description, let alone confident prediction of the child's language development. Anything is still possible at age two, but there are already alerting signs.

Next, from say two to four or five years, comes the period of extremely rapid growth in mastery of verbal variety, syntactic or grammatical structure, and semantic content or meaning—the manipulation of language and capacity for metalinguistic awareness, that is, awareness of language as language. At this stage structure, including morphemic and syllabic and eventually phonemic segmentation, become increasingly important. The child has achieved basic linguistic acculturation, at least in his mother tongue which he now manages more easily than most non-native speakers ever will.

From the complex welter of developmental patterns we can perhaps usefully partial out at this point specific language learning factors from those of the more general category of learning disabilities, as I attempted to do in a 1978 paper on the subject. At this point one might focus on difficulties specific to the language function, as shown in the Listening and Speaking quadrants of Figure 1. Perhaps we can appropriately call the difficulty here Dyslexia I.

By what we generally call school age, six or thereabouts, the child has normally progressed through Erikson's (1964) first three psychosocial stages; Basic Trust, Autonomy, and Initiative should be well established. He is ready to enter the period of developing competence and confidence in the achievement of skills, the years psychoanalysts call the latency period, and Piaget (1926/1953) designates the age of 'operational thinking', with all of the accompanying changes in orientation and functions described by White (1979). The youngster is, in the normal course, ready to tackle the sensory, integrational, more abstract intellectual tasks required in becoming literate, (the Reading and Writing quadrants of Figure 1) which will occupy him intensively for several of his pre-adolescent years and demand varying degrees of attention and effort throughout the rest of his life.

We are all familiar with the vastness of the literature on reading and writing disabilities produced in the years since Orton's (1925) focusing paper and the subsequent literature treating theories and findings about causes, characteristics, diagnostic assessments and treatment efforts. One recent bibliography of some 2400 annotated items confined to 'dyslexia', with varying definitions (Evans, 1982), is less than complete and reaches only into 1976. Buried in this plethora of print are some very significant findings, together with some material that is interesting and promisingly worth watching, and a very great deal that, to put it politely, we can readily do without. To encompass what is relevant as theory and useful in practice from the work going on in the several disciplinary fields makes me, for one, wish, after nearly fifty years at work on it, for an extra lifetime or so, preferably running concurrently with this one.

About our lexic (language learner-user), be he *eu*, *dys*, or in between, there is so much to say that I cannot even summarize it, except as did Alfred, that real and oft-quoted (see Rawson, 1972) ten-year-old, 'I can think OK. What's wrong is just my words. I forget them and I can't manage them'. He may have had problems with spoken language, remediated or not (our Dyslexia I), or there may have been no difficulties to speak of in his early years, and yet he may find the graphic cipher on the spoken code inordinately difficult to master without expert help. We might call this Dyslexia II, or the common reading disability where the Latin root *legere*, *to read*, is sometimes used, although it needs to be enlarged to include problems in spelling, handwriting, and written expression in a variety of forms. We have much clinical and some statistical evidence to show that, with the right help, the learner can become competently literate at levels commensurate with his other abilities and his appropriate life-style expectations, even if his IQ reaches in the 190s or his achievements eventually result in a Nobel prize. Truly, what the linguistically facile seem to absorb with little or no trouble and the rest of us can reach with reasonable effort, the dyslexic can usually aspire to if he gets the right help—as have many young people my colleagues and I have followed into adulthood (see Rawson, 1968; Finucci *et al.*, 1983).

For the briefest and simplest, and yet I think sound, summary, of all this, I refer you to the Orton Dyslexia Society's approved statement, 'What is Dyslexia?' (1981). It defines, describes, prescribes and predicts as well as could be managed in four pages.

If our school-age child reaches adolescence without diagnosis, or with no or inadequate treatment, he is probably in bad trouble, perhaps of several kinds. He is in desperate need of diagnosis and treatment, both educational and therapeutic, to stave off disaster or to reduce disability to manageable difficulty and free him for development. He has more to learn and to unlearn than if he had come to us earlier, but, on the other hand, his greater maturity, capacity for abstract thinking, and responsible motivation, appropriately used, can speed up his rate of progress.

Is adolescence or adulthood too late for diagnosis and, especially, for educational treatment of this kind? By no means! I have seen, and sometimes participated in, such 'rescues'; cases which attest to the truth of the adage 'It is never too late to start; and it is always too soon to stop, as long as the will is there—or can be re-awakened'. We can also take advantage of the 'spiral of growth' phenomenon, discussed in Whitehead's (1929) *Aims of Education*, repetition on progressively higher levels.

Whatever his age, the dyslexic person may expect to go through essentially the same stages of learning, tailored to his personal needs and capacities. The appropriate constraints are contained in the injunction to 'Teach the language as it is to the person as he is', which includes: (1) teaching expertly; (2) one's language, well known as language; (3) to a human-type learner (*homo symbolicus*); (4) with due regard for his uniqueness as an individual.

If the student has had appropriate help earlier, he may (or may not) need further sorts of tuition as he responds to the demands of secondary school, college and adult life, especially in more demanding academic subjects. Perhaps, too, he should have available support services and adaptation of some requirements (for example, oral or untimed tests), and we should expect to see him again as he brings us at least one of his sons as have many of our 'graduates', but now in time for nearer-optimum results.

Always appropriate in all our relationships is caution about being sure that our client shall continue to be for us a whole person and not become lost in those fractions of him that we must examine and work with. Both the student and his mentors should remain conscious that dyslexia, rather than pointing to a defect or a deficiency, indicates a *kind of mind*, inherent and persistent.

It may well be a very fine mind, intelligent and especially creative, which its owner can make work better and better, for himself and for us, through a continuing life of unique personal and social fulfillment.

The 'diversity model', to which I subscribe, (Rawson, 1981) points, on the whole I believe, to strength in the human race, in its adaptability to a world of change and increasingly challenging demands to which the intelligence and creativity so often found among dyslexic persons can make highly significant contributions.

REFERENCES

Erikson, E. H. (1964), *Childhood and Society*. New York, W. W. Norton.

Evans, M. M. (1982), *Dyslexia: An Annotated Bibliography*. Westport, CT, Greenwood Press.

Finucci, J. M., Pulver, A. E., Isaacs, S. D., and Childs, B. (1983), The natural history of specific reading disability. *Educational Outcomes*. Submitted for publication.

Orton, S. T. (1925), "Word-blindness" in school children. *Archives of Neurology and Psychiatry* 14, 581–615.

Orton Dyslexia Society (1982), What is dyslexia? Baltimore, MD, The Orton Dyslexia Society. [Four-page position statement.]

Piaget, J. (1926/1959), *The Language and Thought of the Child*. London, Routledge & Kegan Paul.

Rawson, M. B. (1968), *Developmental Language Disability: Adult Accomplishments of Dyslexic Boys*. Baltimore, MD, The Johns Hopkins University Press. Second printing (1978), Cambridge, MA, Educators Publishing Service.

Rawson, M. B. (1972), Language learning differences in plain English. *Academic Therapy* 7, 4, 411–419.

Rawson, M. B. (1975), Developmental dyslexia: educational treatment and results. In: D. D. Duane and M. B. Rawson (Eds.), *Reading, Perception, and Language*. Baltimore, MD, York Press.

Rawson, M. B. (1978), Dyslexia and learning disabilities: their relationship. *Bulletin of the Orton Society* 28, 43–61.

Rawson, M. B. (1981), A diversity model for dyslexia. In: G. Th. Pavlidis and T. R. Miles, *Dyslexia Research and its Applications to Education*. Chichester, John Wiley.

Spier, P. (1980), *PEOPLE*. Garden City, NY, Doubleday.

Vygotsky, L. S. (1934), *Thought and Language* (in Russian). English translation (1962) by E. Hanfman and G. Vakar. Cambridge, MA, MIT Press.

White, S. (1970), Some general outlines of the matrix of developmental changes between five and seven years. *Bulletin of the Orton Society* 20, 41–57.

Whitehead, A. N. (1929), *The Aims of Education*, New York, Macmillan.

CHAPTER 2

Sampling Issues in Learning Disabilities Research: Markers for the Study of Problems in Mathematics

BARBARA K. KEOGH and BEATRICE C. BABBITT
University of California, Los Angeles, USA

INTRODUCTION

Replicability and generalizability continue to be useful criteria for judging products of scientific enquiry. Indeed, objective, public replication is a fundamental tenet of modern science, and the generalizability of findings might be viewed as one indicator of value. Given their importance, it is somewhat discouraging that much of the ongoing research in the learning disabilities (LD) field is unreplicated and is of limited generalizability. Despite the popularity of LD as a research topic, and despite an increasingly voluminous literature, LD continues to be a subject which is conceptually muddied and operationally diverse. In a recent review Farnham-Diggory (1980) noted, 'We are not sure what the precise symptoms of learning disabilities are, what causes them, or how they manifest themselves in schoolwork, and we are not sure how to fix them' (p. 570). There is considerable accuracy in this rather pessimistic assessment of the state of the art, as even cursory review of the literature will attest.

Inconsistent findings may be a function of task, of operational definition and measurement, or of sampling. All are threats to external validity. Farnham-Diggory (1980) emphasizes the importance of task, arguing that laboratory tasks differ from each other and differ also from the tasks which children are expected

The mathematics sections of this chapter were prepared for presentation at the International Conference on Dyscalculia, sponsored by the International Academy for Research in Learning Disabilities (IARLD), held in Brussels, Belgium, September 7–9, 1983.

to do in school. Thus, it should not surprise us that findings differ across studies and that children perform differently in the laboratory and in the school room. Definition and techniques of measurement also may influence findings. We might agree that visual perception is related to beginning reading skill, but we might find quite different results if we operationally define visual perception as performance on the Bender Gestalt Test, as ability to recognize nonsense figures presented at high speed, or as ability to match visually presented words without time constraints. Certainly external validity relates to the nature of the task and to the techniques employed in any given study.

External validity may also be viewed from a somewhat different perspective, as it is reasonable that limited replicability and generalizibility relate to sampling practices (Keogh and MacMillan, 1983). Said directly, results may differ because subjects differ. The LD label is broad, and it subsumes many different kinds of problems (Kirk and Elkins, 1975; Norman and Zigmond, 1980). In addition to variation in symptom patterns and referral conditions, in many LD studies the range of individual differences on fundamental subject characteristics (e.g. chronological age, IQ) is broad, and the possible impact of this variation on the study focus is unknown. It should come as no surprise that findings do not replicate or that there is limited generalizability of results across studies. In many instances samples are composed of different kinds of LD subjects. It is the sampling aspect of external validity that we address in this paper.

SAMPLING AND RESEARCH DESIGNS

As noted by Cronbach (1957) almost thirty years ago, the demonstration of treatment effects (read intervention in special education) assumes similarity of subjects or homogeneity of sample. In the experimental method the investigator attempts to reduce sample variance and to avoid threats to the internal validity of the study so that it is possible to infer that outcomes or changes are caused by the treatment or intervention. We might like to infer, for example, that a certain reading program improved learning disabled (LD) children's reading skills, or that social skills training leads to better interpersonal competencies. We might also like to be able to state with confidence that Program A is better than Program B for changing arithmetic skills, or that Yoga is more effective than Zen in improving attention of hyperactive children. In the strictest sense, to test treatments or to compare among treatments, we must be assured that subjects in the various conditions are similar, and that their assignment to groups was random. Even superficial examination of the LD research literature suggests that neither of these conditions is met regularly.

MacMillan (1983, personal communication) has suggested that the issue of sampling is also important in descriptive research where the investigator may use a causal-comparative design to contrast the attributes of a selected group of handicapped individuals with a 'normal' control group (probably more accurately described as a comparison group). In such designs the goal is to describe similarities and differences between or among selected groups, to determine if the various samples were drawn from the same population. As emphasized by Keogh and MacMillan (1983), in many cases inferences about between-group differences are drawn neglecting large within-group variability; and, samples may not accurately represent the populations targeted by the investigator. Sampling threats to external validity, thus, deserve serious consideration.

Sampling and External Validity

Review of the research literature in the LD field suggests that most study samples are drawn from predefined populations or groups, e.g. special education classes or programs, clinic rosters, case registers. In their discussion of sampling issues in research on mental retardation, MacMillan, Meyers, and Morrison (1980) refer to these subjects or samples as 'system-identified'. That is, research subjects are drawn from a pool of individuals who have been identified by someone else for some other purposes, usually to provide needed services or treatments. The number and characteristics of system-identified individuals, thus, reflect the criteria and practices of the selecting system. Importantly for this discussion, criteria and selection practices may vary according to geographic location, time of selection, or richness or paucity of resources. For example, in school districts with many resources, extensive special services are often provided and many pupils may be identified as eligible for services. In districts where resources are curtailed, fewer services are available and fewer pupils will be identified.

Identification and selection are not just a matter of resources, of course, but may also reflect the perspective of the identifying agency. To illustrate, in one clinic LD may be defined as a neurologically based condition, and identification and selection may depend upon a neurologist's diagnosis. In another clinic LD may be defined as a language-based problem, and only children with signs of language disabilities may be selected. While there would likely be some overlap in samples, there might well be differences which pose a threat to generalizability or replication of findings and to inferences about 'LDness'.

Keogh and MacMillan (1983) note, too, that because LD is in large part an exclusionary definition, identification as LD depends in part on the criteria for identification as something else. Thus, the time of selection may be important in understanding the composition of LD research samples. The relationship between LD and mild mental retardation is illustrative. In the 1960s the definition of mild mental retardation (EMR) included a cutoff point of one standard deviation below the mean, an IQ of 85; relatively high functioning children were eligible for special education services as EMR under the definition. With the change in the AAMD definition, setting a cutoff point of two standard deviations below the mean, an IQ of 70, many children formerly identified as EMR became eligible for services under the LD rubric. Indeed, examination of current samples in LD research suggests that many LD subjects are within the IQ range 70 to 85 (Norman and Zigmond, 1980). To confound the sample issue further, in a recent review of children served in federally funded Child Service Demonstration Centers, Mann *et al.* (1983) found that the majority of programs served children below the IQ cutoff of 70. While the provision of services to all children with special educational needs is to be applauded, one implication for researchers is that selection of system-identified subjects poses a serious potential threat to external validity, and that within-sample variation must be taken into account.

The characteristic heterogeneity within and across samples in LD research received detailed documentation in the UCLA Marker Variable Project (Keogh *et al.*, 1978, 1980, 1982). This project was carried out from 1977 to 1980 through a grant from the Field Initiated Research Program of the then Bureau of Education for the Handicapped (BEH) of the US Office of Education. As part of the Project a systematic, comprehensive review of the empirical research on learning disabilities was conducted to identify operational criteria used for subject selection and description. Prior to a computer search, a hand search of 23 journals identified disciplines or professions contributing to LD research and allowed specification of terms used to label and describe samples. Four search systems (ERIC, ECEA, PA, and MEDLINE or Index Medicus) yielded 4618 LD citations. Data-based articles were categorized according to discipline of journal and to age of subjects studied. This categorization yielded a 15-cell discipline by age matrix. A random but proportional selection of 408 articles within the matrix ensured a representative literature.

Detailed sample information abstracted from the 408 articles included sample size, demographics, source of subjects, terms used to label subjects, tests and assessment techniques, specific inclusionary or exclusionary criteria, and type of study. The abstracting procedures provided a detailed mapping of the research literature in LD and documented the variations and inconsistencies in labels, symptoms, assessment techniques, and diagnostic tests. The abstracting procedure identified two kinds of problems. First, sample descriptions were often fragmented and superficial, with little information reported in common. Second, descriptions frequently identified such different kinds of subject variables that comparability and generalizability were limited.

Investigators frequently failed to provide even basic background information (e.g. race/ethnicity, socioeconomic status, age, primary language). Consistent with the multidisciplinary nature of the field, samples were described in terms of a wide range of selected functions, including emotional, attentional, perceptual-motor, neurological, learning, and linguistic status. Many different tests and assessment procedures were used to select and/or describe subjects. The variations and inconsistencies in subject selection criteria and practices led to the study of many different subject groups, all bearing the LD label. Clearly these differences pose a serious threat to inferences drawn from LD research.

It is important to emphasize that sampling issues become increasingly important as the content of LD research changes, especially when topics under study lack conceptual or definitional clarity. Investigators now study a wide age range of subjects (infancy through adulthood) and focus on a broad range of problems. For example, while historically effort was directed at the study of reading and reading problems, there is increasing interest in problems in arithmetic or mathematics. Indeed, a recent meeting of the International Academy for Research in Learning Disabilities (IARLD), held in 1983 in Brussels, was devoted to the topic of dyscalculia. A brief review of selected published research on dyscalculia, or problems in mathematics (Keogh and Babbitt, 1983), will illustrate the importance of sample information in understanding this complex topic.

RESEARCH ON PROBLEMS IN MATHEMATICS*

As background we cite findings from the National Assessment of Educational Progress (1980). This was a large-scale, large-N study (over 70 thousand subjects) which provided normative data on the performance of 9-, 13-, and 17-year-olds enrolled in public or private schools in the United States (Technical Report, 1980). These investigators reported differences in mathematics performance related to ethnicity, grade in school, sex, size and type of community, region of the United States, and level of parental education. For the 17-year-olds, differences in mathematics performance were also found based on the highest level of coursework taken. In addition, differences in performance were reported for the mathematical process studied: mathematical knowledge, skills, understanding, and application. The National Assessment studies provide information about arithmetic performance of pupils in regular school programs but allow only limited inferences about subgroups with problems. Certain groups were excluded from the study: non-English-speaking persons, those identified as nonreaders, persons physically or mentally unable to respond, persons in institutions, or those attending schools established for the physically handicapped or mentally retarded. Nonetheless, this study identified important subject differences to be considered in research on this topic.

Sex differences in mathematics achievement identified in the National Assessment of Educational Progress (Carpenter *et al.*, 1978) were also corroborated by findings in the California State Assessment of Mathematics

---

* The analysis and discussion of sampling problems in research in problems in mathematics may also be found in the unpublished proceedings of the Colloque International Consacré à la Dyscalculia, distributed by the Centre d'Étude des Troubles d'Apprentissage, Université Libre de Bruxells, 1983.

Study done in 1978. Pupils in grades 6 and 12 were tested on mathematics items selected from various content areas and differing in complexity. Girls did consistently better than boys in computation with whole numbers, fractions, and decimals as well as on one-step word problems. However, boys consistently scored higher on word problems involving multiple steps or requiring more reasoning ability.

Fennema's (1981) analysis of the results of two national studies support the findings that females tend to score higher than males in computation and in selected cognitive tasks (e.g. recall), while males score higher on more complex mathematics and analytical tasks. Fennema (1981) refers to this as the cognitive complexity of the items or tasks. Explanations for differences in performance include lack of confidence by females, teacher's expectations, effects of attributions, spatial visualization skills, and enrollment in mathematics-related classes such as chemistry and physics. The National Assessment data also suggest differences in mathematical competence relative to ethnicity, urban–rural living status, and level of parent education. Finally, a recent report on mathematics curricula and mathematics achievement in Japan, Taiwan, and the United States documents cross-national differences (Stigler *et al.*, 1982).

At the very least the findings from these large-scale studies support the need for detailed sample description including proportion of males and females according to age groups. The findings also emphasize the need for specification of components of the mathematical measures used in a given study, e.g. computation, mathematical reasoning. Finally, the large-scale studies underscore the need for sample information which includes SES, ethnicity, and national identification. In the published studies of arithmetic problems to date the sample descriptions have been limited, although the studies are often well designed and well carried out and subject selection was appropriate for the study purposes. From the generalization issue the problem is not *what* is reported. Rather, it is *what is not* reported that limits interpretation.

The difficulty in aligning findings across studies or in drawing generalizations when sample information is missing may be illustrated in a brief review of eight recently published journal articles dealing with problems in arithmetic. All investigators reported number of subjects; six of eight included number by sex. However, chronological age information was less precise, three studies providing values of means or medians, one reporting standard deviation, and six reporting only ranges. Locale (rural, urban, suburban) and grade placement of subjects were indicated in five studies, but only three included information about ethnicity or socioeconomic status of subjects, and none reported language background. While five of eight investigators provided some information (usually means) about the general intellectual status of the sample, only one included information about reading. Although arithmetic was the focus of the studies, detailed information about arithmetic achievement and competence was missing in three of the eight studies. Given the findings from the National Assessment Study which document the influence of sex, SES, locale, and reading ability on performance in arithmetic, such basic sample information is important and necessary.

Sampling differences limit interpretation even when the studies focus on specific subsets of problems in mathematics. Gerstmann's (1940) well-known clinical syndrome identified four primary symptoms — finger agnosia, disorientation for left and right, agraphia, and dyscalculia. Gerstmann's work was based on case studies of adult patients who had suffered cerebral accident and/or who had brain tumors, and who had been shown at autopsy to have localized lesions. To be emphasized is that these were adults with known cerebral damage.

Strauss and Werner (1938) in the *American Journal of Orthopsychiatry*, also reported relationships between arithmetic disability and finger agnosia. Their subjects were 14 males, age range 9–15 (mean 12-5), who were in the Wayne County Training School in Michigan. The mean IQ for the group was 68, and the range of IQs was 61–86. The mean reading achievement age was 9.2 years, and the mean arithmetic age was 7.9 years. By many criteria these subjects would have been considered mentally retarded and as evidencing a general cognitive or developmental delay. This is in direct contrast to Gerstmann's subjects, who had been adequately functioning adults before their cerebral trauma.

In 1966 Kinsbourne and Warrington reported a series of seven case studies which in their opinion exemplified the developmental Gerstman Syndrome. Children ranged in age from 8-5 to 15 years. There were five girls and two boys. Nothing is reported of subjects' socioeconomic status or educational history, but their ethnic background is assumed to be Caucasian. In common, the children evidenced symptoms of finger agnosia, right/left disorientation, dyscalculia, dysgraphia, constructional apraxia, and dyslexia. For the most part the WISC verbal IQs were at least 20 points higher than the performance IQs, and the WISC block design and object assembly subtests were lower than the WISC digit span and vocabulary. What is interesting in the Kinsbourne and Warrington findings is that in addition to specific problems with arithmetic processing, these children also had relatively severe reading disabilities. This is in contrast to the earlier Strauss and Werner work, where the mean arithmetic achievement age was approximately a year and a half below that of the reading age for the dyscalculic group.

Finally, in recent work Saxe and Shaheen (1981) applied Piagetian theory to an analysis of Gerstmann's Syndrome. Their subjects were two Caucasian males, ages 8 years 11 months and 9 years 6 months. For Subject One the verbal IQ was 108, performance IQ 91, full scale 100; reading at age expectancy, his arithmetic was at a pre-school level. He was described as highly distractible, evidencing temper tantrums and parallel play. His history was negative for head injuries, major surgery, or neurological symptoms. The second subject was

9 years 6 months of age. His verbal IQ was 82, performance IQ 80, full scale 81. He was active/cooperative, but had a history of delayed motor milestones and hypotonia. From the case studies Saxe and Shaheen concluded that acalculia was not an isolated deficit but was one manifestation of a general cognitive developmental delay. They propose that arithmetic skills, in contrast to reading skills, are dependent on Piaget's stages of development, and suggest that their subjects had not begun a transition to concrete operational reasoning. This interpretation is, of course inconsistent with that of the other investigators who took a clear syndrome perspective.

When the specific syndrome literature is placed within the context of the developmental studies, it is clear that there are serious problems in interpretation. It is difficult to draw inferences and make comparisons among the Gerstmann, Strauss and Werner, Kinsbourne and Warrington, and Saxe and Shaheen findings because of differences in age and in developmental status of subjects. Even within these studies the range of subject characteristics confounds what may be the defining, criterial attributes of the condition under consideration. The problem is not limited to research addressing the Gerstmann Syndrome, of course, as a brief look at current studies of problems in mathematics shows.

In the 1978–83 period the content of two LD journals addressed a selected set of mathematical problems: characteristics of 850 LD-mathematics youths in kindergarten through sixth grade (Cawley et al., 1979); WISC-R arithmetic subtest performance of learning disabled sixth graders (Levy, 1981); remediation of systematic inversion errors in subtraction of LD students, ages 9-0 to 11-2, who were below grade level in reading and at or below grade level in mathematics (Blankenship, 1978); automatization of basic arithmetic facts of 120 LD students ranging in age from 8-0 to 13-2 (Garnett and Fleischner, 1983); personal-social characteristics of seventh and eight grade students identified as low in mathematics but at or above grade level in reading (Badian and Ghublikian, 1983); program effects for students 18 months or more below grade level in math with ages ranging from 8-3 to 13-2 years (Trembley et al., 1980); and, visual-spatial and verbal skills of first through fifth grade LD students identified as discrepant in mathematics performance (McLeod and Crump, 1978). Reported age range of subjects varied from 7 to 14 years, reported grade level ranged from kindergarten through eighth; subjects were from major urban centers and rural areas of the United States; sample size varied from 9 to 850; ethnicity was reported in three studies, one sample containing both black and white students, the other two only white children.

A similar pattern of subject differences may be found in the literature on development of arithmetic skills. Wang, Resnick, and Boozer's (1971) description of the sequence of early mathematical behaviours was based on a sample of public school kindergarten children, the sample skewed to the lower end of the socioeconomic (SES) distribution. In contrast, Gelman and Tucker's (1975) study of young children's conception of numbers was carried out with middle class children of higher SES. It is interesting to note that most of the developmental studies limit sample description to chronological age, grade level, sex, and sometimes social class and ethnicity. Little is known about other possibly important subject attributes: intelligence, reading readiness, or reading levels, opportunity for instruction, etc. As the possible contribution of these variables, including SES, to number understanding and mathematical competence is uncertain, it is difficult to synthesize the findings or to draw inferences to other children or to questions of dysfunction. If Rutter and Yule's (1975) work on reading problems generalizes to arithmetic, then SES and its many correlates must be taken into account. Many of the studies to date contain interesting and important findings relating to LD and mathematic problems. Too often, however, differences in subjects preclude interpretation across studies.

There is no need to belabor the sample-variation issue further. Rather, the task is to identify procedures which will clarify rather than confound the inferences we can draw from research and intervention on learning disabilities, including problems in mathematics, emerging from different investigative groups in many countries. Clearer findings and more powerful interpretations involve more adequate subject description. We suggest that routine use of a marker system of subject description is one step towards achieving this.

A MARKER SYSTEM FOR SAMPLE DESCRIPTION

The notion of markers is not unique to LD, but rather has been proposed in research on a number of topics. Bell and Hertz (1976) working in the child development area, defined a marker variable as 'a background variable (not necessarily the focal variable in the study) that is sufficiently relevant to the measure being used by most studies in a defined research area that it facilitates the general alignment of findings between one study to another' (pp. 8, 9). Focusing on learning disabilities, Keogh *et al.* (1978) suggested that markers 'reflect the constructs which define and characterize a particular field, and thus provide both operational comparability and conceptual organization' (p. 7). Simply said, markers may be viewed as common reference points, benchmarks, or 'empirical anchors' which provide information about subjects and samples. Markers allow identification of similarities and differences across studies and provide a way to align findings, sometimes to aggregate findings.

A marker system seems especially promising in LD research given the likely continued reliance on system-identified samples. It should be emphasized that adoption of a marker system does not influence how subjects are selected nor does it determine the source of subjects. It does provide a comprehensive and systematic way to describe samples.

The use of a marker system would be a major step in reducing some of the conceptual confusion which currently characterizes LD research, and might also allow us to align data from studies from different countries and from different research groups. The use of a marker system would in no sense limit an investigator nor restrict the nature of his/her sampling procedures. What it would do, however, would be to make sampling procedures, sources, and subject characteristics explicit and public, thus clarifying what may be sampling effects on our understanding of LD problems. We illustrate by applying the marker notion to the study of problems in mathematics.

MARKERS IN RESEARCH ON MATHEMATICS PROBLEMS

Our argument for the need for functional markers to describe both research and intervention samples in the study of mathematics problems stemmed in large part from the review of the learning disabilities research conducted as part of the UCLA Marker Variable Project (Keogh et al., 1982). The content of that Project demonstrated clearly that relatively little is known about arithmetic or mathematical competence or problems. It was also clear that intervention or therapeutic efforts directed at dyscalculia were very different; many lacked solid data to confirm the appropriateness or effectiveness of particular practices.

Given the lack of conceptual clarity about the etiology, natural course of development, and remediation of problems in mathematics, we suggest that a broad band set of markers, coupled with specific theoretically linked markers, be applied to research on this topic. The four sets of broad band markers (Keogh et al., 1982) are: Descriptive, Substantive, Topical, and Background. These are listed in Table 1.

Table 1. Markers by Category

Descriptive markers	Topical markers
Number of subjects by sex	Activity level
Chronological age	Attention
Grade level	Auditory perception
Race/ethnicity	Fine motor coordination
Source of subjects	Gross motor coordination
Socioeconomic status	Memory
Language background	Oral language
Educational history	Visual perception
Educational placement	
Physical and health status	
Substantive markers	Background markers
Intellectual ability	Month/year of study
Reading achievement	Geographic location
Arithmetic achievement	Locale
Behavioural and emotional adjustment	Exclusionary criteria
	Control/comparison group

Source: Keogh, B. K., Major-Kingsley, S., Omori-Gordon, H., and Reid, H. P. (1982), *A System of Marker Variables for the Field of Learning Disabilities*. New York, Syracuse University Press.

Alignment of findings from different studies or research groups would be facilitated if investigators routinely reported sample information on all *Descriptive and Background Markers*. These markers address basic sample information. A number of questions related to SES, culture, gender, and ethnicity could be addressed with this information.

Substantive markers provide additional information directly relevant to mathematics. In specific, based on the literature to date, detailed information on substantive markers of intellectual ability (including discrepancies between verbal and performance IQs or specific subtest patterns), and reading achievement, is necessary. Aiken's (1972) review documenting the consistently significant relationship between reading and arithmetic makes essential inclusion of reading achievement information when studying arithmetic problems. Recalling Farnham-Diggory's (1980) point on task differences, information about the arithmetic components studied is also essential. Arithmetic markers would specify computation and analytic components of a task and define level of complexity.

Topical markers of fine motor coordination (including handwriting skills and problems), visual perception, language, and memory also appear relevant in the study of arithmetic problems, as all have been proposed as possible correlates or causes of problems. Selected topical markers, coupled with agreed-upon markers theoretically linked to particular subgroups studied, would provide information which might help clarify the syndrome notion already discussed. Researchers studying the Gerstmann's Syndrome might routinely include markers for finger gnosis, right–left orientation, spelling, and constructional apraxia. It should be emphasized that determination of sample comparability is made easier when both the content of the marker (e.g. intelligence, constructional apraxia) and the technique used to assess it (e.g. WISC-R, Kohs Block) are reported (Keogh, 1984). Detailed information about measures is critical when tests or techniques are researcher-developed for a particular study.

In a recent issue of *Thalamus*, the IARLD Bulletin, Pelham (1983) summarized many of the research problems which have confounded the findings about the impact of psychostimulant medication on the academic performance of hyperactive pupils. Included in his discussion was the imprecision of the definition of the condition and the range of individual differences found within most hyperactive groups. Although dyscalculia and problems in mathematics are just beginning to receive the amount and kind of attention they deserve, certain similarities to hyperactivity are apparent. At best, dyscalculia is a condition which lacks conceptual clarity. More complete and objective subject description may allow the development of a coherent database which can address these theoretical concerns and uncertainties. Such description may also lead to the identification of meaningful subgroups of mathematical problems, a direction consistent with the need for the LD field as a whole (Keogh and Babbitt, 1983; McKinney, 1984).

Some work in subgroup delineation has already begun. Badian (1983), for example, proposes a model for the classification of subtypes of developmental dyscalculia. The four subtypes are alexia and agraphia for numbers, spatial dyscalculia, anarithmetria (combining addition, subtraction, and/or multiplication operations in a single calculation), and attentional-sequential dyscalculia. Subtypes are proposed as a means of reducing sample heterogeneity in research on dyscalculia and, hence, obtaining more reliable and interpretable results. Such a delineation, however, depends upon a precise description of the population of mathematics disabled students from which the subgroups are generated. Badian (1983) particularly emphasizes the need to know if subjects are deficient in mathematics only or are also deficient in other skills such as reading. Badian's work provides an important step in reducing some of the confusion which has characterized research on problems in mathematics. Such sample specification is needed in LD research as a whole.

FINAL COMMENTS

We suggest that the term, learning disabilities, is best viewed as a broad band label for a variety of symptom combinations and etiologies. We argue, too, that various subconditions within the broad label are likely to be differently responsive to particular treatments. From both a theoretical and an applied or programmatic perspective, then, the delineation of subgroups within this large category is essential (McKinney, 1984).

The routine use of markers to describe subjects is one way to go about refining the broad category, and in our view the use of common markers is feasible. In a field test of the marker system described in Table 1, Keogh et al. (1982) found that most investigators of learning disabilities knew far more about their samples than they reported in publication. Lack of sample description was more a matter of convention than of limited information. When presented with a reasonable format most investigators could supply detailed sample information.

We expect that the specific content or form of markers will change as we know more about the condition(s) we study. Some markers will likely be added, and others may be modified or even dropped. Given the current state of the art, however, the use of a marker system would allow determination of comparability of findings across studies, would allow alignment of data from different research groups, and would allow specifications of consistent and consensual subgroups of subjects and symptoms. This would be a major step in the scientific understanding of learning disabilities.

REFERENCES

Aiken, L. R., Jr. (1972), Language factors in learning mathematics. *Review of Educational Research* **42**, 359-385.

Badian, N. A. (1983), Dyscalculia and nonverbal disorders of learning. In H. Mykelbust (Ed.), *Progress in Learning Disabilities*, Vol. 5. New York, Grune & Stratton.

Badian, N. A., and Ghublikian, M. (1983), The personal-social characteristics of children with poor mathematical computation skills. *Journal of Learning Disabilities* **16**, 154–157.

Bell, R. Q., and Hertz, T. W. (1976), Toward more comparability and generalizability of developmental research. *Child Development* **47**, 6–13.

Blankenship, C. S. (1978), Remediating systematic inversion errors in subtraction through the use of demonstration and feedback. *Learning Disability Quarterly* **1**(3), 12–22.

California Assessment Program (1978), *Student Achievement in California Schools* (annual report).

Carpenter, T., Coburn, T. B., Reys, R. E., and Wilson, J. W. (1978), *Results from the First Mathematics Assessment of the National Assessment of Educational Progress*. Reston, VA, National Council of Teachers of Mathematics.

Cawley, J. F., Fitzmaurice, A. M., Shaw, R., Kahn, H., and Bates, H., III (1979), LD youth and mathematics: a review of characteristics. *Learning Disability Quarterly* **2**(1), 29–44.

Cronbach, L. J. (1957), The two disciplines of scientific psychology. *American Psychologist* **12**, 671–684.

Farnham-Diggory, S. (1980), Learning disabilities: a view for cognitive science. *Journal of the American Academy of Child Psychiatry* **19**, 570–578.

Fennema, E. (1981), The sex factor. In: E. Fennema (Ed.), *Mathematics Education Research: Implications for the 80's*. Alexandria, VA, Association for Supervision and Curriculum Development.

Garnett, K., and Fleischner, J. E. (1983), Automatization and basic fact performance of normal and learning disabled children. *Learning Disability Quarterly* **6**(20), 223–230.

Gelman, R., and Tucker, M. F. (1975), Further investigations of the young child's conception of number. *Child Development* **46**, 167–175.

Gerstmann, J. (1940), Syndrome of finger agnosia, disorientation for right and left, agraphia and acalculia. *Archives of Neurology and Psychiatry* **44**, 398–408.

Keogh, B. K. (1984), A marker system for describing LD samples. In: S. Ceci (Ed.), *Handbook of cognitive, social, and neuropsychological aspects of learning disabilities*, Hillsdale, Lawrence Erlbaum, 1986.

Keogh, B. K. and Babbitt, B. C. (1983), Functional markers for use in research on dyscalculia: a technique for subgroup specification. Paper presented at the International Academy for Research in Learning Disabilities Conference in Brussels, Belgium.

Keogh, B. K. and MacMillan, D. L. (1983), The logic of sample selection: Who represents what? *Exceptional Education Quarterly* **4**(3), 84–96.

Keogh, B. K., Major, S. M., Reid, H. P., Gandara, P., and Omori, H. (1978), Marker variables: A search for comparability and generalizability in the field of learning disabilities. *Learning Disabilities Quarterly* **1**, 5–11.

Keogh, B. K., Major, S. M., Omori, H., Gandara, P., and Reid, H. P. (1980), Proposal markers in learning disabilities research. *Journal of Abnormal Child Psychology* **8**(1), 21–31.

Keogh, B. K., Major-Kingsley, S. M., Omori-Gordon, H., and Reid, H. P. (1982), *A System of Marker Variables for the Field of Learning Disabilities*. New York, Syracuse University Press.

Kinsbourne, M., and Warrington, E. K. (1966), The developmental Gerstmann syndrome. In: J. Money (Ed.), *The Disabled Reader*. Baltimore, Johns Hopkins Press.

Kirk, S. A., and Elkins, J. (1975), Characteristics of children enrolled in child service demonstration centers. *Journal of Learning Disabilities* **8**, 630–637.

Levy, W. K. (1981), WISC-R arithmetic subtest performance of mathematically handicapped and nonmathematically handicapped LD students as a function of presentation response behaviors and vocabulary interactions. *Learning Disability Quarterly* **4**, 393–400.

MacMillan, D. L., Meyers, C. E., and Morrison, G. M. (1980), System identification of mildly retarded children: implications for interpreting and conducting research. *American Journal of Mental Deficiency* **85**(2), 109–115.

Mann, L., Davis, C., Boyer, C., Metz, C., and Wolford, B. (1983), LD or not LD that was the question. *Journal of Learning Disabilities* **16**(1), 14–17.

McKinney, J. D. (1984), The search for subtypes of specific learning disability. *Journal of Learning Disabilities* **17**(1), 43–51.

McLeod, T. M., and Crump, W. D. (1978), The relationship of visuospatial skills and verbal ability to learning disabilities in mathematics. *Journal of Learning Disabilities* **11**, 237–241.

National Assessment of Educational Progress (1980), Mathematics technical report: summary volume (Rep. No. 09-MA-21). Washington, DC, US Government Printing Office.

Norman, C. A., Jr., and Zigmond, N. (1980), Characteristics of children labeled and served as learning disabled in school systems affiliated with child service demonstration centers. *Journal of Learning Disabilities* **13**(10), 542–547.

Pelham, W. (1983), The effects of psychostimulants on academic achievement in hyperactive and learning-disabled children. *Thalamus* **3**(1), 1–48.

Rutter, M., and Yule, W. (1975), The concept of specific reading retardation. *Journal of Child Psychology and Psychiatry* **16**, 181–197.

Saxe, G. B., and Shaheen, S. (1981), Piagetian theory and the atypical case: an analysis of the developmental Gerstmann syndrome. *Journal of Learning Disabilities* **14**, 131–136.

Stigler, J. W., Lee, S., Lucker, G. W., and Stevenson, H. (1982), Curriculum and achievement in mathematics: a study of elementary school children in Japan, Taiwan, and the United States. *Journal of Educational Psychology* **74**, 315–322.

Strauss, A., and Werner, H. (1938), Deficiency in the finger scheme in relation to arithmetic (finger agnosia and acalculia). *American Journal of Orthopsychiatry* **8**, 719–725.

Trembley, P. W., Caponigro, J. D., and Gaffney, V. T. (1980), Effects of programming from the WRAT and the PIAT for students determined to have learning disabilities in arithmetic. *Journal of Learning Disabilities*, **13**, 291–293.

Wang, M. C., Resnick, L. B., and Boozer, R. F. (1971), The sequence of development of some early mathematics behavior. *Child Development* 1767–1778.

CHAPTER 3

Methodological Issues in Research with the Learning Disabled: Establishing True Controls

DENNIS F. FISHER
Behavioral Research Directorate, US Army Human Engineering Laboratory, Aberdeen Proving Ground, MD 21005, USA

and

IRENE ATHEY
Dean, Graduate School of Education, Rutgers, The State University, New Brunswick, NJ 08903, USA

It is apparent from the voluminous literature that has appeared in the last decade on dyslexia and learning disabilities that these phenomena and their ramifications are still poorly understood. Moreover, these disabilities seem to manifest themselves in as many different forms as there are students who are disabled (Fisher, 1984). The breadth of topics in the present volume seems to exhibit even further the plethora of definitions and explanations coming from fields as widely diverse as neurophysiology and pedagogy of the learning disabled. For example, the issues range from etiology (Geschwind, Chapter 5, this volume) to subtypes (Kinsbourne, Chapter 12, this volume), laterality (Bryden, 1982), and such seemingly unrelated topics as lesions, perceptual deficits, etc.

There can be little doubt that this lack of convergence among researchers who study the problems of learning disabilities is detrimental to advancement of the field as a whole. However, another primary cause of confusion is the history of inadequate methodological practices. One particularly unfortunate outcome

---

The model of dyslexia discussed in this chapter involves the simplest possible case — homogenous distribution of characteristics. For further examination of subtypes as described in other chapters in this volume, division of Normal readers and their Age and Reading level matched controls must all be done on the basis of that subtype.

of these methodological problems is that many researchers and educators draw inappropriate interpretations from the data or attach undue importance to the many epiphenomena that sometimes exhibit themselves in these research efforts.

A number of issues raised by Fisher and Frankfurter (1977) concerning the non-experimental nature of much of the research continue to be discussed. Conspicuous among these is the problem of obtaining reliable information about the learning disabled without benefit of a suitable control group of normal students (Fisher, 1979, 1980, 1981). How can meaningful conclusions about hypothesized deficits be drawn when the performance of the disabled group is not compared to that of a normal functioning group? In the course of writing this chapter, one of us (DFF) had occasion to review three manuscripts submitted to different psychology and reading journals, all supposedly describing processing characteristics of the learning disabled. The first was a case study comparing a fifth grade normal reader with a disabled counterpart. The second study compared learning disabled college students with a group of normal college students, and the third simply provided a descriptive account of disabled college students on three independent measures. Unfortunately, none of these studies was adequate to test any hypothesis whatsoever. In the first two, the outcome of the so-called hypothesis was predetermined by the very definition used to select the samples, while the third had no controls with which to establish a baseline for comparison. The critical question that none of these studies addressed was: *How do learning disabled individuals differ from their matched normal counterparts?*

In this chapter we hope to demonstrate the advisability, if not the necessity, of including two normal reading control groups, one matched to the LD readers by age to control for the experience factor, the other matched by achievement to control for the proficiency factor. Together, these two groups allow for a comparison of processing breakdown *vs.* developmental lag; either alone provides an incomplete profile.

While various hypotheses of perceptual, memorial, linguistic, and visual, e.g. peripheral retinal prescreening, processing guided this study, it is more important to reiterate the original primary concern which was to employ a rigorous sampling procedure that would permit valid conclusions to be drawn from the data. In this procedure, priority is given to establishing the developmental sequence of skill acquisition in the population of normal readers, with special attention to the processing of perceptual and linguistic information. The LD sample under consideration is then matched to two different subsets of this population, one by age, the other by reading level (IQ is controlled throughout). The LD sample is thus required to engage in two sets of activities, the first of which provides the basis for comparison with the age level counterparts, the other with their reading grade level counterparts. The latter tasks are, of course, at a level two to three years below the age-appropriate tasks.

The variables of interest in the present study were speed of processing and accuracy on perceptual, memory, and linguistic tasks. The skills selected have been historically and intuitively recognized as precursors of successful reading achievement. While the list of skills assessed cannot in any way be considered exhaustive, it does contain a representative cross-section of skills that were deemed adequate to provide a valid and interesting profile of processing capabilities. The skills examined included:

(a) *Letter recognition* where letters appeared in either upper or lower case, in isolation or in groups.
(b) *Word recognition* as measured on graded word lists.
(c) *Memory span* for letters and for words presented in visual or auditory mode.
(d) *Sentence reading time* for normal and anagrammatic sentences.
(e) *Pictograph processing* on both a learning and performance task.

   To facilitate the reader's understanding of the testing sequence and the data analyses while observing the constraints of space and attention span, the sections on method and results will include only those analyses needed to establish the methodology and to present the major findings. Normative data for 28 subjects in grades 1–5 that were needed to establish the pool from which the control Ss were drawn were eliminated from the present discussion.

METHOD

Subjects

From each of the first five grades at the Prospect Mill and Churchville Elementary Schools in Harford County, Maryland, 14 males and 14 females were selected to form the normal group. These Ss were judged by their classroom and reading teachers to be reading at or above their normal reading grade level. The mean age in months at each grade level for the total group and for males and females separately was: Grade 1, 78.79 (M 78.79, F 78.79); Grade 2, 91.14 (M 91.00, F 91.29); Grade 3, 101.93 (M 103.6, F 100.33); Grade 4, 114.04 (M 113.5, F 114.6); and Grade 5, 128.25 (M 128.64, F 127.86). Another group of 27 males and 5 females (hereafter referred to as the 'disabled reader' group) also from Harford County and undergoing or awaiting special remediation at the John Archer School served as the experimental group. The mean age of these Ss was 118.7 months and all were reading at more than two years below grade level. These Ss were matched individually to two samples of Ss from the normal group by reading level (mean age 89.94 months) and by age (mean age 118.4 months) with sex ratios held constant across all three groups. These groups will be referred to as the RL and AL group, respectively.

Measures

Achievement measures used were scores from the Metropolitan Achievement Test for Grades 1 through 3 and the Iowa Basic Skills for Grades 4 and 5.* The

---

* Owing to state and county restrictions on standardized testing, scores reported were taken from tests administered by school officials for use as performance level determinants.

mean percentiles for the first three grades were 89.93, 86.2 and 83.5 on the Metropolitan and mean IQ of 113.75 and 112.4 on the Iowa. The RL group had a mean percentile score of 85.4 on the Metropolitan, while the AL group had a mean IQ of 107.3 on the Iowa. The disabled reader group had a mean IQ score of 103.4 on the Iowa. No sex differences were found on any of these measures.

Procedure

All Ss in both normal groups participated in the following individually administered tasks at least once, while the disabled group participated twice, once on tasks at their reading grade level, and once on tasks at their age grade level.

Letter Recognition

Ss were required to identify upper and lower case letters presented both individually and in full alphabet array. Time taken to complete each task was measured to the nearest second. For the full alphabet array, upper and lower case were recorded separately.

Letter Span

Six sequences of eight randomly selected letters were typed on 4 × 6 cards. Three of these sequences were presented visually and three aurally at the rate of approximately two items/second. The sequences were randomized between Ss and between visual and aural presentations. Responses were recorded and scored for correct sequencing as well as for total letters reported.

Vocabulary Level

Harris and Jacobson's *Basic Elementary Reading Vocabularies* (1972) was used to construct a word list that would tap the vocabulary skills from preschool to Grade 6 with about 10–12 words per grade level. Ss were required to read the entire list until they missed two consecutive words. The grade level represented by the last word was designated as the reading vocabulary level.

Word Span

Memory span for words was examined both visually and aurally by having Ss view or listen to sequences of seven words taken from the vocabulary list of the Scott-Foresman *Reading Unlimited* (1976) at two contiguous grade levels. For example, if the child was reading at the 4.5 level, both fourth and fifth grade sequences were chosen. Of the three visual and three aural sequences, one of each was used for practice. Exposure was at the rate of approximately two items/second. Responses were recorded for correct word sequences and for total number of words reported in each modality.

Sentence Reading

Sentences were chosen and slightly modified from the Scott-Foresman *Reading Unlimited* (1976), a program in use in the Harford County schools. Five sentences were chosen at each grade level and presented in normal and in anagram form. One example from Grade 2 and one from Grade 5 are provided for purposes of illustration:

> Some of the children were afraid of the big cat
> Children of the afraid some cat of the were big
> They walked past some hippies who were tossing a frisbee
> Some walked were hippies who a frisbee tossing they past

Times taken to read the sentence were recorded.

Pictographs

Graded sentences (one at each of the five grade levels) were chosen and modified, e.g. through removal of quotation marks, slight word changes, etc.). An example of a pictographic sentence may be seen in Figure 1.

For each reading grade level a long sentence was chosen from which component sentences could be generated. For example, at Grade 2 the sentence 'The man and the boy came to the bridge over the river and walked across' was broken into 'The man and the boy walked across the bridge' and 'The bridge went over the river'. The subject first learned a list of pictures corresponding to the words. The above sentence required 12 different pictographs to be learned: man, and, boy, came, to, bridge, that, went, over, river, walked, across. The number of exposures (trials) required to learn the complete list of pictographs to a criterion of two errorless repetitions was recorded. Following the learning phase of the task, subsets of the pictographs were displayed and the subject was required to read the new pictographic sentence. Next, the subject received the full

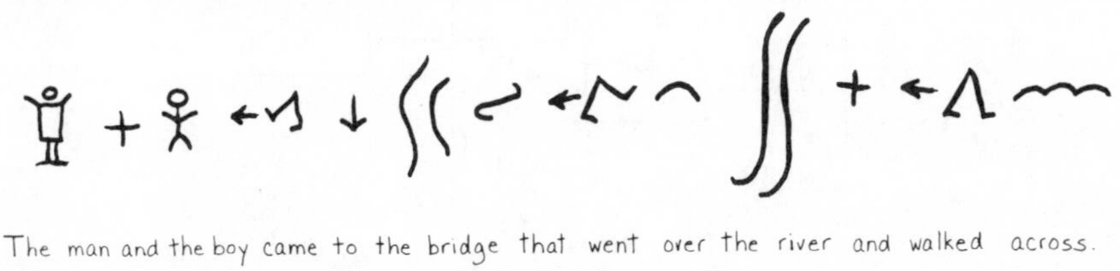

The man and the boy came to the bridge that went over the river and walked across.

Figure 1.

set of individual pictographs and was asked to construct a new sentence of any length desired. The time taken to construct the new sentence, the number of pictographs used, and the linguistic validity of the constructed sentence were recorded.

RESULTS

Normal and Disabled Reader Comparisons

In this section, the results of data analyses comparing normal and disabled readers are reported. Comparisons among reading level group (RL), disabled readers (DR) and age level (AL) are reported as between-subjects effects. A schematic of the origin of these groups appears in Figure 2.

Letter Identification

The number of letters recognized (individual *vs.* full array) by each group was entered into an analysis of variance. The main effect of groups ($F(2, 93) = 6.82$, $ms = 1.8$, $p < 0.01$) was found to be significant, with 25.37, 25.66, and 25.82 letters recognized by the DR, RL, and AL groups, respectively. In addition, the main effect of type of presentation was significant ($F(1, 93) = 7.76$, $ms = 0.9$, $p < 0.01$) with means of 25.48 and 25.75 for individual *vs.* full array, respectively. No other main effects or interactions were significant. The DR identified fewer letters correctly than did the RL or AL, but the magnitude of that difference does not seem to be large enough to be a contributing cause of the disability.

The time required to read upper and lower case full arrays again revealed a highly significant main effect ($F(2, 93) = 27.7$, $ms = 51.4$, $p < 0.001$) with means

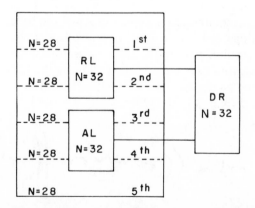

TOTAL NR = 140

Figure 2.

Table 1. Time to read letters (seconds)

Groups	Case	
	Upper	Lower
RL	18.72	21.22
DR	21.80	23.28
AL	13.38	13.40

of 22.55, 19.97, and 13.39 seconds required to read the alphabet by the DR, RL, and AL groups, respectively. In addition, the main effect of case proved to be significant ($F(1, 93) = 10.37$, ms 8.2, $p < 0.001$) with means of 17.97 and 19.3 seconds for upper and lower case, respectively. Although the interaction of Groups × Case only reached the 0.10 significance level ($F(2, 93) = 2.99$, $ms = 8.2$), these data are reported in order to illustrate developmental trends (Table 1), since they show the DR group to be more closely aligned with RL than with AL on speed of letter identification. Further supporting evidence in support of the developmental lag hypothesis is provided by the main effect.

Memory Span for Letters

In these analyses, the three groups were compared on the number of letters recalled by scoring technique (ordered *vs.* total) and by presentation mode (visual *vs.* aural). The following effects were found to be statistically significant: (1) *Groups* ($F(2, 93) = 13.49$, $ms = 2.5$, $p < 0.001$); (2) *Scoring technique* ($F(1, 93) = 412.4$, $ms = 0.8$, $p < 0.001$); (3) *Presentation mode* ($F(1, 93) = 4.99$, $ms = 1.2$, $p < 0.05$); (4) *Groups × Scoring technique* interaction ($F(2, 93) = 5.35$, $ms = 0.8$, $p < 0.01$); and (5) *Groups × Scoring technique × Presentation mode* interaction ($F(2, 93) = 3.13$, $ms = 0.8$, $p < 0.05$). The data for this three-way interaction are shown in Table 2. From this table, it can be seen that the DR group showed a greater similarity on the memory span task to the RL group (younger children) than to their AL counterparts. No other main effects or interactions proved significant.

Vocabulary Level

The groups differed on vocabulary as seen in the main effect ($F(2, 93) = 92.65$, $ms = 1.8$, $p < 0.001$) with means of 2.0, 3.4, and 6.5 for DR, RL, and AL, respectively. Here the DR group demonstrated a sight vocabulary equivalent to the second grade level, significantly lower than that of their RL counterparts.

Table 2. Memory span for letters

	Scoring technique				
	Ordered			Total	
Groups	Visual	Aural	Modality	Visual	Aural
RL	2.45	1.59		3.34	4.03
DR	2.54	1.67		3.64	3.62
AL	2.98	2.33		4.74	4.96

Table 3. Memory span for words

	Materials level	
Reader type	Reading	Age
Normal	2.44	2.55
Disabled	1.57	0.9

Word Span

For these and all subsequent analyses the DR were given tasks corresponding to both their RL and AL equivalents, e.g. a DR of 118 months with reading skills at the Grade 2 level was exposed to words from both Grade 2 and Grade 5 word lists. For these analyses the type of word list (RL *vs.* AL) and reader type are between effects, while scoring technique (order *vs.* total) and presentation mode (visual *vs.* aural) are within-effects. With degrees of freedom of 1 and 124, all effects were significant at the 0.01 level except where otherwise indicated. Significant effects included: (1) *Materials* (RL *vs.* AL), $(F = 6.43, ms = 1.5, p < 0.05)$; (2) *Reader type* (normal *vs.* disabled), $(F = 137.2\ ms = 1.5)$; (3) *Materials × Reader type* $(F = 13.24,\ ms = 1.5)$; (4) *Scoring technique* $(F = 669.04,\ ms = 0.8)$; (5) *Scoring technique × Reader type × Materials* interaction $(F = 19.23,\ ms = 0.8)$; (7) *Presentation mode* $(F = 27.12,\ ms = 1.3)$; (8) *Presentation mode × Reader type* interaction $(F = 68.87,\ ms = 1.3)$; (9) *Presentation mode × Material × Reader type* interaction $(F = 8.77,\ ms = 1.3)$; (10) *Scoring technique × Presentation mode* interaction $(F = 138.05,\ ms = 0.4)$; (11) *Presentation mode × Scoring technique × Material* interaction $(F = 5.97,\ ms = 0.4, p < 0.05)$; (12) *Presentation mode × Scoring technique × Reader type* interaction $(F = 19.23,\ ms = 0.4)$; and (13) *Presentation mode × Scoring technique × Reader type × Material*, a four-way interaction $(F = 4.86,\ ms = 0.4,\ p < 0.05)$ as shown in Figure 3. This interaction shows the superiority of visual processing of normal readers over DR on *both* RL and AL materials.

In brief, memory span remains fairly constant for normal readers on graded material. However, the span for the DR was smaller than even the youngest

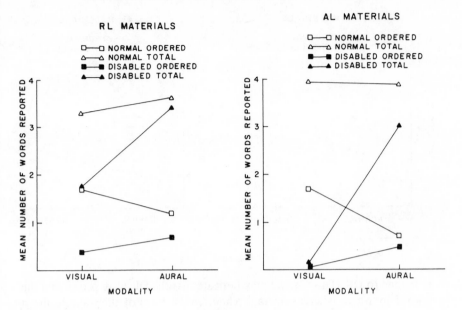

Figure 3.

readers on the most elementary materials, and was reduced to less than one word when AL materials were given. This reduced span seems to be one of the most dramatic differences between normal and disabled readers. Figure 3 shows that, for the DR group, scores are very low for both types of material. It seems likely that the deficiencies are not simply 'visual' or 'aural', but involve higher order cortical processing, possibly at the articulatory encoding level.

Sentence Reading

Normal and DR readers were exposed to regular and anagram sentences. The analyses will be reported separately, since only 23 of the 32 DR readers could read AL materials, whereas 29 of the 32 DR group could read the RL materials. For RL sentences significant effects for time taken to read were: *Reader type* ($F(1, 56) = 20.09$, $ms = 48.6$, $p < 0.001$) with means of 6.67 and 12.47 for normal and DR, respectively; and *Reader type × Sentence type* interaction ($F(1, 56) = 9.45$, $ms = 0.87$, $p < 0.01$) as shown in Figure 4(a). Only 23 of the 32 DR could read the AL materials. Significant effects noted were: *Reader type* ($F(1, 44) = 76.61$, $ms = 26.9$, $p < 0.001$); *Sentence type* ($F(1, 44) = 5.02$, $ms = 3.8$, $p < 0.05$); and *Reader type × Sentence type* interaction ($F(1, 44) = 4.6$, $ms = 3.8$, $p < 0.05$); as shown in Figure 4(b). Here it can be seen that, although the DR read the sentences more slowly than the normal readers, the introduction of anagram sentences was much more detrimental to the performance of normal

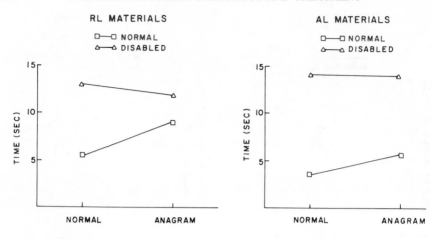

Figure 4.

readers than to DR. This finding may indicate that the DR were processing the text word by word, whereas normal readers, regardless of their age, utilized the contextual features of the sentences to facilitate their reading. One possibility is that word-by-word readers, as the Dr seem to be, ignore linguistic structure in both types of sentences. The characteristics of their pictographic sentence construction may shed more light on that possibility.

Pictographs

(a) *Trials to learn pictographs*. This analysis included material type (RL *vs.* AL) and reader type (normal *vs.* DR) as between-effects. Material type proved to be a significant main effect ($F(1, 124) = 4.65$, $ms = 4.9$, $p < 0.05$) indicating that, although RL materials took 3.65 trials and AL materials required 4.47 trials to learn, the number of trials did not vary as a function of reading ability. No other main effects or interactions proved significant.

(b) *Time to read pictographs*. Statistically significant effects were found for: *Material type* ($F(1, 124) = 113.17$, $ms = 42.5$, $p < 0.001$); *Reader type* ($F(1, 142) = 27.38$, $ms = 42.5$, $p < 0.001$); and *Material type × Reader type* interaction ($F(1, 124) = 24.08$, $ms = 42.5$, $p < 0.001$). The data for this two-way interaction are shown in Table 4. Although normal readers required as many trials to learn the lists as disabled readers, recoding pictographs into meaningful sentences proved more difficult for the DR as the sentences became progressively more complex.

(c) *Sentence construction*.

(1) *Time*. As before, materials type and reader type were compared on time taken to construct new sentences from familiar pictographs. Significant main

Table 4. Time (seconds) to read pictographic sentences

Reader group	Materials	
	Reading level	Age level
Disabled	8.0	20.69
Normal	7.75	12.42

Table 5. Pictographic sentence construction

(a) Time (seconds	(b) Length (words)	(c) Type Freq[a]			
Groups		0	1	2	3
RL (Dis—57.00)	5.47	3	5	5	19
(Nor—53.47)	5.81	2	5	5	22
AL (Dis— 80.53)	5.13	13	2	8	9
(Nor—121.22)	9.41	1	0	8	23

[a] 0 = nonsense; 1 = syntactically correct; 2 = semantically correct; 3 = all correct.

effects were: *Reader type* ($F(1, 124) = 17.03$, $ms = 3915.3$, $p < 0.01$) and *Material type × Reader type* interaction ($F(1, 124) = 4.0$, $ms = 3915.3$, $p < 0.05$). The data for this interaction are shown in Table 5(a).

(2) *Length.* The only significant effect in the analyses of sentence length was that of reader type ($F(1, 124) = 5.35$, $ms = 32.0$, $p < 0.05$), while the interaction of material type × reader type approached significance ($7F(1, 124) = 3.88$, $ms = 32.0$, $p < 0.05$). The data for this interaction are shown in Table 5(b).

(3) *Complexity.* Results of the analysis of sentence complexity as a function of material type and reader type are displayed in Table 5(c). It is apparent that the degree of linguistic awareness is dependent upon reader type and difficulty of the materials. The linguistic awareness of the DR seems more akin to that of the younger reader, and is indeed quite similar to that of the first grade readers.

In brief, these data indicate that the more advanced normal reader, in constructing new sentences, was willing to trade speed in order to produce longer, linguistically appropriate sentences. The DR showed little linguistic sensitivity when manipulating the AL materials to form new sentences. It is evident that DR and younger normal readers have achieved about the same ability level in using elementary materials for this purpose. This lack of linguistic awareness and shorter memory span for both letters and words observed in the DR subjects may well be the primary contributing factors to their reading disability.

SUMMARY AND DISCUSSION

A major purpose of this chapter has been to encourage the use of appropriate control groups in the conduct of research on the learning disabled. The tasks used in this study assessed a variety of cognitive and linguistic processing skills that could be used in the development of comparative group profiles.

Both normal and disabled readers know the letters of the alphabet by the time they enter the first grade, but disabled readers were found to be much slower at reading alphabet sets. The difficulty here may be one of phonological recoding, an output rather than an input problem. Disabled readers and their reading level counterparts performed equally on memory for ordered letter span, with both groups exhibiting a slight advantage for visual over aural model. Older normal subjects performed better than younger or disabled readers, with less differential between the two modes. On total recall measures the trend was reversed with both older and younger normal readers now exhibiting an advantage in the aural mode, while no such advantage was evident for the disabled readers. This finding suggests that a deficiency in phonological recoding processes may be the source of the perceived language dysfunction.

Word span tasks involve both memory and phonological recoding capabilities. When confronting words requiring complex phoneme–grapheme translation, normal readers perform equally well on total recall in both the visual and the aural mode. On ordered recall measures, however, the visual mode proved to be somewhat advantageous, suggesting that spatial ordering skills are slightly superior to temporal ordering skills. Among the disabled readers, difficulty of material affected only performance in the visual, but not the aural mode, which was essentially similar to that of the normal readers. Generating grapheme-to-phoneme correspondence from a spatial array proved extremely difficult for these disabled readers and probably interfered with memory. Some support for this thesis may be seen in their performance on easy words where order was not critical, for here the DR were able to salvage two of the six words on the list. Also, translation was not so necessary when the grapheme was presented in the aural mode.

Younger and older normal readers showed the same trends in reading times for regular and anagram sentences, the latter requiring much longer times in both cases. On the other hand, disabled readers, while requiring more time than normals to read either type of sentence, did not exhibit any significant difference between the two types. Clearly, for normal readers, meaning is a major factor in increasing the speed with which text is processed. For disabled readers, at least three possibilities may account for the finding: (1) reading of both types of sentence proceeds word by word, the grapheme-to-phoneme translation requiring the same amount of time whether the words are in order or scrambled; (2) context is not used to make predictions or to read units larger than a single word; (3) in anagram sentences, the textual array itself is confusing, with words competing for attention to such an extent that visual prescreening is impeded.

Learning new symbols in the form of pictographs did not appear to present an insurmountable problem for disabled readers. In fact, there were no differences among the groups on the number of trials needed to learn the lists. When the new symbols were arranged in horizontal arrays, however, it took the disabled readers 67 per cent longer than normal readers to read grade the level pictographs. When the task required the construction of new sentences from reading level pictographs, the DR produced sentences about five words in length and showed insensitivity to syntactic and semantic aspects equal to that of their reading level counterparts. Not so when constructing grade level sentences. Normal readers produced sentences twice as long as those of disabled readers, and only 9 of 32 DR produced sentences that were syntactically and semantically acceptable. Linguistic awareness seemed to be quite undeveloped in these subjects, suggesting a maturational lag in conceptual processing.

Disabled readers bring to the task of reading a far greater experiential base than their younger normal reading counterparts, but many fewer visual and verbal reading-relevant experiences than their age-level cohorts. Although the maturational lag hypothesis has of late fallen into some disrepute, the findings of the present study could be interpreted as providing some support for this hypothesis, though other interpretations are also possible.

The data sets presented in this chapter provide a much more accurate picture of the disabled reader by virtue of the comparisons made possible by having two control groups, one matched for age, the other for reading ability. The expense and effort of adding the second control group are far outweighed by the value of the additional information it provides, and the practice is to be encouraged in future research on dyslexia and learning disabilities.

Information on the etiology and symptomatology of learning disabilities is as yet incomplete. We have much to learn about the general characteristics of this group, characteristics that are liable, in any event, to be transformed by individual differences among cases. Two subjects of the same IQ and reading level may well be performing below their expected level for totally different reasons. Naturally, this variability will affect the kinds of pedagogical recommendations that are appropriate in each case. Similarly, attempts to match the 'educational opportunity' of LD subjects will be doomed to failure unless these individual differences are taken into account. Notwithstanding these cautions, the search for generalizations must proceed through the rigorous pursuit of research that observes the kind of controls and attention to validity that we have advocated in this chapter.

ACKNOWLEDGEMENT

The authors wish to thank Phyllis Mitchell for her assistance with the data collection.

REFERENCES

Bryden, M. P. (1982), *Laterality: Functional asymmetry in the intact brain*. New York, Academic Press.

Fisher, D. F. (1979), Dysfunctions in reading disability: there's more than meets the eye. In L. Resnick and P. Weaver (Eds.), *Theory and Practice in Beginning Reading*, Vol. 1. Hillsdale, NJ, Lawrence Erlbaum Associates.

Fisher, D. F. (1980), Compensatory training for disabled readers: research to practice. *Journal of Learning Disabilities* 13, 134–140.

Fisher, D. F. (1981), Compensatory training for disabled readers, II: Implementing and refining. *Journal of Learning Disabilities* 14, 451–454.

Fisher, D. F. (1984), Learning disabilities. In R. Corsini (Ed.), *John Wiley Encyclopedia of Psychology*. New York, John Wiley.

Fisher, D. F., and Frankfurter, A. (1977), Disabled readers can locate and identify letters: where's the perceptual deficit. *Journal of Reading Behaviour* **IX**, 31–43.

Harris, A. J. & Jacobson, M. D. (1972). *Basic Elementary Reading Vocabularies*. New York, Macmillan Co.

Reading Unlimited. (1976) New York: Scott Foresman.

Neurological Aspects

CHAPTER 4

Animal Studies and the Neurology of Developmental Dyslexia

ALBERT M. GALABURDA
The Neurological Unit and Charles A. Dana Research Institute, Beth Israel Hospital, 330 Brookline Avenue, Boston, Mass. 02215, and the Department of Neurology, Harvard Medical School, Boston, Mass. 02115, USA

It is now almost 100 years since a physician in the United Kingdom wrote a letter describing a student of his who, despite normal intelligence and adequate motivation, showed difficulty in learning to read and write adequately (Morgan, 1896). Subsequently, an ophthalmologist from Glasgow described several similar cases which came to be known under the descriptive title of Congenital Word Blindness (Hinshelwood, 1917). As these early discoveries came during a time when neurological explanations were being sought for a variety of disorders (usually acquired) affecting language, the initial explanations for 'Congenital Word Blindness' were also neurological. Thus, Hinshelwood and others thought the condition was the result of incomplete or abnormal ontogenetic development of the left angular gyrus, an area the lesions of which, when acquired later in life, were apt to produce difficulties in reading and writing. In spite of these early theories, no neurological documentation was ever gathered, and slowly these theories gave way to psychological explanations for developmental reading disability.

There is no uniform agreement as to the nature of developmental dyslexia. In all probability this general description relates to a group of children who, because of a variety of reasons, exhibit difficulty in learning to read and write efficiently despite normal intelligence, standard education, adequate motivation, and absence of psychiatric illness. Most workers in the field are aware that many dyslexic children have mild neurological accompaniments (Critchley, 1964). Furthermore, although dyslexia is mainly defined behaviorally, there are clearly some non-behavioral, biological associations (Galaburda and Kemper, 1979; Geschwind and Behan, 1982). Thus dyslexics vary behaviorally, i.e. there are

39

different subtypes of dyslexia, and also biologically, i.e. there are left-handers and right-handers, there are boys and girls, there are those with and those without family history and those with or without eye movement disturbances, EEG abnormalities, etc. Recent discoveries have shown that definable neuroanatomical substrates may be present in dyslexic children (Galaburda, 1983). Related studies have suggested differences in the anatomy of brain asymmetries among some dyslexics (Hier *et al.*, 1978). These realizations provide the impetus for the development of animal models in which to study the mechanisms underlying brain asymmetry as well as its breakdown during development. In the following paragraphs, I will attempt to show that certain aspects of language and reading in humans may share neurological substrates with experimental animals. Thus manifestations of brain asymmetry in animals, and the demonstration that brain asymmetry may develop abnormally in non-human species are biological data of significant potential usefulness for human studies.

ASYMMETRY IN ANIMALS

Cerebral lateralization (or cerebral dominance) refers to the differential proficiency of each cerebral hemisphere for the acquisition, performance and control over certain specific neurological functions. In humans, the most striking example of cerebral lateralization is illustrated by the left hemisphere's predominant control over language function. The few studies on developmental dyslexia that have dealt with its biological substrates have suggested that the condition may represent a disorder in the manifestation of cerebral lateralization (Witelson, 1977). First the demonstration of normal cerebral lateralization in experimental animals, and, second, the discovery of abnormal animal asymmetry, are a principal goal in any study of dyslexia based on animal models.

The first mention of brain asymmetry in non-human primates appeared in 1892 (Cunningham). In that report, the author noted asymmetry in the sylvian fissures of the mangaby, the chimpanzee, the orangutan and the baboon brain, but not in the brain of the macaque monkey. These asymmetries were similar to those seen in the human brain, i.e. one of the fissures (the right) tended to be shorter and curved upward whereas the other (the left) was longer and straighter (LeMay and Culebras, 1972). Similar findings were made in chimpanzees by Fisher (1921) as well as by LeMay and Geschwind (1975) and Yeni-Komshian and Benson (1976).

The human brain tends to show a prominence of the left occipital area (LeMay and Kido, 1978). This frequently produces an indentation of the inner table of the skull known as petalia. Left occipital petalia is more than five times as common in the human as right occipital patalia. Henschen (1926) found left occipital petalia in old male gorillas. Likewise, John Daniels III presumably a right-handed mountain gorilla, showed left occipital petalia. LeGros Clark

(1927) found a similar petalia in four and the opposite effect in one of eleven gorilla skulls.

The sylvian asymmetries in humans have been correlated with language lateralization. The discovery in non-human primate brains of asymmetries that are similar to those that have been reported in humans, may help to answer one of the questions about language capacity in non-human primates that has been heretofore difficult to resolve. If the communicative sounds made by monkeys and apes could be abolished by unilateral lesions in those asymmetrical perisylvian regions, it would strongly argue in favor of a preadapted form of language in these animals. Bilateral lesions in non-perisylvian areas would argue against homology between animal communication and human language.

Brain asymmetries have been reported in animals other than primates. Webster and Webster (1975) showed in two separate studies that about 45% of cats have asymmetric fissural patterns between the hemispheres. Furthermore, Kolb et al. (1982) found that 18 out of 25 cats had a heavier right hemisphere. Asymmetries in cortical thickness have been shown to be present in rats, cats, mice and rabbits (Diamond et al., 1975; Diamond et al., 1982; Kolb et al., 1982). Asymmetries have also been found in the total volume of a neocortex (Sherman and Galaburda, 1982) as well as in the thickness and weight of the hippocampus (Diamond et al., 1982; Kolb et al., 1982; Robinson et al., 1983; Valdes et al., 1981). In some of these asymmetries, sex differences have been documented. For instance, the thickness of the cortex is more asymmetric in males than in females, and in some regions it is biased toward the right side only in males. In females, on the other hand, the asymmetry is much less striking and tends to be biased toward the left side. Hippocampal asymmetries are also more striking in males than in females (Diamond et al., 1982).

Webster and Webster (1975) looked for, but were unable to demonstrate, a correlation between asymmetry of fissural patterns in cat brains and pawedness. In general, there have been no consistent findings of anatomical asymmetry in animals that can be correlated to behavioral measures of laterality. In my view, this may relate to the inability to predetermine sites of functional localization in animals. For instance, vocalization in animals may be thought to be akin to human language and asymmetries may be searched for in high order association cortices. Yet it is equally likely that such vocalization in fact arises in more primitive structures and is received and analyzed also in primitive subcortical auditory centers. In fact, preliminary results from our laboratory have established no correlation between lateralization of species-specific sources and cortical auditory asymmetries in the Japanese macaque monkey (Rosen et al., 1984).

Sherman and Galaburda (1982) on the other hand, have recently shown a relationship between total volume neocortical asymmetry and lateralized behavior. For instance, emotionality, a behavioral measure that can be altered by right hemisphere but not by left hemisphere lesions (cf. Denenberg, 1981), relates to the degree of asymmetry of total neocortical volume. The larger the degree of asymmetry between the two hemispheres, the larger the emotionality of the animal (Sherman *et al.*, 1984). It appears furthermore that the direction of wall-hugging behavior (the tendency for animal to traverse an open field by staying close to one of its walls) is related to the direction of the volume asymmetry, but only when this asymmetry is small in magnitude. Animals with asymmetry of greater magnitude show a diminished amount of movement which makes directionality measures unreliable.

There are many studies documenting the presence of additional postural and motor asymmetries in non-human species. These include measures of handedness, rotational behavior and tail posture in mice, rats, cats, gerbils and hamsters. Some of these asymmetries in behavior have been found to coexist or relate to asymmetries in neurochemical substances in various regions of the brain. For instance, there are asymmetries in dopamine level, dopamine-releasing effects, and dopamine receptors as well as dopamine-related enzyme activity in the striatum, the nucleus accumbens, and the frontal neocortex (cf. Robinson, *et al.*, 1984). By and large these asymmetries show greater catechol activity on the right side. These chemical asymmetries are similar to those occasionally documented in the human brain, which has also shown increased catechol-related activity in the right anterior thalamus (Oke *et al.*, 1980). Furthermore, recent anatomical studies of asymmetry in non-human species have shown that the right hemisphere tends to be predominant over the left, especially in males.

Asymmetries in favor of the right side in human males have been suggested at the level of function, whereby it is believed that on the average men exhibit better so-called right hemisphere skills such as some visual-spatial abilities. That these asymmetrical effects are seen mainly in males may reflect gender differences in sex chromosomes and/or of differences in sex-related hormones. It has been shown that some of these asymmetries can be altered by the manipulation of sex steroids. Thus, Diamond *et al.* (1984) have reported that the typically found right hemisphere preponderance in thickness of the visual cortex in the male rat can be abolished by castration, and that the typical female pattern, consisting of a tendency toward left preponderance, can be turned into the masculine pattern by exposure to male sex steroids soon after birth. These findings suggest that the male effect is to shift asymmetrical development away from left hemisphere and in favor of the right. An extreme instance of this effect, perhaps pathological in nature, might result in incompetency of left hemisphere development such as that illustrated by developmental dyslexia. One useful means to investigate this possibility would be by creating this exaggerated slowing of left hemisphere development in experimental animals and testing for behavioral consequences.

ASYMMETRY OF PATHOLOGY

The discovery that the animal and human brain are asymmetrical with respect to anatomy and chemistry suggests that insults even administered bilaterally or at random in the nervous system, and toxic metabolic events affecting both sides, may in fact have asymmetrical effects. Therefore, just as the injection of amphetamines into the abdomen of a rat produces unidirectional rotation (although the drug is distributed bilaterally in the blood stream), the injection of a toxin that binds to the receptor sites of catecholamines will likely produce asymmetrical pathology. There are several examples in neurology of neurological and systemic diseases that affect one side of the body more often than the other. Thus, the incidence of certain tumors, of certain malformations, as well as some allergic responses may be different on the two sides. Experimental animals may offer additional help in the specification of mechanisms underlying asymmetrical pathology.

Layton and Hallesy (1965) showed that pregnant rats exposed to high levels of acetazolamide developed predominantly unilateral limb deformities (hemimelias). In their experiments, female rat pups were affected more frequently than males, and only the right forelimb was affected in cases of unilateral malformation. The mechanisms leading to this type of malformation are still unknown, but research conducted in our laboratory has shown that the limb deformity may be associated with a unilateral defect in hemisphere development. Malformations in rat pups were produced following the protocol of Layton and Hallesy. In some instances we were able to show that the cortex of the hemisphere ipsilateral to the malformation showed evidence of migration arrest. This developmental arrest was characterized by a primitive appearance of the laminar organization of the visual cortex particularly. In those instances, the deeper layers contained large primitive cells whereas the superficial layers were sparsely populated and the fourth layer scanty, suggesting an arrest at an earlier stage of neuronal migration to the cortex. It is interesting to note that similar malformations have been described in the human (O'Rahilly, 1951). Hemimelia, therefore, occurs spontaneously in the human population, and, in this case, males are affected more commonly than females, although, as in the rat, the right upper extremity is also the most likely single limb to be affected. It is also noted that this type of limb malformation occurs more commonly in the children of mothers taking sex steroids during pregnancy. Both in the human and animal limb deformity a chemical agent is capable of affecting one side of the body and brain preferentially, and in the human case sex steroids play an etiologic role. In humans a smaller right hand may reflect an early left-hemisphere lesion, thus suggesting that left hemisphere abnormalities might accompany the right hemimelia in the human males. This possibility would again support the notion that sex-steroid related malformations affect the left hemisphere more than the right. It is easy to see that the specification of the mechanisms involved in limb malformation in animals may shed light on the mechanisms responsible for left hemisphere impairment in developmental dyslexia.

Thus far, three brains of dyslexic individuals have been examined in our laboratory, and an additional brain was reported from another center. All of these brains have shown abnormalities dating back to the period of neuronal migration to the cerebral cortex. The anomalies affect the left hemisphere more than the right hemisphere. In the first case, reported by Drake (1968), mention was made of ectopically located cells, abnormality of folding of the parietal cortex, and thinning of the corpus callosum. The second case (Galaburda and Kemper, 1979) disclosed an instance of micropolygyria and multiple instances of neuronal ectopias and cortical dysplasias involving the cortex of the left hemisphere. A subsequent case (Galaburda, 1983) showed similar dysplasias and ectopias involving predominantly the left cerebral cortex of the brain of a 14-year-old dyslexic boy with familial dyslexia. A recent study (Galaburda et al., 1985) of the brain of a 19-year-old man with developmental dyslexia as well as a congential attentional deficit has shown multiple dysplasias and ectopias involving the cortex of both hemispheres, but most severely the superior temporal gyrus and inferior frontal gyrus of the left hemisphere.

The discovery of instances of ectopia and dysplasia in the brains of dyslexic individuals has suggested that these lesions must have been formed during the period of neuronal migration and could not therefore have been acquired after birth. This dispels fears regarding possible traumatic, toxic and other environmental effects in the newborn, infant or childhood periods. Studies on experimental animals helped to confirm the migration theory. Thus, Dvořák and co-workers (1977, 1978) have shown that it is possible to produce the whole gamut of abnormalities from mild neuronal ectopias, cortical dysplasia, through verrucous dysplasia, and micropolygyria in newborn rodents while still in the period of neuronal migration to the cerebral cortex. The same experiments performed either before or after this period failed to produce the desired pathology. Irrespective of the behavioral consequences of these lesions in the rodents, the anatomical knowledge obtained from these experiments can be used to clarify the possible chronology of the lesions in developmental dyslexia.

'DYSLEXIC' LESIONS IN AUTOIMMUNE MICE

Recently Geschwind and Behan (1982) published a report linking left-handedness with the increased incidence of certain immune-related disorders. Among left-handers there was an increased incidence of learning disabilities (especially developmental dyslexia), migraine headaches, and certain immune disorders particularly of the bowel and thyroid. This clinical observation prompted the design of a pilot study on an experimental animal that regularly develops immune diseases (Sherman et al., 1983). The New Zealand Black mouse was developed initially for cancer research and was soon noted to develop a disorder which is similar to human systemic lupus erythematosus, an immune-mediated disease affecting females in their reproductive years. We have looked at 38 brains of NZB, its F1 hybrid NZB/W, and the NZW and C57 Black control mice. Approximately 25 per cent of the experimental animals show abnormalities in cortical development characterized by neuronal ectopia, and their appearance under light microscopy is strikingly similar to the ectopic collection of cells seen in the brains of dyslexics. The ectopias are located in layer one of the cortex which is normally virtually devoid of neurons. The most typical location of the ectopias is in the areas surrounding the primary sensory motor cortices of the fronto-parietal region. The anomalies are either completely unilateral, or, when bilateral, affect one side much more strongly than the other. Unlike other reports in the literature (de Vries and Hijman, 1967), our animals have not shown significant collections of inflammatory cells in the choroid plexus, the pial surface, or the perivascular spaces. This may reflect the fact that our animals are young and have not, as yet, developed clinical signs of inflammatory autoimmune disease.

Most of the cortical abnormalities have been seen in 30-day-old mice, and occur similarly in males and females. No particular side is affected more frequently than the other. On the other hand, additional studies are being carried out now on larger numbers in order to see if in fact there is a sex or side preference for the location of the neuronal ectopias. These preliminary findings suggest that the New Zealand mouse and some of its hybrid forms may be a suitable model for the study of mechanisms underlying cortical ectopias as seen in the brains of dyslexics. The model will be much stronger if one is also able to document behavioral accompaniments to the neuroanatomical abnormalities. Two short papers in the literature have documented learning abnormalities in this population of mice. One paper reported that, in association with increased brain-reactive antibodies, NZB mice showed learning deficits on a conditioned avoidance response task (Nandy *et al.*, 1983); another study found deficits in a variety of associational and memory tasks in the NZB mice (Spencer and Lal, 1983).

ASYMMETRIES IN DEVELOPMENT

Thus far, asymmetries have been demonstrated in the anatomy of the nervous systems of non-human animals as well as in certain aspects of their behavior. Asymmetries have also been shown in pathological tendencies and the relevance of these findings is particularly clear in the ectopic collections of neurons seen in the autoimmune mice and in the brains of dyslexic individuals. Underlying all of these observations is the notion that, at least in the dyslexic person, the left hemisphere appears to be more vulnerable to developmental neuropathology. This lateralized vulnerability may be in fact the result of the asymmetrical development of the nervous system. Thus, it has been noted that the human brain develops more quickly on the right side than on the left side. For example, it has been noticed in several studies that the folding of the cortex surrounding the sylvian fissure is visible earlier on the right side than on the left (Hervé, 1888; Fontes, 1944; Chi et al., 1977). In the case of the cortex containing the auditory representations in the sylvian fossa, the sulci and gyri are visible sometimes two weeks earlier on the right as compared to the left. This would suggest that the left hemisphere is developing over a longer period of time and is thus vulnerable over a longer period to the noxious effects capable of altering its development. We recently reported that the right frontal lobe of the rat brain grows faster than the left during the early post-natal period (DeBassio et al., 1982). Thus after measuring the growth of the olfactory migratory stream to the bulb, we noted that the initial growth of the right stream was faster than the left and then slowed down, whereas the initially more slowly growing left migratory stream continued to grow beyond the period during which the right had already stopped. Although a repeat study in our laboratory has not confirmed this initial observation, a recent study by Narang (1977) showed in the rabbit that the right optic nerve myelinates earlier than the left, and that this earlier myelination was accompanied by the earlier opening of the right eye in the neonatal period.

The few observations available at this time indicate that the left hemisphere, both in humans and some animals, develops more slowly than the right. Although the asymmetry in cortical folding clearly manifests itself during the period following neuronal migration, when the neurons are growing and establishing connectivity, and the cortex is folding, it is possible that the hemispheric asymmetry in developmental rates in fact is present during or even before the period of neuronal migration. The effect of sex steroids, particularly male hormones, on the development of the asymmetry of the hemispheres (see above) suggests that male sex steroids could be acting to retard the growth of the left hemisphere. This would explain the asymmetries in favor of the right side for certain portions of the cortex of the male rat. This might also help explain the observation that, on the average, those functions associated with left hemisphere function, i.e. language, are on the average less well developed in males than in females. A corollary to this hypothesis would state that the testosterone effect, when present in an extreme form, could result in the abnormal retardation of left hemisphere development. This could possibly lead to abnormal cortical development and the presence of ectopias, dysplasias and primitive patterns of cortical connections. In the latter situation a left hemisphere could be produced which is incapable of handling effectively the linguistic tasks required for reading and writing, hence developmental dyslexia. This hypothesis would also explain the excessive incidence of dyslexia among boys, as compared to girls, and the greater representation of left-handers among dyslexic populations.

As noted by Geschwind and Behan (1982) male steroids also have effects on the development and manifestations of the immune system. It is conceivable that the postulated enhanced testosterone effect among dyslexics not only produces abnormalities in the development of the left hemisphere, but also abnormalities in the development of the immune system. It is even conceivable that the neuronal migration anomaly seen in the left hemisphere of dyslexics is a result of immune mediated phenomena affecting the apparatus required for proper neuronal migration. These hypotheses require experimental confirmation.

The discovery of an animal model showing disordered neuronal migration similar to that seen in the dyslexic brains offers a way by which to study the mechanisms involved in the formation of these anomalies as well as the relationship between these anomalies and lateralized behavior. Furthermore, such an animal can offer the possibility to study the relationships among cortical development, lateralized brain development, and the development of immune functions and their interaction with sex steroids. It appears, therefore, that the three neurological principles coming to bear on developmental dyslexia, i.e. asymmetry, immunity, and sex differences, can all be studied in experimental animals because of the recent demonstrations of normal and abnormal asymmetry in non-human species.

ACKNOWLEDGEMENTS

This work has been supported by NIH grants NS14018 and NS07211, the Wm. Underwood Co., the Powder River Company, the Essel Foundation, and a biomedical research award from the Beth Israel Hospital.

REFERENCES

Chi, J. G., Dooling, E. C., and Gilles, F. H. (1977), Gyral development of the human brain. *Annals of Neurology* 1, 86–92.
Clark, W. E. LeGros (1927), Description of cerebral hemispheres of the brain of the gorilla. *Journal of Anatomy* 61, 467–475.
Critchley, M. (1964), *Developmental Dyslexia*. London, Heinemann.
Cunningham, D. J. (1892), Contribution to the surface anatomy of the cerebral hemispheres. *Cunningham Memoirs* 7, 372.
DeBassio, W. A., Kemper, T. L., and Galaburda, A. M. (1982), Asymmetric olfactory migratory stream in the rat. *Society for Neuroscience Abstracts* 8, 326.
Denenberg, V. H. (1981), Hemispheric laterality in animals and the effects of early experience. *Behavioral Brain Sciences* 4, 1–49.
Diamond, M. C., Johnson, R. E., and Ingham, C. A., Morphological changes in the young, adult and aging rat cerebral cortex, hippocampus and diencephalon. *Behavioral Biology* 14, 163–174.
Diamond, M. C., Murphy, G. J. Jr, Akiyama, K., and Johnson, R. E. (1982) Morphological hippocampal asymmetry in male and female rats. *Experimental Neurology* 76, 553–565.
Diamond, M. C. (1984), Age, sex and environmental influences on anatomical asymmetry in rat forebrain. In: Geschwind, N., and Galaburda, A. M. (Eds.), *Biological Foundations of Cerebral Dominance*. Cambridge, Mass., Harvard University Press.

Drake, W. E. (1968), Clinical and pathological findings in a child with a developmental learning disability. *Journal of Learning Disabilities* **1**, 9–25.

Dvořák, K., and Feit, L. (1977), Migration of neuroblasts through partial necrosis of the cerebral cortex in newborn rats. *Acta Neuropathologica* **38**, 203–212.

Dvořák, K., Feit, L., and Juránková, Z. (1978), Experimentally induced focal micropolygyria and status verrucosus deformis in rats: Pathogenesis interrelation. *Acta Neuropathologica* **44**, 121–129.

Fisher, E. (1921). Reported by Yeni-Komshian and Benson (1976).

Fontes, V. (1944), *Morfologia do Cortex Cerebral*, Boletin do Instituto de Antonio Aurelio da Costa Ferreira: Lisbon.

Galaburda, A. M. (1983), Developmental dyslexia: Current anatomical research. *Annals of Dyslexia* **33**, 41–53.

Galaburda, A. M., and Kemper, T. L. (1979), Cytoarchitectonic abnormalities in developmental dyslexia: A case study. *Annals of Neurology* **6**, 94–100.

Galaburda, A. M., Sherman, G. F., Rosen, G. D., Aboitiz, F., and Geschwind, N. (1985), Developmental dyslexia: Four consecutive patients with cortical anomalies. *Annals of Neurology* **18**, 222–233.

Geschwind, N., and Behan, P. (1982), Left-handedness: Association with immune disease, migraine, and developmental learning disorder. *Proceedings of the National Academy of Sciences (USA)* **79**, 5097–5100.

Henschen, S. E. (1926), On the function of the right hemisphere of the brain and its relation to the left in speech, music, and calculation. *Brain* **49**, 110–123.

Hervé, G. (1888), *La Circonvolution de Broca*. Paris, Delahaye et LeCrosnier.

Hier, D. B., LeMay, M., Rosenberger, P. B., and Perlo, V. P. (1978), Developmental dyslexia. *Archives of Neurology* **35**, 90–92.

Hinshelwood, J. (1917), *Congenital Word Blindness*. London, Lewis.

Kolb, B., Sutherland, R. J., Nonneman, A. J., and Whishaw, I. Q. (1982), Asymmetry in the cerebral hemispheres of the rat, mouse, rabbit and cat: The right hemisphere is larger. *Experimental Neurology* **78**, 348–359.

Layton, W. M., and Hallesy, D. W. (1965), Deformity of forelimb in rats: Association with high doses of acetazolamide. *Science* **149**, 306–308.

LeMay, M., and Culebras, A. (1972), Human brain: Morphologic differences in the hemispheres demonstrable by carotid arteriography. *New England Journal of Medicine* **287**, 168–170.

LeMay, M., and Geschwind, N. (1975), Hemispheric differences in the brains of great apes. *Brain, Behavior and Evolution* **11**, 48–52.

LeMay, M., and Kido, D. K. (1978), Asymmetries of the cerebral hemispheres on computed tomograms. *Journal of Computer Assisted Tomography* **2**, 471–476.

Morgan, W. P. (1896), A case of congenital word-blindness. *British Medical Journal* **2**, 1378.

Nandy, K., Lal, H., Bennett, M., and Bennett, D. (1983), Correlation between a learning disorder and elevated brain-reactive antibodies in aged C57B1/6 and young NZB mice. *Life Sciences* **33**, 1499–1503.

Narang, H. K. (1977), Right-left asymmetry of myelin development in epiretinal portion of the rabbit optic nerve. *Nature* **266**, 28.

Oke, A., Keller, R., Mefford, I., and Adams, R. N. (1980), Lateralization of norepinephrine in human thalamus. *Brain Research* **188**, 269–272.

O'Rahilly, R. (1951), Morphological patterns of limb deficiencies and implications. *American Journal of Anatomy* **89**, 135–167.

Robinson, T. E., Becker, J. B., and Camp, D. M. (1983), Sex differences in behavioral and brain asymmetries. In: Myslobodsky, M. S. (Ed.), *Hemisyndromes: Psychobiology, Neurology, Psychiatry*. New York, Academic Press, pp. 91–128.

Robinson, T. E., Becker, J. B., Camp, D. M., and Mansour, A. (1984), Variations in the pattern of behavioral and brain asymmetries due to sex differences. In: Glick, S. D. (Ed.), *Cerebral Lateralization in Non-Human Species*, New York, Academic Press.

Rosen, G. D., Petersen, M. R., Aboitiz, F., and Galaburda, A. M. (1984), Auditory lateralization in Japanese macaques and its relationship to cortical and subcortical asymmetries. *Society for Neuroscience Abstracts* 10, 313.

Sherman, G. F., and Galaburda, A. M. (1982), Cortical volume asymmetry and behavior in the albino rat. *Society for Neuroscience Abstracts* 8, 627.

Sherman, G. F., Galaburda, A. M., and Geschwind, N. (1983), Ectopic neurons in the brain of the autoimmune mouse: A neuropathological model of dyslexia? *Society for Neuroscience Abstracts* 9, 939.

Sherman, G. F., Hasselmo, M. E., and Galaburda, A. M. (1984), Early experience, sex, and hippocampal asymmetry in the albino rat. *Society for Neuroscience Abstracts* 10, 313.

Spencer, D. G. Jr, and Lal, H. (1983), Specific behavioral impairments in associational tasks in mice with an autoimmune disorder. *Society for Neuroscience Abstracts* 9, 96.

Valdes, J. J., Mactutus, C. F., Cory, R. N., and Cameron, W. R. (1981), Lateralization of norepinephrine, serotonin and choline uptake into hippocampal synaptosomes of sinistral rats. *Physiology and Behavior* 27, 381-383.

Vries, M. J. de, and Hijman, W. (1967), Pathological changes of thymic epithelial cells and autoimmune disease in NZB, NZW, and (NZB×NZW) F1 mice. *Immunology* 12, 179-196.

Webster, W. G., and Webster, I. H. (1975), Anatomic asymmetry of the cerebral hemispheres of the cat brain. *Physiology and Behavior* 14, 867-869.

Witelson, S. F. (1977), Developmental dyslexia: Two right-hemispheres and none left. *Science* 195, 309-311.

Yeni-Komshian, G. H., and Benson, D. A. (1976), Anatomical study of cerebral asymmetry in the temporal lobe of humans, chimpanzees and rhesus monkeys. *Science* 192, 387-389.

CHAPTER 5

Dyslexia, Cerebral Dominance, Autoimmunity, and Sex Hormones

NORMAN GESCHWIND*
James Jackson Putman Professor of Neurology, Harvard Medical School; Director, Neurological Unit, Beth Israel Hospital; Professor of Psychology, Massachusetts Institute of Technology

Nearly a century has passed since developmental dyslexia was first recognized. Over this period it has been linked to the concept of cerebral dominance, but the importance of this connection has not always been fully appreciated. Many theories have been offered to explain this common and disturbing condition, but they have often failed to take into account the clues as to causation that a closer consideration of cerebral dominance might have made available. Within a space of less than 10 years, however, new investigations have begun to lay bare the foundations for this condition in disturbance of the processes which lead to asymmetrical structure and function of the brain.

It need not be surprising that the concept of cerebral dominance has been so often linked to that of dyslexia. Developmental difficulty in the acquisition of the comprehension and production of the written word is a disorder of acquisition of a set of language functions. It is, therefore, reasonable to consider how the knowledge of the biology of language might contribute to an understanding of this particular failure of the acquisition of linguistic competence.

The history of the understanding of the linkage of the brain to language begins, as is well known, with one of the great discoveries of the nineteenth century, i.e. Paul Broca's finding that brain lesions in aphasics lay in nearly all cases on the left side of the brain. In the wake of this initial discovery many investigators in the last half of the nineteenth century began to search for the neurological substrates of many conditions in which one or another aspect of

* Deceased

51

language was impaired as a result of an acquired brain lesion. In the years 1891 and 1892 the great French neurologist Jules Dejerine described the brain lesions which were responsible for the loss of the capacity to understand written language.

Of particular importance from the point of view of the understanding of dyslexia was the description by Dejerine (1891) of the post-mortem findings in a case of acquired alexia with agraphia. In this condition a person who had previously been capable of reading and writing loses these abilities while retaining his capacities for the production of spoken language and for the comprehension of the utterances of others (Benson and Geschwind, 1969). The loss of reading and writing is best described as a return to the state of illiteracy. Thus, like the illiterate, these patients, retain normal visual function and are able to describe objects in the environment with great accuracy. On the other hand they are incapable of comprehending the written word. Although they can use their limbs quite normally for other activities they are no longer capable of writing. Even the act of copying the printed word is slow and the patients copy words of their own language as slowly as a native reader of English might copy a text in a strange alphabet such as Chinese or Russian.

The analogy with a return to illiteracy is, however, even closer than is suggested even by these striking facts. Thus, like the illiterate, patients, can repeat a word spoken to them but they cannot spell it. If a word is spelled to them they can repeat the letter names but they are not able to say what word they form. When letters are drawn on their hand or when they palpate anagram letters, they are incapable of deciding what word they represent. They have thus lost not only the capacity to understand and produce visual language but also all capability of carrying out those performances which depend on a knowledge of written language.

The lesion in this remarkable condition, as has been verified many times since Dejerine's original description, illustrates again the laterality of language function. There is destruction within the cortical area lying at the junction of the temporal, parietal and occipital lobes on the left side.

These facts were known to many of the early students of dyslexia such as Orton. The conjecture immediately presented itself that the brain disturbance in those children who were suffering from an inability to acquire reading might lie in the same location as the acquired lesion which led to the loss of these acquired abilities in the adult. The possibility that there was some disturbance in the left angular gyrus region in the dyslexic thus arose naturally as one of Orton's hypotheses as to the cause of this condition.

The evidence that dyslexia had some special relationship to cerebral dominance extended, however, even beyond the suggestive parallelism between the acquired disorders of reading and the developmental failure to acquire this talent. In his very first paper, in which he describes the childhood dyslexics he had observed for the first time in his career in rural Iowa, Orton (1925) pointed out that there was an elevated rate of left-handedness both in the dyslexics themselves and in their families. He also pointed out in this very first paper that there appeared to be an elevated frequency of stuttering among the dyslexics, i.e. specific reading disability was linked to another condition in which there was an elevated frequency of left-handedness.

There was another extremely important clue as to the underlying cause of dyslexia which was commented on by Orton in this pioneering initial publication and which has been found repeatedly over the years. Although dyslexia could occur in both sexes there was a dramatic preponderance of males. In this way, also, it resembled stuttering, in which the male preponderance is even more striking.

Orton made only one incorrect guess in his original discussion as to theoretical possibilities as to the cause of childhood dyslexia. He assumed that there would be no visible abnormality in the malfunctioning zone within the left hemisphere but that the disturbance would be 'functional'.

These three findings, i.e. the resemblance of childhood dyslexia to acquired alexia with agraphia, the elevated frequency of left-handedness among dyslexics, and the male predominance of this condition, contained the seeds of a biological theory of this condition as well as of other related disorders such as stuttering and delayed speech. The clues were, however, not immediately seized upon. There were many who were understandably suspicious of too facile an extrapolation from acquired disorders of the adult to the developmental disorders of childhood. One major argument, which I also accepted for a long time, against the possibility of a unilateral disturbance in the brain confined to the left side, was based on the well-known fact that there was typically very good recovery from the language disorders produced by unilateral brain lesions in early childhood. If there was such excellent recovery from an early childhood lesion than a disturbance taking place even earlier, i.e. at birth or in intrauterine life should be compensated for even more dramatically.

It is now clear, however, that anomalies of formation of the cortex at the junction of the temporal and parietal lobes are indeed present in a significant proportion of dyslexic brains, and these anomalies may be found only on the left side. (Galaburda and Kemper (1978) described these findings in one case and since then they have also been found in others.)

It has also become clear that the expectation that a lesion or a disturbance of formation of a language region on the left side which takes place in intrauterine life is not responded to in the same manner as a lesion acquired after birth. In the case of the post-natal damage to a language area on the left there is a shift of language to the opposite side at the expense of the normal right hemisphere functions. It is now clear, however, from the work of such investigators as Goldman and Galkin (1978) that a cortical lesion sustained before birth leads to enlargement of the corresponding region of the opposite side as well as of some other cortical regions. Thus, the pre-natal lesion may lead to impairment of the function normally represented in the area of cortex which is disturbed, but in compensation there is superior development of cortical regions mediating other functions.

It is clearly of importance to attempt to understand the mechanisms which lead to this intrauterine delay of development, such as is represented in the anomalous cortical structure described by Galaburda and Kemper. Clues as to this mechanism have now come from another surprising source. Left-handedness is associated in elevated frequency not only with the learning disabilities of childhood such as dyslexia, stuttering and autism, but also with an elevated frequency of disorders of the immune system and migraine (Geschwind and Behan, 1982). As should become clear by the end of this chapter, these surprising associations offer what I believe to be important clues as to the ultimate mechanisms of disturbance of formation of the brain in childhood dyslexia and related disorders. It is perhaps worth recounting what led to these observations. In November 1980 the Orton Dyslexia Society held its annual meeting in Boston. Preceding this meeting a special symposium took place on 'Sex differences in dyslexia' organized by Richard Masland with my assistance. In the course of this conference one of the speakers discussed the familial patterns of dyslexia. In discussing this paper I pointed out that it might be useful to look not only for dyslexia in other family members, as well as other cognitive impairments, but also to look for diseases of any nature whatsoever. Immediately following the session many members of the audience, themselves either dyslexics or close relatives of dyslexics came up to me to tell me about their familial medical histories. I was immediately struck by the high frequency of two sets of conditions. The first group consisted of disorders of the immune system and the second of migraine headaches.

A brief digression is appropriate here concerning the term 'disorders of the immune system'. As is well known the immune system is a very complicated array of organs such as the thymus gland and the lymph nodes and of circulating cells, including lymphocytes as well as other components of the blood. The major function of this system is to combat infection by bacteria viruses, or parasites. In a system of such complexity it is not surprising that something can go wrong in the complex pattern of control. There are at least two major ways in which the system can go awry. Attack may be mounted against harmless, noninfective substances such as cat hair or ragweed pollen that are in themselves innocuous and do not disturb the majority of people. In some people, however, the immune system attacks these substance as if they were invading organisms. The anomalous misdirected immune responses of this type are the cause of the childhood allergies such as asthma, eczema, or hayfever.

The immune system can also go wrong in another way. Normally, the system has been very cleverly designed so that it does not attack foreign substances which are found in the blood stream of the fetus during intrauterine life. In other words any substances which is present at that time is recognized as 'self' rather than as foreign. As a result of this mechanism the immune system in later life does not attack components of the person's own body. Something can, however, upset this mechanism so that the immune system does attack components of the organism itself. Immune attack may thus take place against the lining of the joints, thus producing immune arthritis, against the skin, producing many forms of immune dermatitis, or against the thyroid gland leading to autoimmune thyroiditis, one of the most common conditions of this type and the leading cause of diminished thyroid function. In other cases, the immune system can attack various parts of the gastrointestinal tract leading to disorders such as ulcerative colitis, regional ileitis (Crohn's disease), or celiac disease. Indeed, there is probably no structure within the body which may not be the target of autoimmune attack in susceptible individuals.

Following my discussions with many of the attendants at that meeting I began to watch carefully for this set of associations among those with childhood learning disorders. I was soon struck by the fact that the association appeared to be a much broader one, i.e. it was not an association primarily with the developmental disorders of childhood, but more broadly with left-handedness. Before long I had collected accounts of several families in which over generations one found individuals with left-handedness, developmental disorders, immune diseases, and migraine. All of the conditions might be present in one individual but in other cases they were distributed over different family members. Thus, one might observe a strongly left-handed dyslexic who had right-handed relatives with immune disease. On the other hand some members of the family might be left-handed while there were right-handed members with learning disabilities or with any of the other conditions mentioned.

Another brief digression is appropriate at this point concerning left-handedness. Most students of dyslexia and of stuttering will be aware that while many authors have stressed the existence of an elevated frequency of left-handedness in these conditions others have denied the association. There are several reasons for the existence of these discrepancies. In the first place it is important to devote considerable care to the assessment of manual dominance. Many investigators have relied only on the hand used for writing. This is, however, treacherous for several reasons. While Americans are probably more tolerant than any other people in the world concerning the use of the left hand it is still not rare to find individuals particularly in the older generation who were forced to use the right hand for writing against their natural inclinations to use the left. Secondly, there are many individuals who will write with the right hand but carry out a large number of activities with the left. One should recall that the most common single pattern of handedness is one in which the individual uses his right hand for just about every task. About 70 per cent of the population fall into this category. Approximately 10 per cent are frankly left-handed, i.e. they write with the left hand and do most other activity with this hand. There are, however, about 20 per cent of individuals who do several tasks with the left hand but write with the right hand. This intermediate group is often referred to as ambidextrous. There are several pieces of evidence that they are quite different from the 70 per cent majority who are overwhelmingly right-handed, but if the writing hand alone is used as an index of handedness they will be classified with the majority rather than with the non-right-handed minority. It is thus important to obtain some quantitative measure of handedness. I would like to point out that there is at the present time no really good test for handedness. Space does not permit me to go into a full discussion of this topic. Despite this fact, however, it is far better to use some quantitative measure rather than to rely on the use of the writing hand alone.

It is sometimes argued that it is legitimate to use the writing hand alone because there is a high correlation between the writing hand and scores obtained on formal batteries. It is true that there is a high correlation but this does not alter the fact that reliance on the hand with which writing is carried out leads to important errors. It is easy to see the reason. Approximately 70 per cent of the population carry out nearly all activities with the right hand, and this group almost universally uses the right hand for writing. On the other hand in the remaining 30 per cent a significant number of activities are carried out with the left hand but about two-thirds of this group are also right-handed writers. When one considers the larger group one finds a correlation of nearly one between the writing hand and the score on the handedness battery. The remaining 30 per cent, the group of major interest, is one in which the correlation is much lower.

As a result of the many observations mentioned above which had led me to hypothesize that there was a strong connection between left-handedness and immune disorders in migraine I decided that it was necessary to carry out a formal study. I therefore enlisted the help of Peter Behan, who had trained in neurology with me and who was now one of the senior neurologists at the University of Glasgow and a leading expert on immunological aspects of neurology.

Let me now specify how we planned this study. We realized that a major difficulty in other studies which had considered handedness as one variable was that of specifying a cut-off point for left-handedness. In our studies we made use of the Oldfield (1971) battery for handedness which had been validated in a Scottish population. On this test the subject receives a score called a laterality quotient which extends from + 100, i.e. complete right-handedness to − 100, i.e. complete left-handedness. Oldfield had chosen a score of 0, i.e. the score achieved when the respondent indicated equal use of the right and left hands in his reply to the ten questions. We decided, however, to begin our studies by taking only subjects with extreme scores, i.e. + 100 or − 100. In this manner we believed that one would be observing individuals who by any criterion would be regarded as strongly right-handed or strongly left-handed and we would thus avoid the possible confounding effect of including subjects with intermediate scores i.e. individuals whose predominant handedness might not be so easily determined. We placed a large group of questionnaires in the shop Anything Left-Handed in London which sells items for left-handers. In order to obtain our strongly right-handed

Table 1. First study, Part 1: Immune and learning disorders in left- and right-handers

| | Immune disorders | | | Learning disorders | | |
	LH	RH	p	LH	RH	p
	No. (96)	No. (96)		No. (96)	No. (96)	
Subjects	27 (10.7)	10 (4.0)	<0.005	24 (9.5)	2 (0.8)	<0.005
1st degree relatives	48	25	<0.01	21	7	<0.01
2nd degree relatives	45	23	<0.01	11	1	<0.001

LH = left-handers (N = 253); RH = right-handers (N = 253). The first row indicates the number and percentage of subjects suffering from one of the indicated disorders. The second and third rows indicate the number of relatives suffering from these disorders

control group our assistants administered questionnaires to a large group of individuals in the general population of Glasgow. We received 253 responses from individuals with laterality quotients of −100, and out of our general population group we selected 253 individuals with laterality quotients of +100 who were selected for the purpose of matching our sinistral group for age and sex.

The results of this study are seen in Table 1. Our questionnaire contained not only the Oldfield Handedness Battery but also a number of questions concerning familial and personal history of health and function. As can be seen from Table 1 this pilot study appeared to provide strong verification of our hypothesis. The rate of immune disorders was 2.5 times as high in our strongly left-handed group as in the right-handed group. Similarly, we found a much higher rate of immune disease in the relatives of our left-handers than in those of our right-handers. Another aspect of the study was the responses to the questions concerning the developmental learning disorders, i.e. dyslexia and stuttering. As can be seen from the table the rate of these disorders was more than ten times as high in our strongly sinistral group as in the strongly dextral and the rate of these conditions was also much higher in the relatives of the left-handers.

We realized that the results of the first study, dramatic as they were, raised some important questions. The left-handers who had gone to the shop in London and responded to our questionnaires were, of course, a self-selected group and one had to take cognizance of the possibility that we might get cooperation more readily from those who had the disorders mentioned in our questionnaire. We, therefore, decided to carry out a second study to which this objection could not be raised.

In the second study our interviewers administered questionnaires to a large number of individuals in the general population of Glasgow. We then selected questionnaires in which the laterality quotient was −100 or +100. In this study we had 247 left-handers and 647 right-handers. In addition, in this study, we did not accept the diagnosis of immune disease unless it had been made in a teaching hospital in Glasgow. It should be pointed out that many patients with

Table 2. First study, Part 2

| | Immune disorders | | | Learning disorders | | |
	LH	RH	p	LH	RH	p
	No. (96)	No. (96)		No. (96)	No. (96)	
Subjects	13 (5.3)	15 (2.3)	<0.025	27 (10.9)	8 (1.2)	<0.001
1st degree relatives	58	102	<0.025	19	24	<0.025
2nd degree relatives	19	18	<0.005	2	4	a

LH = left-handers ($N = 247$); RH = right-handers ($N = 647$).
[a] Numbers too small for calculation of p.

autoimmune disease will be diagnosed and treated entirely outside the hospital setting. This is true of autoimmune hypothyroidism and of rheumatoid arthritis. We did not, in this study, use any of the figures on such diagnoses but included only those individuals who had been diagnosed either in one of the hospital clinics or on an inpatient service. Although this cut down the absolute number of patients with immune disease it did insure a much more uniform standard of diagnosis.

As can be seen from Table 2 the results in this study were essentially similar to those of the first study. As we have already noted the absolute number of patients with immune disorder was smaller because of the exclusion of those who had not been seen in one of the hospitals, but we found that the strongly left-handed individuals again had about 2.5 times as many cases of autoimmune disease as the right-handed individuals. Furthermore, we again found a higher rate of immune disease in the relatives of the sinistrals than those of the dextrals.

The data on childhood learning disorders in this study provided an important check on our first study. We found almost the identical figures for the percentage of learning disabilities in the two groups in this study as we did in the first study. Thus, roughly 10 per cent of our strong sinistrals had suffered from one of the childhood learning disorders and the rate among the sinistrals was again about ten times as high as the rate in the dextrals.

On the basis of these two studies we could be quite confident that the rates of immune disorder and learning disability were much higher among the strong left-handers than among the strong right-handers. We do not place as much stress on the higher frequencies of these disorders in the relatives of the left-handers for two reasons. In the first place there is obviously a very high rate of error in questions concerning illness in family members. Secondly, individuals who have immune disease are much more likely to be aware of its presence in other family members than those who do not.

Since the time of publication of our original paper we have completed another large series comparing strong left-handers and strong right-handers and our results again confirm those found in the first two series.

Another question immediately presents itself. There are many different types of autoimmune disease and it is therefore reasonable to ask whether all of them are more frequent among strong left-handers than strong right-handers. Obviously, some of these disorders are common, such as autoimmune hypothyroidism or rheumatoid arthritis, while others are very rare. Our study could not, therefore, answer this question in regard to the full range of immune diseases. We were struck, however, by the fact that certain immune disorders appeared in apparently high frequency among our patients with personal sinistrality. We were impressed by the large number of patients with autoimmune diseases of the thyroid, or with autoimmune disorder of the gastrointestinal tract, i.e. ulcerative colitis, regional ileitis, and celiac disease. We, therefore, felt another important step was that of studying groups of patients with different diseases in order to ascertain the frequency of left-handedness in these groups compared to that in the general population.

At the time of the publication of our paper we did not have available to us large groups of individuals with the disorders that had appeared most often. We did, however, have some patients groups available to us. Because the numbers were small we now used as our criterion of left-handedness a score below zero. Our control studies of a large group of individuals in the general population of Glasgow gave similar figures to those which Oldfield had found, i.e. about 8 per cent of the general population scored less than zero. We found an elevated rate of left-handedness among patients with severe migraine and also a trend in a smaller group of patients with myasthenia gravis. On the other hand, we did not find an elevation in our study of a group of patients with rheumatoid arthritis.

Studies now in progress are permitting us to look more deeply into these issues. We have found results which confirm our initial impressions. Thus, the rate of left-handedness among patients with immune thyroid disease or immune disease of the gastrointestinal tract is two to three times that of general population controls. In addition, the rate of left-handedness is significantly elevated among those with the childhood allergies, with migraine, and with myasthenia gravis. Our results in this series again seem to be compatible with those of our earlier study of patients with rheumatoid arthritis, i.e. the rate of left-handedness found does not differ significantly from that of the general population.

It is also of interest that in the studies which are now in progress we have looked separately at dyslexia and stuttering. Both are much more frequent in strongly left-handed individuals than in the strongly right-handed but this effect is found in our preliminary studies to be stronger for dyslexia than for stuttering.

I would also like to mention preliminary results obtained from another study carried on in Boston which has been conducted primarily by Steven Schachter. In this study Schachter and I were interested in ascertaining over what parts of the range of laterality scores the rates of learning disability were high and low. In this study we used a somewhat different scoring method which will be presented in our publication. We found that the rate of childhood learning disorders was about 10 per cent in all ranges of laterality scores from − 100 to + 70. This group comprises about 30 per cent of the population. Above + 70 the rate drops rapidly to 3 per cent or less. These preliminary results are of particular interest since they support the belief that those individuals who carry out more than two or three tasks with the left hand are similar to those who are very strongly left-handed. It can easily be seen why the use of the writing hand as a measurement of handedness would lead to misleading results since the roughly 20 per cent of individuals whose scores lie between 0 and + 70 usually write with the right hand. Our tentative hypothesis, therefore, which will require much further study, of course, is that a cut-off score of about + 70 will probably separate the roughly 30 per cent of the population with anomalous dominance from the 70 per cent with standard dominance.

Let me now turn to the implications of these results. In the first place I believe that by comparing the rates of learning disabilities in strongly left-handed and strongly right-handed individuals we have clearly documented the increased risk of the left-hander for learning disorders. The ratio of 10 to 1 found in our studies in all three series clearly seems to exclude any possibility of chance variations. We believe that other studies which have not confirmed an increase in sinistrality among the learning disabled have possibly run into difficulties because of the inclusion of the middle group who write right-handed but clearly show their deviance from full right-handedness when a full quantitative laterality test is used. I believe that with the development of still better measures of laterality the results will be even clearer than the dramatic ones I have presented here. These results also help to explain data which have existed in the literature over a long period documenting the association of childhood learning disabilities with immune disorders. The literature on stuttering has over more than 50 years contained evidence for a high rate of allergies in this population. I believe that this type of finding in the past has, however, often led to an incorrect conclusion concerning the significance of associations of this type. The high frequency of food allergies among hyperactive children has led some to conclude that food allergy is the cause of hyperactivity and that treatment for it will abolish it. Similarly, the documentation that a bowel disorder similar to celiac disease is common among children with autism led some investigators to conclude that some cases of autism were caused by celiac disease.

The data presented here, however, suggest a quite different interpretation. It is my belief that all of the examples just cited are special cases of the increased frequency of immune disorders in groups in which there is an elevated frequency of left-handedness. As I shall soon point out it is likely that left-handedness, learning disability, and immune disease all stem from a common cause but one does not cause the other.

There are certain other explanations that one can reject. It might be tempting to argue that a high rate of migraine among dyslexics or of allergies among stutterers might simply reflect the effects of the stresses resulting from frustration.

There are, however, powerful arguments against this interpretation. As I have already pointed out these conditions are more frequent among left-handers even when they do not have learning disabilities. It is furthermore clear from examination of the family constellations that these conditions may occur in different individuals, e.g. the example given above of a left-handed dyslexic with two close right-handed relatives with immune disorders, who do not themselves suffer from learning disorders. The case of childhood autism is particularly illuminating since, as Coleman (1976) showed, not only is there a high rate of bowel disorder among the autistic individuals themselves but there is also a high rate of autoimmune thyroid disorder among the parents who are, themselves, never autistic.

Let me very briefly sketch the outlines of a theory of these associations. It is impossible to present this in adequate detail at this time, since the supporting data which already exist, and the experimental data now being obtained, are extremely extensive.

One must accept that any adequate theory of the genesis of anomalous brain dominance must explain certain facts. Thus, many, but not all, studies have shown that left-handedness is more common in males than females, e.g. in the Oldfield studies the figure are 10 per cent and 6 per cent respectively. Secondly, one must account for the elevated rate of left-handedness among the learning disabled, i.e. among dyslexics, stutterers, the autistic, and the hyperactive, and also in cases of Tourette syndrome. Furthermore, one must take into account the strong male predominance of these conditions.

There are some major pieces of evidence which must enter into this discussion. Asymmetry is present in the brain even *in utero*, indeed as early as three months. Several pieces of evidence show that right hemisphere development is in general proceeding more rapidly than that on the left side. One may well ask whether this is the result of influences which speed up growth on the right or of influences which delay growth on the left. I believe that an important clue is given by the findings of Galaburda and Kemper (1978) in the dyslexic brain. The anomaly in that case and in a second case now being prepared for publication is present only on the left side. This anomaly reflects a disturbance of development on the left side, and in particular the presence of many nerve cells which have not reached their targets strongly suggests that in these cases there is some influence delaying growth on the left.

The hypothesis I wish to advance is the following. The basic pattern of the brain is one in which there is strong asymmetry in favour of the regions controlling language and manual control on the left side. The growth of the left side exposed *in utero* to testosterone show a rapid rise of antibodies against their own thyroid glands immediately after birth.

In brief, the theory outlined here suggests that there is some common factor *in utero* which delays the growth of the left hemisphere and the development of the immune system and thus increases the rate of left-handedness, learning disabilities and immune disorders. I will not go into further detail here. Further pieces of evidence for this theory are given in Geschwind and Behan (1982) and the evidence will be presented in greater detail in a paper now being prepared by Galaburda and myself.

I would, however, like to turn briefly to some of the many implications of these findings for the study of dyslexia and other learning disorders. In the first place this theory indicates the possibility eventually of preventing these conditions by appropriate control of the chemical atmosphere of the fetus *in utero*. Much more experimentation will be required but this seems to be a reasonable goal. A second and most important implication of the theory is that it clearly points the way to studies in animals. It would have been regarded as inconceivable only a few years ago that one could have studied the problems of the childhood learning disabled by animal experiments. Yet the studies reported here enable us to look specifically at the development of the brain and of other organs and indicate experimental approaches to modifying how the brain is put together. It should thus be possible to learn in detail how the abnormalities in dyslexia and in other learning disorders are created. The possibility of animal experimentation indicates the way to study other problems. We know that all dyslexics are not similar to each other. The theory presented here suggests the possibility that delays at different periods in fetal life may lead to a wide variety of patterns of alteration in the final brain structure. Experiments to modify brain structure in one particular region can readily be carried out in animals but obviously much less readily in humans.

There is another important set of issues which should now be open to experimentation. Most students of dyslexia are familiar with the heated arguments which have arisen concerning the relationship of alterations in such functions as eye movements and the behavior of the vestibular system in children with retarded reading. The theory presented here opens up a possibility of delaying development at critical periods so that one can reproduce the kinds of abnormalities in eye movements which have been found by several investigators (Pavlidis, 1981a, 1981b). It should furthermore be possible in principle to find out whether these alterations in eye movements are unalterably linked to changes in particular cortical structures or whether they simply represent independent alterations which accompany these cortical changes in many cases but are in no way closely linked to cortical dysfunction. It should be pointed out that, as in other fields of investigation, studies in animals may lead to observations which will suggest investigations in humans not previously carried out. They may thus eventually enrich the armamentarium of studies which will be available for the diagnosis of dyslexia and the elucidation of its underlying disorders.

ACKNOWLEDGEMENTS

From the Dana Research Center, Beth Israel Hospital, Boston, the Department of Neurology of the Harvard Medical School, and the Aphasia Research Center,

V.A. Hospital and Boston University School of Medicine. Supported in part by grants from the National Institutes of Health ININCDS 06209 and NS17018 and from the Orton Research Fund and the Essel Foundation.

REFERENCES

Benson, F., and Geschwind, N. (1969), The alexias. In: P. J. Vincken and G. W. Bruyn (Eds.), *Handbook of Neurology*, Vol. 4. Amsterdam, North Holland, pp. 112–140.

Coleman, M. (Ed.) (1976), *The Autistic Syndrome*. New York, Elsevier/North Holland.

Dejerine, J. (1891), Sur un cas de cécité verbale avec agraphie suivi d'autopsie. *Mém. Soc. Biol.* **3**, 197–201.

Diamond, M., Dowley, G. A., and Johnson, R. E. (1981), Morphologic cerebral cortical asymmetry in male and female rats. *Exp. Neurol.* **71**, 261–268.

Galaburda, A. M., and Kemper, T. L. (1978), Cytoarchitectonic abnormalities in developmental dyslexia: a case study. *Annals of Neurology* **6**, 94–100.

Geschwind, N., and Behan, P. (1982), Left-handedness: association with immune disease, migraine and developmental learning disorder. *Proc. Natl. Acad. Sci. USA* **79**, 5097–5100.

Goldman, P. A., and Galkin, T. W. (1978), Prenatal removal of frontal association cortex in the fetal rhesus monkey: anatomical and functional consequences in postnatal life. *Brain Research* **152**, 451–485.

Oldfield, R. C. (1971), The assessment and analysis of handedness: The Edinburgh Inventory, *Neuropsychologia* **9**, 97–113.

Orton, S. T. (1925), 'Word-blindedness' in school-children. *Arch. Neuro. Psych.* **14**, 581–615.

Pavlidis, G. Th. (1981a), Do eye movements hold the key to dyslexia? *Neuropsychologia* **19**, 57–64.

Pavlidis, G. Th. (1981b), Sequencing, eye movements and the early objective diagnosis of dyslexia. In: Pavlidis, G. Th. and Miles, T. R. (Eds.), *Dyslexia Research and its Applications to Education*. Chichester, John Wiley.

CHAPTER 6

Neurodiagnostic Tools in Dyslexic Syndromes in Children: Pitfalls and Proposed Comparative Study of Computed Tomography, Nuclear Magnetic Resonance, and Brain Electrical Activity Mapping

DRAKE D. DUANE
Department of Neurology, Mayo Clinic, Rochester, MN 55905, USA

Recent technologic advances have provided the means for more detailed study of the relationship between the central nervous system and behavior in the intact, living human. Among the behavioral syndromes that have been of interest to neuroscientists is that of underperformance in reading, commonly referred to as 'dyslexia'. The recent literature implies that these new tools provide diagnostic information in dyslexic subjects. However, there is reason to reflect on the validity of these reports before considering any test other than tests of reading ability and intelligence as 'diagnostic'. More careful replication of such studies may not only clarify the role of these neurodiagnostic tools in dyslexia but also establish the clinical characteristics of the childhood dyslexias.

This review will encompass computed tomography of the head and brain electrical activity mapping as they have been applied to childhood-onset (constitutional) dyslexia. Additionally, the radiation-free technique of nuclear magnetic resonance will be considered as a potential anatomic display of the brain of the dyslexic person. Because dyslexia is not uniform in its presentation, these measures will be considered in relation to at least three types of clinically relevant dyslexic syndromes — namely, dyslexia/pure, dyslexia/plus attention-deficit disorder, and dyslexia/plus overt oral language disorder. Finally, a study will be proposed by which a rational conclusion regarding the relationship between these brain investigations and the clinical phenomenon of dyslexia may be reached, including the question of what constitutes an appropriate control population.

BRAIN ASYMMETRY, PATHOLOGY, AND DYSLEXIA

A consistent and provocative observation is that of the physical asymmetry of the human cerebral hemispheres. Autopsy studies have confirmed differences in width and surface area between the right and left hemispheres, most striking in the superior temporal region—specifically, the temporal plane (planum temporale). These anatomic studies have examined subjects ranging in age from 31 weeks of gestation through senescence, and they repeatedly record a wider left temporal plane in 65 per cent, a wider right temporal plane in 11 per cent, and equality of the two sides in 24 per cent (Chi, Dooling, and Gilles, 1977; Geschwind and Levitsky, 1968; Wada, Clarke, and Hamm, 1975; Witelson and Pallie, 1973). Because of the documented importance of the left temporal plane in language as well as the proclivity for left hemisphere language lateralization among right-handers (98 per cent) and left-handers (70 per cent), it was speculated that the observed asymmetry favoring the left hemisphere might be related causally to the left hemispheric language lateralization (Galaburda *et al.*, 1978).

Morphologic analyses of adult-onset acquired reading disorders, referred to as 'alexias' (Benson and Geschwind, 1969), document, virtually uniformly, the presence of a lesion posteriorly in the left hemisphere. Clinical (Orton, 1928) and neuropsychologic (Witelson, 1977) observations in childhood developmental reading disorders suggested that at least some might be causally associated with inefficient functional capacities presumed to be 'left hemispheric'.

In 1968, Drake briefly noted gross anatomic anomalies in the left posterior cortex at autopsy of a child with a history of developmental reading disorder. Subsequently, Galaburda and Kemper (1979) performed a more detailed gross and microscopic analysis of the brain of a 20-year-old left-handed dyslexic who had died from an accidental fall. Sequential intelligence and academic skill level tests confirmed a specific reading disability. There was no history of a complication during pregnancy or delivery; the subject's history did include delay of speech development in childhood. The family history was positive for reading underperformance. During life, the patient was considered to be an artisan. Routine electroencephalograms made after nocturnal seizures at age 16 were essentially normal. Dichotic digits showed right ear superiority, suggesting left hemispheric language lateralization. At post-mortem examination, although the left hemisphere was wider than the right, the temporal planes were of equal size. Microscopically, polymicrogyria and disordered cortical cellular arrangement (dysplasia) were observed only in the left hemisphere, particularly in regions acknowledged to be language areas. The frequency with which such findings occur in the non-dyslexic population remains to be determined, as well as the consistency of their occurrence in dyslexics as a group. A. M. Galaburda (personal communication, 14 February 1984) has found similar cortical anomalies in two other dyslexia cases studied post mortem. However, selected sectioning of the brain of a 62-year-old dyslexic has suggested bilateral temporal cortical cellular anomalies (Witelson, 1983a), but not the same type described by Galaburda and Kemper (1979).

While these cellular issues are being resolved, clinicians and researchers have expanded their efforts to correlate results of *in vivo* tests of the central nervous system with dyslexic behavior.

COMPUTED TOMOGRAPHY AND DYSLEXIA

Computed tomography (CT) is an established neurodiagnostic radiologic tool for visualization of the brain without trauma and with an acceptable level of radiation hazard. It has been reported that cerebral hemispheric asymmetries, particularly in respect to the width of the two hemispheres, are observable within the general population (Galaburda *et al.*, 1978; LeMay, 1976). These asymmetries are not identical to the post-mortem asymmetries found in the temporal plane. The reported studies suggest a relationship between cerebral asymmetry by CT and hand preference. Right-handers were characterized as demonstrating a longer left hemisphere posteriorly, a wider left hemisphere posteriorly, and a wider right hemisphere anteriorly. Reversal of this asymmetry pattern or absence of asymmetry by CT scan was reported as distinguishing left-handers. However, the proportions of left- and right-handers demonstrating the purported asymmetries were not identical in the two studies cited, and the numbers of subjects in whom the various dimensions were measured were dissimilar between and within these two studies, presumably due to technical difficulties limiting measurement in all cases.

Weinberger *et al.* (1982) claimed anatomic support of the CT findings of asymmetry on the basis of volumetric measurements of the frontal and posterior poles of the right and left hemispheres in an autopsy survey. However, (a) the number of cases was much smaller, 40, than the number investigated by CT, 223, (b) the sample was derived from the Yakovlev collection but the selection method was not given, and (c) for the adults there was no information as to handedness in life. These data, however, did suggest that in 80 per cent of the specimens examined the right frontal area was larger than the left and the left occipital region was larger than the right. These volumetric asymmetries were consistently observed between 20 weeks of gestation and 98 years of age. Notably, the absolute measurements varied considerably between adults and between infants and fetuses. Despite its limitations, this study, like that of Chi *et al.* (1977), suggests that hemispheric asymmetry may be established as early as the completion of the second trimester of gestation and is reasonably considered to be an innate biologic human trait.

Because left-handedness is generally conceded to be more common among dyslexics than among non-dyslexics and a major thesis as to the cause of dyslexia has been left hemispheric malfunctioning, it is not inappropriate or unexpected that attempts would be made to establish to what extent hemispheric asymmetry patterns detected by CT might differ between dyslexic and non-dyslexic populations. There are three studies that relate specifically to this problem.

The first of these is that by Hier *et al.* (1978). These authors suggested that 'reversed asymmetry'—i.e., right wider than left posterior hemisphere by CT scanning—was observed more commonly in their dyslexic sample than chance would predict (in this instance, 10 of 24 dyslexic subjects). Seven of their 24 subjects had equal hemispheric widths by CT. The study sample consisted of 22 males and 2 females with ages ranging between 14 and 47 years (mean, 25 years). Eighteen were right-handed and 6 were left-handed. All had age-appropriate measures of intelligence (Wechsler Adult Intelligence Scale [WAIS] or Wechsler Intelligence Scale for Children [WISC]). Four of the 24 were diagnosed at centers other than the one where the study was conducted. The criterion for designation as dyslexic was performance on the Gray Oral Reading Test below the fifth grade level *or* a history of reading at least 2 years below grade level while in school. Twelve of the 24 met the criterion on the basis of history. A history of a delay in 'speech in phrases' beyond age 3 was obtained in 5 of the 24 subjects.

The observation was made that a wider right hemisphere than left by CT was associated with lower verbal than performance IQ (9 of 10 subjects) and with a history of a delay in speech (4 of 5 subjects). The conclusion was drawn that the presence of a wider right hemisphere carries a five-fold increased risk for the occurrence of dyslexia although the mathematics for such a statement are not clear. All subjects were said to have had normal results on neurologic examination but in no instance was there mention of the extent of educational experience.

Additional limitations of the study include lower verbal than performance IQ in 5 of the 6 subjects with equality of hemispheric width and in 5 of the 8 subjects with wider left than right hemisphere, a wide spread in verbal IQ scores (71 to 124) and in performance IQ scores (75 to 120), variable degrees of differences between the IQ scores (2 to 20), lack of any other measure of academic skill, broad age range, no comment on history of birth trauma or familial occurrence of dyslexia, use of history as a marker of reading level, and, potentially, nonuniformity of sex or hand preference in the population studied. Furthermore, those with persistent speech production deficits may have scored lower on a test of oral reading than they would have on one of silent reading. No measure of the extent of depressed reading comprehension is available, although the expectancy would be that, with the measured low grade of performance orally, reading comprehension similarly would be adversely affected. Finally, because there was no control population, an average of previous CT studies of a nondesignated population of adults was used for comparison purposes.

The report of the second study (Rosenberger and Hier, 1980) refers to the target population as exhibiting 'learning disability', an unfortunate term for a medical study because of the recognized heterogeneity of that population (National Joint Committee on Learning Disabilities, 1981). All 53 of the subjects selected for study were investigated at the same institution. All but 1 had been referred for evaluation because of academic difficulties, yet all were described as having shown achievement deficit of at least two grade equivalents in reading skill 'at some point in their school careers'. The means of determining reading achievement were not specified, and whether the achievement tests were uniform is speculative. The sample consisted of 39 males and 14 females. The age range was 6 to 45 years but no mean was reported. Forty-five of the subjects were right-handed and 8 were left-handed. Subjects were selected 'in part' because of discrepancy between verbal IQ and performance IQ. All were examined by age-appropriate Wechsler Intelligence Scales, and the mean discrepancy was reported as 15.8 ± 8.7 points. History of delay in speech, defined as 'speaking in phrases' after age 36 months, was noted in 22 of the subjects. Thirty-eight of those studied had a relative with a history of reading or speech disorder. Results of neurologic examinations were construed as essentially normal, although 11 were described as showing 'some degree of left-right confusion'.

Twenty-two of the 53 subjects demonstrated 'reversed' asymmetry—i.e., right parietal-occipital width wider than left. This 42 per cent incidence contrasted with a 25 per cent incidence of reversed asymmetry in a 'control' population (100 subjects who had had CT scans for 'other reasons' but about whom there was no information as to age, sex, hand preference, intelligence, reading skill level, or speech and language performance). Analysis was predicated on the basis of reversed asymmetry in 22 subjects who were contrasted with the 31 subjects in whom there was either equality of posterior hemispheric width or wider left than right posterior hemisphere width. Mean full-scale IQ scores were approximately equivalent in the two categories of cerebral asymmetry. Those subjects with wider right than left had a mean disparity of approximately 16 points favoring performance IQ. Both groups of asymmetry had a standard deviation of approximately 17 points in verbal IQ and 13 points in performance IQ. Similar results were derived when the verbal comprehension and perceptual organization factor derived from the Wechsler Intelligence Subtest Scores were compared with the two patterns of asymmetry—i.e., lower verbal comprehension factor tended to be associated with wider right than left posterior hemisphere by CT scanning. Twelve of the 22 subjects with reversed asymmetry and 11 of the 31 without reversed asymmetry had a history of delay in speech development. Analysis of those with reversed asymmetry and normal speech development compared to delayed speech development suggested that delayed speech development was crucial to the results obtained. Omission of those subjects with a history of language delay resulted in an inability to distinguish between the 'learning disabled' subjects and the 'control' subjects by means of reversed asymmetry.

The conclusion drawn was that reversed asymmetry constituted a risk factor for language delay and later academic failure. However, many of the criticisms noted in the discussion of the Hier *et al.* study (1978) also apply to this report, such as lack of specification of educational experience, broad age range, mixed sexes, mixed hand preference, and poor specification of controls or other attributes of the study population such as current speech and mathematics skills, socioeconomic level, geographic location, and maximal or minimal constraints of IQ scores; and no consideration of relationships among educational experience, measured intelligence, and specific measures of reading ability was recorded. Interestingly, mean verbal IQ was higher in the 8 left-handers than in the 45 right-handers. Contrariwise, right-handers demonstrated a mean performance IQ said to be statistically significantly greater than that of the left-handers. However, the standard deviations among left-handers were almost 23 points in verbal IQ and almost 17 points in performance IQ. Based on the above, it is difficult to reach a meaningful conclusion regarding CT cerebral asymmetry and reading disability.

In contrast with the preceding two studies, that by Haslam *et al.* (1981) offers some distinct advantages. The target population was 26 males 9 to 13 years old (mean, 11.7 years). All 26 were right-handed. Consequently, sex and hand preference were controlled, and the age range was narrow. Furthermore, a minimum criterion for intelligence was established: full-scale IQ on the WISC-R more than 80. The criterion for developmental dyslexia was a reading performance 2 years or more below expectancy with the Denver Reading and Spelling Test. Additionally, an attempt at subtype classification of dyslexia was made by utilizing the classification of Boder (1971). This aspect of the study responds in part to the concerns raised in the literature regarding the nonuniformity of reading underachievement (Benton, 1978; Duane, 1983).

Among those designated as dyslexic, 'soft neurologic signs' were said to have been observed in 50 per cent. However, no specifics were given as to what constituted soft neurologic signs. Some abnormality of pregnancy or delivery was noted in 46 per cent of the 26 dyslexic boys, although the nature of the abnormality also was not specified. A history of language delay was noted in 6 of the dyslexic subjects but no specifics were reported as to the criteria for language delay. The control group used was 8 right-handed males with a mean age of 9.8 years, presumably controlling for equality of reading performance. The control group was described as demonstrating normal school performance and being normal on neurologic examination, without further elaboration. No comment was made for either group as to the presence or absence of family history of reading underperformance, nor was there a comment regarding pregnancy and delivery or speech development historically in the control population. Controls had been referred because of a complaint of headache. Using hemispheric measurement criteria comparable to those in the preceding two studies, it was observed that, in the control group, 7 had a wider left than right posterior hemisphere, 1 had equality, and none showed reversed asymmetry. In the dyslexic population, 12 of the 26 showed the presumptive 'normal' pattern of left wider than right, 11 had equality of left and right, and 3 had right wider than left.

When classified by the Boder subclassification, 10 were considered nonspecific, 8 were dyseidetic, and 8 were dysphonetic. One student in each of these three categories demonstrated reversed asymmetry of the posterior parietal occipital region. The 6 with a history of language delay were equally distributed in all Boder subtypes; 4 of these 6 showed the typical pattern of left wider than right posterior hemisphere, 1 each showed equality, and 1 showed right wider than left. These authors could find no correlation of dyslexia with reversed asymmetry, verbal IQ, or history of speech delay. Indeed, the data suggest a higher frequency of relative symmetry of the two hemispheres in dyslexics. This is a point of interest because symmetry had been described previously as more common in the left-handed population (Galaburda et al., 1978). Citing other authors, Haslam et al. (1981) suggested that perhaps reading disability and hemispheric symmetry or asymmetry are genetically determined. Yet, no reference was made in this study to attempts to determine if there were relatives with reading disabilities in either the control or the dyslexic population, and no relatives underwent CT scanning.

Because of the age range selected, it is reasonable to assume that the subjects were prepubescent and had been attending school regularly. It is reasonable to assume that the academically achieving students were of average intelligence, but a specific determination would have been reassuring so that comparability of IQ would have been established between the dyslexic and non-dyslexic groups. Finally, it would be reassuring to know that the socioeconomic backgrounds were comparable within and between the two groups and that other academic skills and attentional control behaviors were comparable. Because of the large number of dyslexic students classified as 'nonspecific', it is not clear whether one can refute the idea that dysphonetic dyslexia is associated with reversed asymmetry.

The authors are correct in asserting that CT scans are not routinely indicated as a diagnostic tool in the assessment of students with specific reading disability unless there is evidence from the history or clinical examination raising the question of newly developing and potentially progressive central nervous system disease. Furthermore, there is not sufficient evidence from the above three studies to state that CT scanning is without merit in the further investigation of dyslexic subtypes or in correlating such results with other investigative (research) noninvasive instruments or procedures.

BRAIN ELECTRICAL ACTIVITY MAPPING
AND DYSLEXIA

Although numerous attempts have been made to correlate electroencephalo-graphic (EEG) patterns with dyslexia, virtually all of these have suffered

suffered serious methodologic or technical flaws (Conners, 1978; Duane, 1981). The solitary exception is in identifying the rare phenomenon of reading epilepsy. The technique of brain electrical activity mapping (BEAM) eventually may be of some utility. This procedure combines the spectral analysis of routine EEG recordings under various circumstances as well as averaged evoked responses, both visual and auditory, into a visual display that is unique and appealing. The initial report of its application in dyslexia was made recently (Duffy *et al.* 1980).

This study was performed on 8 boys ranging from 9 to 10.7 years old. Four were described as right-handed, 2 as left-handed, and 2 as ambidextrous. Full-scale IQ ranged between 94 and 114. However, the report did not specify which intelligence test was used nor were the verbal and performance IQ scores reported. The designation 'dyslexia' was based on the criterion of 1.5 years or more below expectancy on the Gray Oral Reading Test. The authors took into account educational experience as well as intelligence. These students were classified 'dyslexia/pure' as defined by Denckla (1978)—i.e., no evidence of associated attention-deficit disorder was found as confirmed by a low Conners Rating Scale score and normal results on neurologic and psychiatric examinations. The controls in this study included 10 boys whose ages (9 to 10.5 years) and socioeconomic status were similar to those in the dyslexic group, who were above the 50th percentile on the Raven Coloured Progressive Matrices, and who achieved at the fifth grade level on the Gray Oral Reading Test. In the control group, 7 were right-handed, 2 were left-handed, and 1 was ambidextrous. No comment is offered for either the dyslexia/pure or the control group as to the presence or absence of family history or reading disability, complications of pregnancy or delivery, or language development milestones. The issue of family history and birth trauma should not be neglected because Denckla (1977) has pointed out that, in many instances, one or the other may be positive and not uncommonly, both. Of interest is whether these historical data have any influence on any of the central nervous system or behavioral measures used with the dyslexic population.

The investigators concluded that the computer program was able to separate dyslexics from non-dyslexics. Combining the results of the ten conditions under which power spectral analysis was carried out and the three conditions under which averaged evoked potentials were sampled suggested that dyslexics differed from the controls in the left posterior hemisphere and in the paramedian frontal region.

However, there are a number of constraints that do not allow the judgment that BEAM is *diagnostic*. Each point generated on the video screen is an arbitrarily selected point in time which, in reality, represents group rather than individual comparisons. Furthermore, the data base upon which the computer comparison is made is predicated on the average performance of three dyslexics compared with the average performance of three controls. At no point is there a comparison of any individual dyslexic with any individual control. Furthermore, there have yet to be reported longitudinal follow-up tracings to verify the consistency of the results within an individual or, less important, within either group.

F. W. Sharbrough (personal communication, June 1983) has suggested that the statistical techniques used in this analysis are both powerful and complex. However, with such techniques, at times it is difficult even for expert statisticians to be certain that all of the appropriate conditions are satisfied to allow for valid application of these techniques. Furthermore, when any statistical technique is applied, apparently impressive results in small, highly selected groups (in this case, all boys with 8 dyslexics and 10 non-dyslexics in the original training group and 3 dyslexics and 3 non-dyslexics in the test group) must be interpreted cautiously. In particular, general acceptance and application of the technique should be contingent on replication of the results, preferably at different centers and in larger training and test groups.

MAGNETIC RESONANCE IMAGING

The technique of magnetic resonance (MRI) has been available since the 1940s. However, only in the last 8–9 years have attempts been made to apply this technique to biologic systems (Partain et al. 1983). After the introduction of a radiofrequency pulse generated within a magnetic field, hydrogen nuclei will spin; the time required for them to return to their original position is the basis of the measurement. The return to the original position is measured in two axes, longitudinal and transverse. The time to return in the former is referred to as the T_1 relaxation time; this value is approximated on the inversion recovery (IR) images seen on the screen or photographic plate. The transverse relaxation time is referred to as T_2 and is approximated by images obtained by using continuous spin echo (SE) pulse-sequence techniques. Images that reflect inversion recovery are visually reminiscent of the images generated by CT. However, in this instance, no irradiation is required. Spin echo images appear more homogeneous but are sensitive to selective changes, particularly in the white matter, as may be observed in disease states such as multiple sclerosis.

An obvious advantage is the absence of any irradiation, and no known hazard to humans has been identified within the electromagnetic fields now in use. The MRI is more sensitive to alterations in white matter water content. Although post-mortem studies as yet have not identified aberrations in the white matter of the central nervous system of a dyslexic, the microscopic techniques that have been used thus far are limited in their assessment of white matter but focus exquisitely upon cortical and neuronal cellular detail. Recent post-mortem observations of corpus callosum cross-sectional area suggest relative increases in females compared to males and in left-handers compared to right-handers (Witelson, 1983b). In vivo study of this interhemispheric region in dyslexia would be of interest. Additionally, MRI provides sections of the brain sagittally (i.e., cut through the middle and seen from the side) including the low portion of the brain (i.e., the brainstem, cerebellum, and upper spinal cord) which is not readily achievable with present CT techniques.

However, the instrument has disadvantages. In its present form, the gantry has a relatively narrow bore and couch which some patients find to be disquieting place. Newer systems will lessen this constraint. The presence of certain metallic objects in the brain, skull, or eyes may be a relative contraindication to use of NMR, because of both the possibility of artifact and the risk of harmfully changing the position of the metal. Other disadvantages include the bulkiness and cost of the instrument, its inability to show bone, and its slow rate of information acquisition.

Another disadvantage is that the experience with MRI still is insufficient to permit us to be fully certain of its application. Can we detect changes in conditions in which central nervous system anatomic changes are either putative or at best subtle? A large number of individuals with various known disease states, as well as controls, are being investigated with this device to prepare for its routine use in diagnosis. Finally, the various MRI devices in operation in various locations in the United States are not identical in configuration, field, and pulse sequences, so that images may not be comparable from one center to the next. Whether this difficulty will increase or lessen as experience is gained with the instrument remains to be determined. In CT scanning, it has been argued that the change in the construction of the CT device itself may have affected the comparability of earlier and later investigations in dyslexia. Thus, it seems reasonable to consider the application of this safe tool in a rational manner in childhood dyslexia with appropriate controls and the possibilities of integrating such a study with other existing neurologic diagnostic instruments.

PROPOSED DESIGN OF STUDY RELATING
CT, NMR, AND BEAM TO DYSLEXIC SYNDROMES

The above literature review makes it clear that there is uncertainty as to what extent, if any: (a) results of CT examination of the head, in individuals or groups, have any relationship to childhood reading underachievement; (b) BEAM or any other EEG technique distinguishes underachieving from achieving readers; and (c) the radiation-free technique of MRI will provide new information about the brain of dyslexic children. The uncertainties in (a) and (b) relate to limitations in study design. Assuming that the issue of 'during life' anatomy and physiology in dyslexia is worthy of investigation, how might such an investigation be conducted with some assurance that a conclusion can be reached? Furthermore, it is desirable that such investigation also shed light on the behavioral phenomena of dyslexia and influence clinical practice in diagnosis and intervention.

The first issue in any study is defining the target population and an otherwise comparable control population (Keogh et al., 1982). Certainly sex should be controlled. Because of the prevalence of males in the dyslexic population, an initial study perhaps should be confined to males and in all studies it would be imperative to match for sex. Controlling for age and selecting a relatively narrow age band is especially important for studies using such methods as BEAM because there is a well-documented effect of age upon EEG patterns, most striking in the first two decades and beyond the seventh decade.

If dyslexia is construed as having a biologic substrate, it would be especially appealing to use a biologic marker such as levels of sexual development. Tanner (1962) defined the physical stages of sexual maturation in adolescence and these are used widely in medical centers dealing with adolescents (Daniel, 1980). However, in adolescence the most significant factor associated with alterations in manifestations of dyslexia may be the adolescence-related change that drives the social conduct of the emerging adult and emotionally stresses the adults who directly relate to these students (as any junior high school educator or beleaguered parent will attest). Thus far, no reported studies dealing with dyslexia have addressed the sexual maturity of the subject as a boundary factor in subject selection. Studies conducted in a medical center should not neglect this issue. Furthermore, there is the advantage that, if age selection were begun early, age 9, and the upper limit for inclusion were approximately age 13 or Tanner sexual development stage 2, one would have the opportunity for longitudinal investigation with re-examination of the subject at or beyond Tanner stage 4 (adult sexual development is reached at Tanner stage 5). Thus, a potentially important biologic factor quickly determined by an examining physician or paramedical assistant would be included as well as the notation of chronologic age.

The issue of selection on the basis of hand preference is intriguing and complex. Although a higher-than-anticipated frequency of occurrence of left-handedness is associated with reading underachievement, the majority of underachieving readers are right-handed. It would seem prudent to select hand preference in a manner similar to that used by Geschwind and Behan (1982) in which individuals were separated as either being strongly right-handed or strongly left-handed. An initial study should focus on individuals who are strongly right-handed. At some point a comparison in which the variable of handedness is used might clarify whether or not handedness represents behavioral or biological subgroups within the dyslexic population.

In the age group suggested above, the WISC-R (Wechsler, 1974) would be the age-appropriate measure of academic aptitude; however, extremes in intelligence as measured by that instrument constitute the minority rather than the majority of the underachieving reading population. The collaborative experience at this institution has been that the majority of individuals designated as dyslexic, like the general population, fall within 10 to 15 points on either side of 100 on the verbal and performance IQ determinations. To ensure average intelligence in the group, verbal or performance IQ should be 90 or higher and the lower of the two should not be less than 85. Similarly, individuals with extremely high verbal or performance IQs for the region—i.e., in excess of 125—should not be included in the study or control population.

The chief characteristic must be reading failure not explained by visual, auditory, intellectual, experiential, or sociocultural–linguistic factors (primary language should be English). In three of the four studies reviewed above, the Gray Oral Reading Test (Gray, 1963) was used. Reading comprehension may be derived from this instrument or, as is standard practice in the assessment of suspected specific selective academic underachievement, the Woodcock–Johnson reading cluster could be used (Woodcock and Johnson, 1977). Failure on either of these instruments—a score 1.5 standard deviations below the performance predicted on the basis of age, educational experience, and intelligence—would constitute specific reading disability or childhood dyslexia. Such criteria would meet those defined in the Diagnostic and Statistical Manual of Mental Disorders (DSM-III) terminology of developmental reading disorder (American Psychiatric Association, 1980). As long as the data were normalized for a given geographic population, the concerns of Eisenberg (1978) and Rutter et al. (1976) would be addressed.

However, there are other issues that must be addressed in both the study population and the control population. Because these students are assigned the rubric 'specific learning disability', the other academic skills associated with that term should be assessed. Especially, as Denckla (1978) has pointed out, reading disability may coexist with the DSM-III designation of attention-deficit disorder (ADD) with or without hyperactivity. The Conners Teacher Rating Scale (Conners, 1969) and Parent Symptom Questionnaire (Conners, 1970) should be utilized to determine the presence or absence of ADD. A score 2 standard deviations or more above the mean is considered as evidence of ADD with hyperactivity. In the course of psychometric assessment, if the freedom from distractibility factor derived from the WISC-R is more than 2 standard deviations below that predicted, ADD without hyperactivity is suggested. The same obtains when the freedom from distractibility factor is more than 1 standard deviation below relatively congruent verbal comprehension and perceptual organization factors. For this proposed study, the latter will be noted but reliance will be placed upon the more commonly employed Conners scales. Thus, there is an immediate separation of dyslexia/pure (i.e., without ADD) and dyslexia/plus ADD.

Spelling should be assessed, but not used as a criterion for acceptance or rejection, based upon performance on the Wide-Range Achievement Test (WRAT) (Jastak and Jastak, 1978). Arithmetic computation skills should be measured by using the Woodcock–Johnson Test (Woodcock and Johnson, 1977); written expression can be assessed on the Myklebust Test (Myklebust, 1965) or the Test of Written Language (TOWL) (Hammill and Larsen, 1983). In regard to speech, a developmental history should be recorded, articulation should be noted, and particular attention should be paid to the Grammatic Closure Subtest of the Illinois Test of Psycholinguistic Ability (ITPA) (Kirk, McCarthy, and Kirk, 1968), the Test of Verbal Fluency (Borkowski, Benton, and Spreen, 1967), part V of the Token Test (DiSimoni, 1978), and the Clinical Examination of Language Functions (CELF) (Semel and Wiig, 1980). A psychiatric interview is used to confirm the absence of associated psychiatric disease or, for the dyslexia/plus ADD, to confirm the presence of that condition. Social factors to be controlled for are race (Caucasian), socioeconomic class (middle class), and geographic setting.

The medical examination should include a neurologic examination. Soft neurologic signs may be referred to but should not be the basis for inclusion or exclusion from study. Vision and hearing should be within established limits of normal. The medical history should include notes as to the presence or absence of relatives identified as having or suspected to have reading disability, unequivocal complications of pregnancy or delivery, and unequivocal encephalopathic events from which there is no evidence of neurologic sequelae.

There is at least one other dyslexia/plus group that has clinical relevance. Those students with inordinate spoken language deficit present unusual challenges in regard to remediation. Although the many studies of correlates with reading disability have documented an associated more-generalized language deficit (Benton, 1975; Bradley and Bryant, 1983; Davenport et al., in press; Denckla, 1977; Denckla and Rudel, 1976; Duane, 1983; Hallgren, 1950; Johnson and Mykelbust, 1967; Liberman et al., 1980; Mattis, French, and Rapin, 1975; Menyuk and Flood, 1981; Myklebust, 1978; Orton, 1937; Petrauskas and Rourke, 1979; Pirozzolo, 1979; Vellutino, 1977), it appears prudent clinically to separate out a dyslexia/plus group in which performance on tests of spoken language suggests a more severe discrepancy on these measures than on measures of reading. Although these two reasonably could be subdivided further as expressive or receptive, the focus should be upon expressive spoken language in which performance is more than 2 standard deviations below prediction and lower than the performance on tests of reading.

A potential fourth group are those students with a reading disorder and memory disorder. Although not specifically designated in the DSM-III classification or definition of learning disability, there are such students. At times this group overlaps with those students who have reading disability and associated ADD or reading disability and associated profound expressive spoken language disorder. The memory disorder is not explained on the basis of poor verbal labeling. For simplicity, this group need not be specifically separated but, in the course of the psychometric assessment, measures of memory such as the Auditory Verbal Learning Test (Lezak, 1976) should be performed.

In the three broad subclassifications—dyslexia/pure, dyslexia/plus ADD, and dyslexia/plus spoken language disorder—there is the matter of choice of subclassification of the type of reading disability. The easiest to use is that of Boder and Jarrico (1982). With the data obtained, some approximation of other classifications such as those of Mattis *et al.* (1975) and Petrauskas and Rourke (1979) may be attempted. The need for such cross-validation studies of dyslexic subtypes has been pointed out by Benton (1978) and has been addressed, in part, by Lyon (1983).

There should be at least 15 controls, the same number as in each of the three dyslexic subtypes. However, an excess of controls may prove desirable. Criteria for admission should be similar to those for the study population: right-hand preference, ages 9 to approximately 13 years but not beyond Tanner stage 2; similar IQ constraints as in determination of the presence of dyslexia; reading performance no more than 0.5 standard deviation below or more than 1.5 to 2.0 standard deviations above that predicted as is done with the study population. Similarly, performances in spelling, arithmetic, speech, and attention should be roughly congruent with reading performance, none of these being more than 0.5 standard deviation below or more than 1.5 to 2.0 standard deviations above prediction. Socioeconomic status and school attendance should be comparable, and neurologic, general physical, and psychiatric assessments should give normal results. The medical history should be obtained as in the study population, with the same criteria as used for exclusion from the study population.

The subgroup dyslexia/pure should be made up of 15 subjects who meet the above criteria. Arithmetic performance may be less than that predicted but not lower than reading performance. Performance on measures of speech may be lower than predicted but not below that for reading. Attention-hyperactivity as assessed by the Conners Rating Scale must be no more than 1 standard deviation above the mean.

The dyslexia/plus ADD group should include 15 subjects. The other criteria specified above must be met but arithmetic performance may be lower than reading performance but by not more than 0.5 standard deviation. This bending of the criterion is permitted for the ADD group because clinical experience suggests a commonly associated arithmetic underperformance. In the Langley–Porter studies of dyslexia, more than one-third of the students identified on the basis of reading underachievement demonstrated concomitant arithmetic under-achievement (Yingling *et al.*, 1982). The dyslexia/plus ADD group may demonstrate underperformance in speech but no lower than that of reading. Like the dyslexia/pure group, speech performance must not be lower than reading underachievement and must not be more than 2 standard deviations below predicted. On the Conners Rating Scales, scores must be more than 2 standard deviations above the mean for inclusion as dyslexia/plus ADD. As in the other two groups, factor analysis of the WISC-R for the freedom from distractibility factor should be noted but not used initially as a criterion for diagnosis.

The dyslexia/plus speech deficit group should have 15 subjects. All other criteria must be met for the diagnosis of dyslexia as noted above but one or more measures of speech performance as listed above must be disproportionately decreased in contrast to reading and must be at least 2 standard deviations below predicted. Measures of attention and arithmetic skill should be noted but not used as criteria for acceptance or rejection from the group except that the Conners Rating Scales score may not be more than 1.5 standard deviations above the mean. This is an arbitrary decision because some students, particularly those with a receptive spoken language disorder, may be perceived by surrounding adults as restless. Clinical experience suggests that arithmetic performance is variable in this category but a subject should not be accepted if performance in arithmetic is more impaired than that in speech.

Ideally, the subjects in the three dyslexic groups and the control group would be examined by CT, NMR, and BEAM. However, serious consideration must be given to the radiation risk associated with CT scanning in otherwise healthy children. Therefore, to be included in a CT study, controls may have a neurologic complaint but may not have an unequivocal neurologic deficit. The defined study populations offer a unique opportunity to attempt to replicate the work of Duffy et al. (1980). BEAM is a more expensive study than routine EEG, and it is important that the same computer program be applied in all studies. However, approximations of the BEAM procedure can be attempted and perhaps the data could be run through the original computer source for a comparison; this must be done with the stipulation that the identity of the patient would be protected and that the patient's diagnostic designation within the study would not be revealed. Subjects studied by EEG must not be taking any medication known to affect the EEG—e.g., methylphenidate in subjects with dyslexia/plus ADD. This caution applies as well to psychometric, speech, and neurologic examinations. The MRI component at the present time can be readily carried out.

This type of investigation would be the natural continuation of one that was previously suggested in 1981 (Duane, in press). The study could be longitudinal—i.e., the subjects could be reinvestigated after they passed Tanner stage 4. Of interest would be how many of those previously qualifying for one of the three dyslexic groups would still meet those criteria and how many of those previously designated as controls would later meet the criteria for the diagnosis of dyslexia. Such had been the case in a longitudinal study on the Isle of Wight (Rutter et al., 1976) and in the predictive attempts by Satz et al. (1978) in which some students were achieving normally at grade 3 but demonstrated reading failure by grade 5 or 6.

The above study would permit the following questions to be answered. (1) Do measurements of hemispheric width by NMR equate with those made by CT? (2) Do control subjects differ from dyslexia/pure or either of the dyslexia/plus subjects in asymmetry by CT or NMR? (3) Do control subjects differ from dyslexia/pure or either of the dyslexia/plus subjects in the appearance of the white matter? (4) Does MRI reveal cortical anomalies in dyslexia/pure or dyslexia/plus subjects not observable in controls? (5) Do controls differ from dyslexia/ pure or dyslexia/plus subjects by BEAM? (6) Do dyslexia/pure subjects differ from dyslexia/plus ADD subjects by CT, MRI, or BEAM? (7) Do dyslexia/pure subjects differ from dyslexia/plus speech deficit subjects by CT, MRI, or BEAM? (8) Do dyslexia/plus ADD subjects differ from dyslexia/plus speech deficit subjects by CT, MRI, or BEAM?

It is unlikely that the results would permit any of these instruments to be used as *diagnostic* instruments in place of the behavioral measures currently in use. More important would be to determine whether behavioral trends observed at one point in life continue to be observed later in adolescence. If so, do they continue to be associated with underperformance in receptive or expressive written language? Other interesting behavioral questions include the relationship of family history and encephalopathic events to the three dyslexic subgroups and controls, the extent of correspondence between the various previously suggested subclassifications of dyslexia, the effects of medical and educational remedial intervention upon the academic and personality characteristics of the three dyslexic subgroups, and the relative ease or difficulty in obtaining the various subject subgroups as defined above.

It is hoped that this discussion of previous research deficiencies provokes a reassessment of present and future research in dyslexia. The research proposed above attempts to obviate those investigative weaknesses highlighted. More important, such a collaborative interdisciplinary study may favorably affect the delivery of services for this population because the goal is not only a clearer understanding of the relationship between brain function and behavior but also an understanding of how society may assist the intelligent yet struggling reader to achieve to his or her capacity.

ACKNOWLEDGEMENTS

I thank my associates who have kindly collaborated in my clinical practice involving dyslexic and other patients with various learning disabilities. A special note of thanks goes to Norman H. Rasmussen, Ed.D., Section of Psychology, Franklin Earnest IV, M. D., Department of Diagnostic Radiology, Frank W. Sharbrough, M. D., Department of Neurology and Section of Electro-encephalography, and Joseph R. Duffy, Ph.D., Section of Speech Pathology. Many studies performed at the Mayo Institution were done with the advice and collaboration of the Learning Disability Study group chaired by Dr F. L. Yan-Go which includes A. E. Aronson, Ph.D., Speech Pathology, Mrs D. M. Becher, Medical Social Service, R. C. Colligan, Ph.D., Psychology, F. L. Darley, Ph.D., Emeritus staff, Speech Pathology, J. R. Duffy, Ph.D., Speech Pathology, R. H. Feldt, M.D., Pediatric Cardiology, G. S. Gilchrist,

M.D., Pediatrics, R. V. Groover, M.D., Pediatric Neurology, H. R. Martin, M.D., Psychiatry, K. A. Miller, M.D., Pediatrics, R. D. Olsen, M.D., Pediatrics, W. O. Olsen, Ph.D., Audiology, N. H. Rasmussen, Ed.D., Psychology, E. G. X. Rieder, D. O., Child and Adolescent Psychiatry, R. R. Sawtell, M.D., Physical Medicine, Mr K. K. Schreurs, Audiology, and A. H. Schutt, M.D., Physical Medicine.

REFERENCES

American Psychiatric Association (1980), *Diagnostic and Statistical Manual of Mental Disorders* (3rd edn). Washington, D. C.

Benson, D. F., and Geschwind, N. (1969), The alexias. In: P. J. Vinkens and G. W. Bruyn (Eds.), *Handbook of Clinical Neurology*, Vol. 4. Amsterdam, North-Holland.

Benton, A. L. (1975), Developmental dyslexia: neurological aspects. *Advances in Neurology* **7**, 1–47.

Benton, A. L. (1978), Some conclusions about dyslexia. In: A. L. Benton and D. Pearl (Eds.), *Dyslexia: An appraisal of current knowledge*. New York, Oxford University Press, pp. 451–525.

Boder, E. (1971), Developmental dyslexia: a diagnostic screening procedure based on three characteristic patterns of reading and spelling. In: B. Bateman (Ed.), *Learning disorders*, Vol. 4. Seattle, Special Child Publications.

Boder, E., and Jarrico, S. (1982), *The Boder Test of Reading–Spelling Patterns*. New York, Grune & Stratton.

Borkowski, J. G., Benton, A. L., and Spreen, O. (1967), Word fluency and brain damage. *Neuropsychologia* **5**, 135–140.

Bradley, L., and Bryant, P. E. (1983), Categorizing sounds and learning to read—a causal connection. *Nature* **301**, 419–421.

Chi, J. G., Dooling, E. C., and Gilles, F. H. (1977), Left–right asymmetries of the temporal speech areas of the human fetus. *Archives of Neurology* **34**, 346–348.

Conners, C. K. (1969), A teacher rating scale for use in drug studies with children. *American Journal of Psychiatry* **126**, 884–888.

Conners, C. K. (1970), Symptom patterns in hyperkinetic, neurotic, and normal children. *Child Development* **41**, 667–682.

Conners, C. K. (1978), Critical review of 'electroencephalographic and neurophysiological studies in dyslexia'. In: A. L. Benton and D. Pearl (Eds.), *Dyslexia: An Appraisal of Current Knowledge*. New York, Oxford University Press, pp. 251–261.

Daniel, W. A., Jr. (1980), Sex maturity ratings. In: J. T. Y. Shen (Ed.), *The Clinical Practice of Adolescent Medicine*. New York, Appleton-Century-Crofts, pp. 73–79.

Davenport, L., Yingling, C. D., Fein, G., Galin, D., and Johnstone, J. (1984), Narrative Speech Deficits in Dyslexics. *Journal of Clinical and Experimental Psychology* (in press).

Denckla, M. B. (1977), Minimal brain dysfunction and dyslexia: beyond diagnosis by exclusion. In: M. E. Blaw, I. Rapin, and M. Kinsbourne (Eds.), *Topics in Child Neurology*. New York, Spectrum Publications, pp. 243–261.

Denckla, M. B. (1978), Minimal brain dysfunction. In: J. S. Chall and A. F. Mirsky (Eds.), *Education and the Brain* (National Society for the Study of Education. Yearbook, 77th, Pt. 2). Chicago, University of Chicago Press.

Denckla, M. B., and Rudel, R. G. (1976), Rapid 'automatized' naming (R.A.N.): dyslexia differentiated from other learning disabilities. *Neuropsychologia* **14**, 471–478.

DiSimoni, F. (1978), *The Token Test for Children*. Boston, Massachusetts, Teaching Resources Corporation.

Drake, W. E., Jr. (1968), Clinical and pathological findings in a child with a developmental learning disability. *Journal of Learning Disabilities* 1, 486–502.

Duane, D. D. (1981), Toward the demystification of the clinical electroencephalogram. In: W. M. Cruickshank and A. A. Silver (Eds.), *Bridges to Tomorrow* (Selected papers from the 17th International Conference of the Association for Children with Learning Disabilities, Syracuse, New York). New York, Syracuse University Press.

Duane, D. D. (1983). Underachievement in written language: auditory aspects. In: H. R. Myklebust (Ed.), *Progress in Learning Disabilities*, Vol. 5. New York, Grune & Stratton, pp. 177–206.

Duane, D. D., (1985), Written language underachievement: an overview of the theoretical and practical issues. In: F. H. Duffy and N. Geschwind (Eds.), *Dyslexia: A Neuroscientific Approach to Clinical Evaluation*. Boston, Little, Brown & Company, pp. 3–32.

Duffy, F. H., Denckla, M. B., Bartels, P. H., and Sandini, G. (1980), Dyslexia: regional differences in brain electrical activity by topographic mapping. *Annals of Neurology* 7, 412–420.

Eisenberg, L. (1978), Definitions of dyslexia: Their consequences for research and policy. In: A. L. Benton and D. Pearl (Eds.), *Dyslexia: An Appraisal of Current Knowledge*. New York, Oxford University Press, pp. 29–42.

Galaburda, A. M., and Kemper, T. L. (1979), Cytoarchitectonic abnormalities in developmental dyslexia: a case study. *Annals of Neurology* 6, 94–100.

Galaburda, A. M., LeMay, M., Kemper, T. L., and Geschwind, N. (1978), Right–left asymmetries in the brain: structural differences between the hemispheres may underlie cerebral dominance. *Science* 199, 852–856.

Geschwind, N., and Behan, P. (1982), Left-handedness: association with immune disease, migraine, and developmental learning disorder. *Proceedings of the National Academy of Sciences of the United States of America* 79, 5097–5100.

Geschwind, N., and Levitsky, W. (1968), Human brain: left–right asymmetries in temporal speech region. *Science* 161, 186–187.

Gray, W. S. (1963), *Gray Oral Reading Test*. Indianapolis, Bobbs-Merrill Company.

Hallgren, B. (1950), Specific dyslexia ('congenital word-blindness'): a clinical and genetic study. *Acta Psychiatrica et Neurologica Scandinavica (Supplementum)* 65, 1–287.

Hammill, D. D., and Larsen, S. C. (1983), *Test of Written Language*. Austin, Texas, PRO-ED.

Haslam, R. H. A., Dalby, J. T., Johns, R. D., and Rademaker, A. W. (1981), Cerebral asymmetry in developmental dyslexia. *Archives of Neurology* 38, 679–682.

Hier, D. B., LeMay, M., Rosenberger, P. B., and Perlo, V. P. (1978), Developmental dyslexia: evidence for a subgroup with a reversal of cerebral asymmetry. *Archives of Neurology* 35, 90–92.

Jastak, J. F., and Jastak, S. (1978), *Wide Range Achievement Test*. Wilmington, Delaware, Jastak Associates.

Johnson, D. J., and Myklebust, H. R. (1967), *Learning Disabilities: Educational Principles and Practices*. New York, Grune & Stratton.

Keogh, B. K., Major-Kingsley, S., Omori-Gordon, H., and Reid, H. P. (1982), *A System of Marker Variables for the Field of Learning Disabilities*. Syracuse, New York, Syracuse University Press.

Kirk, S. A., McCarthy, J. J., and Kirk, W. D. (1968), *Illinois Test of Psycholinguistic Abilities* (revised edn). Champaign, Illinois, University of Illinois Press.

LeMay, M. (1976), Morphological cerebral asymmetries of modern man, fossil man, and nonhuman primate. *Annals of the New York Academy of Sciences* 280, 349–366.

Lezak, M. D. (1976). *Neuropsychological Assessment*. New York, Oxford University Press, pp. 352–356.

Liberman, I. Y., Shankweiler, D., Camp, L., Blachman, B., and Werfelman, M. (1980), Steps toward literacy: a linguistic approach. In: P. J. Levinson and C. Sloan (Eds.), *Auditory Processing and Language: Clinical and Research Perspectives*. New York, Grune & Stratton.

Lyon, G. R. (1983), Learning-disabled readers: identification of subgroups. In: H. R. Myklebust (Ed.), *Progress in Learning Disabilities*, Vol. 5. New York, Grune & Stratton, pp. 103–133.

Mattis, S., French, J. H., and Rapin, I. (1975), Dyslexia in children and young adults: three independent neuropsychological syndromes. *Developmental Medicine and Child Neurology* 17, 150–163.

Menyuk, P., and Flood, J. (1981), Linguistic competence, reading, writing problems and remediation. *Bulletin of the Orton Society* 31, 13–28.

Myklebust, H. R. (1965), *Development and Disorders of Written Language:* Vol. 1. *Picture Story Language Test*. New York, Grune & Stratton.

Myklebust, H. R. (Ed.) (1978), *Progress in Learning Disabilities*. Vol. 4. New York, Grune & Stratton. pp. 1–39.

National Joint Committee on Learning Disabilities (1981), Learning disabilities: issues on definition. *Perspectives on Dyslexia (Orton Society)* 6, 1, 4.

Orton, S. T. (1928). Specific reading disability—strephosymbolia. *Journal of the American Medical Association* 90, 1095–1099.

Orton, S. T. (1937), *Reading, Writing and Speech Problems in Children: A Presentation of Certain Types of Disorders in the Development of the Language Faculty*. New York, W. W. Norton.

Partain, C. L., James, A. E., Jr, Rollo, F. D., and Price, R. R. (Eds.) (1983), *Nuclear Magnetic Resonance NMR Imaging*. Philadelphia, W. B. Saunders.

Petrauskas, R. J., and Rourke, B. P. (1979), Identification of subtypes of retarded readers: a neuropsychological, multivariate approach. *Journal of Clinical Neuropsychology* 1, 17–37.

Pirozzolo, F. J. (1979), *The Neuropsychology of Developmental Reading Disorders*. New York, Praegar.

Rosenberger, P. B., and Hier, D. B. (1980), Cerebral asymmetry and verbal intellectual deficits. *Annals of Neurology* 8, 300–304.

Rutter, M., Tizard, J., Yule, W., Graham, P., and Whitmore, K. (1976), Research report: Isle of Wight Studies, 1964–1974. *Psychological Medicine* 6, 313–332.

Satz, P., Taylor, H. G., Friel, J., and Fletcher, J. M. (1978), Some developmental and predictive precursors of reading disabilities: a six year follow-up. In: A. L. Benton and D. Pearl (Eds.), *Dyslexia: An Appraisal of Current Knowledge*. New York, Oxford University Press, pp. 313–347.

Semel, E. M., and Wiig, E. H. (1980), *Clinical Evaluation of Language Functions— Diagnostic Battery*. Columbus, Ohio, Charles E. Merrill Publishing Company.

Tanner, J. M. (1962), *Growth at Adolescence* (2nd edn). Oxford, Blackwell Scientific Publications.

Vellutino, F. R. (1977), Alternative conceptualizations of dyslexia: evidence in support of a verbal-deficit hypothesis. *Harvard Education Review* 47, 334–354.

Wada, J. A., Clarke, R., and Hamm, A. (1975), Cerebral hemispheric asymmetry in humans: cortical speech zones in 100 adult and 100 infant brains. *Archives of Neurology* 32, 239–246.

Wechsler, D. (1974), *Wechsler Intelligence Scale for Children—Revised*. New York, The Psychological Corporation.

Weinberger, D. R., Luchins, D. J., Morihisa, J., and Wyatt, R. J. (1982), Asymmetrical volumes of the right and left frontal and occipital regions of the human brain. *Annals of Neurology* 11, 97–100.

Witelson, S. F. (1977), Developmental dyslexia: two right hemispheres and none left. *Science* **195**, 309–311.

Witelson, S. F. (1983a). *Neuroanatomical Asymmetry in the Human Temporal Lobes and Related Psychological Characteristics: Final Report*. (U.S. NINCDS contract number N01-NS-6-2344.)

Witelson, S. F. (1983b). The corpus callosum is larger in left handers. *Abstracts of the Society for Neuroscience* **9**, no. 269.5.

Witelson, S. F., and Pallie, W. (1973), Left hemisphere specialization for language in the newborn: neuroanatomical evidence of asymmetry. *Brain* **96**, 641–646.

Woodcock, R. W., and Johnson, M. B. (1977), *Woodcock–Johnson Psycho-Educational Battery*. Hingham, Massachusetts, Teaching Resources Corporation.

Yingling, D. D., Galin, D., Brown, P., Fein, G., Herron, J., Marcus, M., and Kiersch, M. (1982), *Neuropsychology of Reading Disabilities: Final Report*. (NICHD contact number 1-HD-8-2824.)

Experimental Findings

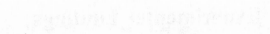

CHAPTER 7

Learning to Read:
Changing Horses in Mid-Stream

DIRK J. BAKKER and ROBERT LICHT
Free University and Paedological Institute, Amsterdam

Readers are faced with a large number of graphic shapes. For the beginning reader this can be disconcerting because clusters of shapes (words) and arrays of clusters (sentences) are meaningful or meaningless depending on the spatial sequence of shapes within clusters and clusters within arrays. Thus, the meaning of 'deer' is different from the meaning of 'reed', whereas 'eder' is meaningless. The phrase 'John is at home' has a very different meaning from its anagram 'is John at home' while another variation 'John home is at' is totally meaningless. However, 'Deer', 'DEER', 'deer', and even 'DeeR', all mean the same, regardless the type, size, and color of the graphic shapes. But 180 degrees of rotation of the 'd' in 'deer' produces 'peer', a word which, though phonetically similar is semantically unrelated to 'deer'. Thus, graphic shapes fail to show 'object' constancy. Novice readers then are faced with complex visuo-perceptual puzzles which they have to solve in order to catch their meaning. Early reading, as a consequence, is a relatively slow process. Slowness, fortunately, is accepted in the first grades of the elementary school and 'accuracy first, speed later' is a frequent advice.

Speed is inherent in reading fluency. This fluent reading is incompatible with visuo-perceptual preoccupation. Perceptual analysis must become automatic and sink below the level of consciousness in advanced reading (Fries, 1963; LaBerge and Samuels, 1974), while semantic and syntactic analyses predominate. The semantic bias may induce a neglect of textual features as evidenced by the frequent omission of the second 'to' by adults reading the notice in Figure 1. Advanced readers bridge the gap between surface (perceptual) and deep structure (meaning) from the meaning side, while less fluent readers bridge the gap from the perceptual side (Smith, 1971).

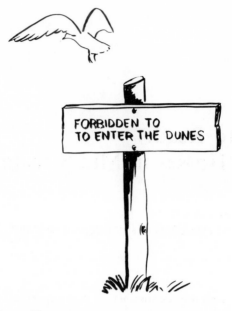

Figure 1. On entering the dunes.

In view of the prominence of visuo-perceptual analysis in early reading and semantic/syntactic analysis in advanced reading it is quite conceivable that reading is primarily mediated by the right cerebral hemisphere at younger school ages and by the left hemisphere at older school ages. This model implies that the lateral location of primary reading mediation shifts from the right to the left hemisphere at some point during development. Both neuropsychological and psychophysiological evidence in support of this hypothesis have been examined (Bakker, 1973, 1979a, 1979b, 1981, 1983; Bakker, Smink, and Reitsma, 1973).

NEUROPSYCHOLOGICAL EVIDENCE

Words are projected onto the right hemisphere when presented in the left visual field and onto the left hemisphere when presented in the right visual field. Carmon, Nachshon, and Starinsky (1976) had letters, words, and numbers flashed in the hemifields of first, third, fifth, and seventh graders of a normal primary school. Oral identification was required. They found a right field advantage (RFA) in older children, absence of field advantage was found in younger children, but the youngest showed a left field advantage (LFA) for single letters.

Broman (1978) examined speed of processing of letters for seven-year old boys and adults and found left and right visual field advantage, respectively.

Using words, Silverberg *et al.* (1980) found a shift in visual field advantage from left to right in second and third graders, respectively. These results suggest that younger and older elementary school children (and adults) use different strategies for the processing of letters and words. The strategies may primarily be generated by the right hemisphere during initial reading and by the left hemisphere during advanced reading.[1] Young children seem to process letters as visual configurations (Carmon *et al.*, 1976). In this connection it is interesting to note that Broman (1978) found LFAs in seven-year-olds both for letters and faces, and that the reaction times to letters were longer than the reaction times to faces in seven-year-olds, but not for adults.

The notion that hemispheric dominance in primary reading control is dependent on the amount of experience with alphabetical material is also suggested by the results of an investigation into the field asymmetry for words printed in a second language. Silverberg *et al.*, (1979) studied the visual half field effects of Hebrew and English words which were flashed to Israeli adolescents who were either in their second, fourth or sixth year of studying English. All groups showed RFA for Hebrew words; field advantage for English words appeared to depend on amount of experience with English: subjects having two years of experience with English showed LFA, those having six years of experience showed RFA.

In conclusion, neuropsychological evidence indicates that beginning readers, in showing LFA to printed words, primarily use their right hemisphere for reading. Advanced readers usually show RFA to printed words which suggests that the left hemisphere is primarily involved in reading. The change of primary hemispheric reading subservience may occur after one year and before two years of reading instruction (Silverberg *et al.*, 1980). A longitudinal electro-physiological investigation was carried out in an effort to find evidence for 'changing hemispheres' in word-elicited brain potentials (Licht *et al.*, in preparation).

PSYCHOPHYSIOLOGICAL EVIDENCE

In searching for psychophysiological evidence for a changing hemispheric subservience during reading, some 50 kindergarten children were randomly selected and followed up for three years (Licht *et al.*, 1982, 1984). The kindergarten children were taught four meaningful words. The number of trials needed to meet the criterion of reading these words correctly was considered the reading acquisition score. Upon completion of this task the same words were flashed in the *central* visual field (50 trials) for oral identification. In addition a Sternberg type of figure matching task (Sternberg, 1969) was presented: the subjects had to indicate by an oral yes or no response whether a nonsense figure did or did not match one of three, two, or one figures which had been presented prior to the target figure.

Event-related potentials (ERP) to words and figures were recorded from left and right temporal (T3, T4) and parietal (P3, P4) locations. Recording was over a period of 1500 ms following stimulus presentation. Responses (ERPs) were averaged over trials, for words and figures separately. The entire procedure was repeated after one and two years, when the children were in the first and second grade of the primary school, respectively.

Averaged brain responses are graphically represented in Figure 2, for grades (kindergarten vs. grade 1 vs. grade 2), hemispheres (left vs. right), locations (temporal vs. parietal), and tasks (word reading vs. figure matching) separately. A principal components analysis revealed five ERP components. One of these components, viz. the one representing the slow positive wave (SW), was found both for word reading and figure matching. An analysis of variance on the factor scores disclosed the SW factor elicited by words to be affected by the interaction of grade, hemisphere and location. This interaction indicates that SW activity increased with age at the temporal sites and decreased at the parietal sites. The interaction also disclosed a striking developmental change in SW asymmetry at the temporal sites. These interaction effects over the temporal areas could not be shown for figures. Another ERP component, viz. the one representing the temporal N2a which peaked around 380 ms (see Figure 2), was found for words only. The N2a component appeared to be affected by grade and hemisphere. This interaction indicates that words elicited greater right than left hemispheric negativity in kindergarten and greater left than right hemispheric negativity in second grade. A multiple regression analysis with factor scores as predictor variables and reading acquisition as criterion, revealed the factor scores of the right temporal components, especially the component representing N2a, to account for a significant proportion of the variance in reading acquisition during kindergarten.

These findings suggest that at least some aspects of reading change hemispheric representation during development. Temporal N2a negativity, uniquely elicited by words and associated with reading acquisition, appeared to be prominent in the right hemisphere during kindergarten, in both hemispheres during the first grade, and in the left hemisphere during the second grade (see Figure 2). Therefore one is inclined to infer that the predominantly left hemispheric subservience of some reading components gets established after one year and before two years of reading instruction. A similar conclusion could be drawn on the basis of previously discussed neuropsychological evidence.

DYSLEXIA

A child starting to learn horseback riding may be faced with a choice of two horses: (A) is a quiet, reliable and 'perceiving' horse, the other, (B) is a fast and skillful horse. (A) would be a good choice to start with, however, in order to become a fast and skillful horseback rider the child should learn to exchange

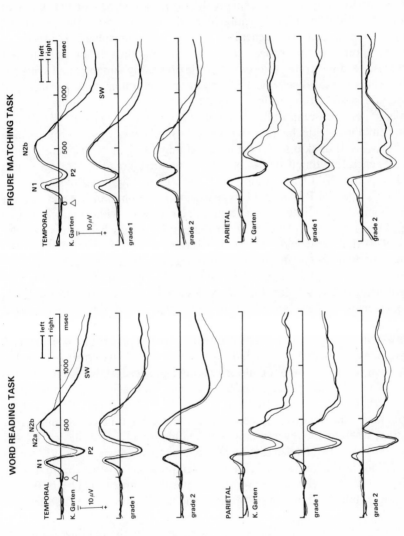

Figure 2. ERPs by task (word reading vs. figure matching), grade (kindergarten vs. grade 1 vs. grade 2), location (temporal vs. parietal), and hemisphere (left vs. right); words and figures were presented in the central visual field.

(A) for (B) at some point during the process of learning to ride. Some children may resist that change and, as a consequence, develop an A-type 'dysamazonia'. Other children may begin by riding horse (B) and a number of accidents and disappointments may result, characteristic of B-type 'dysamazonia'.

The metaphor may serve to explain the possible etiology of two types of dyslexia. A child beginning learning to read should select visuo-perceptual reading strategies, primarily generated by the right hemisphere. However, at some later point of this process the child should shift from right to left hemispheric reading strategies because of the prevailing semantic and syntactic requirements of text processing. In terms of the metaphor: a child learning to read should shift from 'riding the right hemisphere' to 'riding the left hemisphere', or be susceptible to developing a P-type ('P' of perceptual) dyslexia. Another child may 'ride the left hemisphere' from the very onset of the learning to read process, thus skipping the stage of 'riding the right hemisphere'. While untimely generating linguistic (semantic and syntactic) reading strategies such a child runs the risk of developing a L-type ('L' of linguistic) dyslexia.

If it holds true that P-type and L-type dyslexics predominantly generate right and left hemispheric strategies for reading, respectively, what, then, would be the reflections of these strategies in reading style? It has been shown (Diller et al., 1974) that right and left hemiplegics are quite different in the visual scanning of digit-arrays. Right hemiplegics generally are accurate but slow whereas left hemiplegics are inaccurate but quick. These findings suggest that the right hemisphere is a slow but accurate scanner and that the reverse holds for the left hemisphere. If the results of Diller et al. (1974) may be generalized over populations and tasks, one would predict that P-types are relatively accurate but slow readers and that L-types are relatively inaccurate but fast readers. Accuracy may be operationalized in the number of substantive errors (real errors, i.e. the final response is wrong) during reading and speed (slowness) in the total number of words attempted and/or the number of so called 'time-consuming' errors, such as stutterings, fragmentations, and repetitions. Thus, P-type dyslexics may make relatively few substantive and many time-consuming errors in reading, whereas the reverse supposedly holds for L-type dyslexics. P- and L- types thus identified tended to generate asymmetric negativity to printed words (presented in the central visual field) in the temporal areas of the brain (Figure 3).[2] Type of dyslexia (P vs. L) appeared to interact significantly ($p = 0.03$) with Hemisphere (left vs. right temporal) as to the amplitudes of the first negative wave (N1).

When P- and L-type dyslexia is associated with reading strategies predominantly generated by the right and left hemisphere, respectively, one might wonder whether stimulation of the left hemisphere in P-types and stimulation of the right hemisphere in L-types would activate the stimulated hemisphere and subsequently improve reading performance. A pilot study (Bakker et al., 1981) into the effects of hemisphere-specific stimulation through

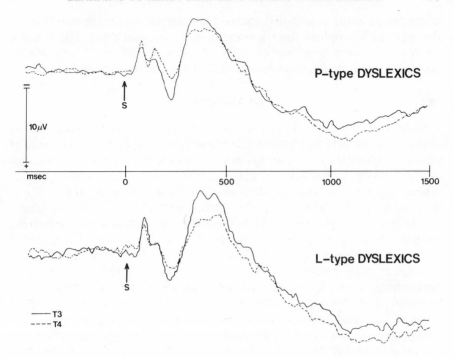

Figure 3. ERPs elicited by words presented in the central visual field of P- and L-type dyslexics.

the visual half-field presentation of words (right field presentation in Ps, left field presentation in Ls) revealed the wave forms of the event-related potentials (ERP) to alter and reading performance to improve on pre- versus post-test comparisons. The changes were in directions predicted by the field of word presentation and the nature of the subtype. In a more recent investigation (for a provisional report see Bakker, 1984) experimental P-type dyslexics received words to read in the right visual field, whereas controls received central field training with words or no special training at all.

Experimental L-types received words in the left visual field, controls in the central visual field whereas some other controls did not receive any special training. Significant Type (P vs. L) × Group (Experimental vs. Control) × Hemisphere (Left vs. Right) × Test (Pre- vs. Post-) interactions were found as to the amplitudes and latencies of some peaks in the parietal and temporal areas. These interactions mainly indicated 'leftening' of activity following left hemisphere stimulation in Ps and 'rightening' of activity following right hemispheric stimulation in Ls. Moreover, between-hemispheric changes of activity tended to correlate with measures of post- vs. pre-test improvement of reading. Since the subtype-differentiating N1-component of the ERP (see Figure 3) was not included in the provisional analysis, a statement about the sensitivity of this wave to hemisphere-specific training is, as yet, precluded. The P and L typology, in conclusion, shows signs of external validity in that neural mechanisms appear to correlate with this classification of dyslexia.

SUMMARY

Evidence is available to indicate that initial and advanced reading are primarily mediated by the right and left cerebral hemispheres, respectively. Outcomes of neuropsychological and psychophysiological investigations suggest that the shift of primary hemispheric subservience occurs in between one and two years of reading experiences. Some children may not be able to make the shift and continue to rely on right hemispheric reading strategies. They thus develop a P-type dyslexia. Some other children predominantly generate left hemispheric strategies from the very onset of the learning to read process. These readers run the risk of developing a L-type dyslexia. P-type dyslexics tend to be relatively slow but accurate readers whereas L-types tend to show the reverse pattern. Some components of word-elicited brain responses have been found to be differently lateralized in P and L dyslexics. Hemisphere-specific stimulation through the visual half-field presentation of words affects the hemispheric distribution of word-elicited brain responses and improves some parameters of reading on post- versus pre-test comparisons. The P/L dyslexia typology thus shows some external validity.

NOTES

1. A similar developmental change in the hemispheric subservience of speech has been suggested by Moscovitch (1977).
2. Right ear advantage (REA) and left ear advantage (LEA) in dichotic listening has been used as an additional criterion in P- and L-classification, in view of the admissibility that REAs do have and LEAs do not have spoken language completely represented in the left hemisphere. Since spoken language is part of reading aloud it may be that REA and LEA cause biases to the generation of left-hemispheric and right-hemispheric reading strategies, respectively. There is some evidence (Bakker, 1979b, 1981) to suggest that REA and LEA correlate with different patterns of reading errors and different hemispheric subserviences of reading (Bakker *et al.*, 1980). The Ps and Ls of Figure 3 were selected both on the basis of type of reading errors and ear preference in dichotic listening to verbal inputs.

REFERENCES

Bakker, D. J. (1973), Hemispheric specialization and stages in the learning to read process. *Bulletin of the Orton Society* **23**, 15–27.

Bakker, D. J. (1979a), Perceptual asymmetries and reading proficiency. In: M. Bortner (Ed.), *Cognitive Growth and Development*. New York, Brunner/Mazel, pp. 134–152.

Bakker, D. J. (1979b), Hemispheric differences and reading strategies: two dyslexias? *Bulletin of the Orton Society* **29**, 84–100.

Bakker, D. J. (1981), A set of brains for learning to read. In: K. C. Diller (Ed.), *Individual Differences and Universals in Language Learning Aptitude*. Rowley, Massachusetts, Newbury, pp. 65–71.

Bakker, D. J. (1983), Hemispheric specialization and specific reading retardation. In: M. Rutter (Ed.), *Developmental Neuropsychiatry*. New York, Guilford, pp. 498–506.

Bakker, D. J. (1984), The brain as a dependent variable. *Journal of Clinical Neuropsychology* **6**, 1–16.

Bakker, D. J., Licht, R., Kok, A., and Bouma, A. (1980), Cortical responses to word reading by right- and left-eared normal and reading-disturbed children. *Journal of Clinical Neuropsychology* **2**, 1–12.

Bakker, D. J., Moerland, R., and Goekoop-Hoefkens, M. (1981), Effects of hemisphere-specific stimulation on the reading performance of dyslexic boys: a pilot study. *Journal of Clinical Neuropsychology* **3**, 155–159.

Bakker, D. J., Smink, T., and Reitsma, P. (1973), Ear dominance and reading ability. *Cortex* **9**, 301–312.

Broman, M. (1978), Reaction-time differences between the left and right hemispheres for face and letter discrimination in children and adults. *Cortex* **14**, 578–591.

Carmon, A., Nachshon, I., and Starinsky, R. (1976), Developmental aspects of visual hemifield differences in perception of verbal material. *Brain and Language* **3**, 463–469.

Diller, L., Ben-Yishay, Y., Gerstman, L. J., Goodkin, R., Gordon, W., and Weinberg, J. (1974), *Studies in Cognition and Rehabilitation in Hemiplegia* (Rehabilitation Monograph No. 50). New York, New York University Medical Center, Institute of Rehabilitation Medicine.

Fries, C. C. (1963), *Linguistics and Reading*. New York, Holt, Rinehart & Winston.

LaBerge, D., and Samuels, S. J. (1974), Toward a theory of automatic information processing in reading. *Cognitive Psychology* **6**, 293–322.

Licht, R., Bakker, D. J., Kok, A., & Bouma, A. (1982), Lateralized electrical activity subsequent to word reading in first grade primary school children. Paper presented at the meeting of the International Neuropsychological Society, Deauville, France.

Licht, R., Bakker, D. J., Kok, A., and Bouma, A. (1984). Hemispheric asymmetry and reading: a three year longitudinal ERP study. Paper presented at the meeting of the International Neuropsychological Society, Houston.

Moscovitch, M. (1977), The development of lateralization of language functions and its relation to cognitive and linguistic development: a review and some theoretical speculations. In: S. J. Segalowitz and F. A. Gruber (Eds.), *Language Development and Neurological Theory*. New York, Academic Press, pp. 193–211.

Silverberg, R., Bentin, S., Gaziel, T., Obler, L. K., and Albert, M. L. (1979), Shift of visual field preference for English words in native Hebrew speakers. *Brain and Language* **8**, 184–190.

Silverberg, R., Gordon, H. W., Pollack, S., and Bentin, S. (1980), Shift of visual field preference for Hebrew words in native speakers learning to read. *Brain and Language* **11**, 99–105.

Smith, F. (1971), *Understanding Reading: A Psycholinguistic Analysis of Reading and Learning to Read*. New York, Holt, Rinehart & Winston.

Sternberg, S. (1969), Memory-scanning: mental processes revealed by reaction-time experiments. *American Scientist* **57**, 421–457.

CHAPTER 8

The Role of Eye Movements in the Diagnosis of Dyslexia

GEORGE TH. PAVLIDIS
Department of Pediatrics, UMDNJ-Rutgers Medical School, Piscataway, NJ 08854, USA

For more than a century eye movements have been found to be a sensitive indicator of the reading process (Javal, 1879; Hue, 1908; Tinker, 1958; Pavlidis, 1985a). Javal (1879) was the first to report that during reading the eyes do not move continuously from left to right along the line, but proceed through a succession of short, fast jumps (saccades) and pauses (fixations). These components have been shown to play a vital, distinct and complementary role in the reading process. The main visual function of the saccade is to bring onto the fovea the image to which the subject is attending.

Information intake during a saccade is severely restricted because shortly before, during, and shortly after the saccade, visual acuity is drastically reduced to avoid smearing of the visual image (Matin, 1974; Volkman, 1976). Visual information is taken in only during fixation. In the course of reading the eyes are in a state of fixation for about 87–95 per cent of the total reading time (Tinker, 1958; Pavlidis, 1981b). The eye movement patterns and characteristics during reading reflect the reader's efficiency and, hence, provide a reliable tool for the study and analysis of the components of the reading process (Taylor *et al.*, 1960; Tinker, 1958).

THE USEFULNESS OF EYE MOVEMENTS

Eye movements correlate highly with reading skill and, therefore, provide a simple, reliable, and objective method for the evaluation of reading efficiency and for the diagnosis of reading difficulties. One of the great advantages of studying eye movements is that they can be embedded in tasks which vary greatly in complexity. For example, the effect of the text's difficulty on the eye movement patterns can be studied. Tasks can be also presented in ways that demand no reading skill (e.g. following patterns of lights); they, thereby, offer an approach in which performance deficiencies due to mechanisms directly related to the reading process can be studied independently of the cognitive factors in reading (e.g. memory, verbal skill). Through the superimposition of the eye fixations onto the text being read, the source and nature of the reading problem can be accurately determined.

Despite its numerous advantages, research on oculomotor behavior has not yet been extensively pursued especially with young children. A chief reason for the scarcity of such studies has been the absence of the appropriate technology that can be used easily and effectively with young children. For example, a frequently used technique with older subjects involves the use of a bite bar (where a person grips a bar with his teeth so as to reduce head movements (Young and Sheena, 1975)). This procedure places uncomfortable motor restrictions on the subject and is inappropriate for use with young children. Over the past several years, however, eye movement technology has improved and alternative methods have been developed which allow the comfortable and accurate recording of children's eye movements (Young and Sheena, 1975; Lloyd and Pavlidis, 1978).

Another inhibiting factor has been the laborious, extremely time consuming, expert analysis of eye movement records. This obstacle has now been overcome thanks to automated, computerized methods for data collection and analysis. These recent advances will facilitate the spread of the use of eye movements for educational, clinical, and neurological evaluations, including dyslexia.

The diagnostic usefulness of eye movements has also been demonstrated in many neurological conditions that include coma (Coakley and Thomas, 1977), schizophrenia and attentional disorders (Holzman et al., 1976; Schwartz et al., 1984), hyperactivity (Bala et al., 1981), and dyslexia (Lesevre, 1968; Griffin et al., 1974; Pavlidis, 1978, 1981a, 1985b).

EYE MOVEMENTS IN DYSLEXIA

Only a brief review of the major studies will be given here as major reviews of eye movements and dyslexia studies can be found elsewhere (Pavlidis, 1981b, 1983a, 1985a). Instead, the interpretations of the results of eye movement studies and the significance of these findings will be discussed.

Eye movement patterns and characteristics are affected by many factors including age (Gilbert, 1953; Taylor et al., 1960), text variables, and reading efficiency (Tinker, 1958; Pavlidis, 1981b). These studies have shown that increased text difficulty leads to an increased number and duration of eye movements of shorter size. The developmental patterns of eye movements and reading follow parallel courses and are highly correlated (Gilbert, 1953; Taylor et al., 1960). Gilbert (1953) and Taylor et al. (1960) found that the younger

Figure 1. *Illustrative eye movement records.*

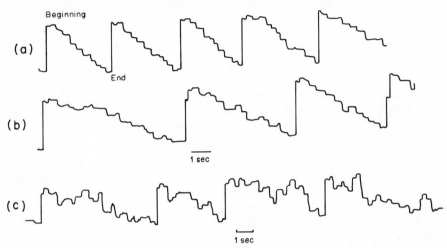

The horizontal lines represent fixations. The vertical lines represent eye movements. The sizes of the lines are proportional to the duration of fixation or to the eye movement size. (a) Eye movement record of a normal reader during reading. It consists of successive similar eye movements and fixations which form a repetitive staircase pattern. The regressions are rare and they are invariably smaller in amplitude than the preceding forward saccade. (b) A retarded reader's eye movement record during reading. It is noteworthy that the eyes make more forward and regressive movements than the normal readers, but the amplitude of his regressions is also smaller than the preceding forward saccades. His eye movements form a prolonged staircase pattern. (c) Dyslexic's erratic eye movement record. Every line has its own idiosyncratic shape, unlike normal and retarded readers' patterns which are consistent throughout. It is often difficult to distinguish the end of one line from the beginning of the next. The regressions are not only very frequent but they also sometimes occur in clusters of two or more. Their amplitude is frequently bigger than that of the preceding forward saccade.

the reader, the higher the number of eye movements made for the reading of the same number of words.

Besides age, reading proficiency also significantly influences eye movement patterns and characteristics. Normal readers make regular eye movements across lines of text that are of more constant size and duration than those made by poor readers (Tinker, 1958; Pavlidis, 1981b; 1985a). An even greater irregularity of eye movement patterns have been found in dyslexics (Figure 1).

There have been very few studies comparing dyslexics to matched controls (Lesevre, 1964, 1968; Griffin, *et al.*, 1974; Goldrich and Sedgwick, 1982; Pavlidis, 1981a, 1981b, 1985b), but many reports of case studies on dyslexia (Zangwill and Blakemore, 1972; Pavlidis, 1978; Pirrozolo and Rayner, 1978; Ciuffreda *et al.*, 1976, 1985; Elterman *et al.*, 1980). In most of the above-mentioned studies the dyslexics' eye movements during reading have been found to be both erratic and idiosyncratic. Dyslexics, for instance, made significantly more eye movements than their matched controls. Their most striking difference was found in the number and percentage of their regressions. Advanced, normal, and retarded readers made anywhere from 10 per cent to 22 per cent while dyslexics made on average about 25–35 per cent regressions. Not only did they make more regressions but also their regressions often occurred in clusters of two or more successive regressions (Figure 1). The dyslexics, unlike other readers, also have highly variable and longer durations of fixations and sizes of eye movements.

The finding that dyslexics exhibit erratic eye movements during reading is almost undisputable. The extent and cause, however, of these erratic eye movements and how they relate to dyslexia is a controversial matter. Part of the debate is due to a misunderstanding of the function of eye movements. Unfortunately, eye movements are sometimes *erroneously* associated only with vision, or their function is falsely attributed to peripheral factors. Those who are unaware of the functional plurality of eye movements do not realize that eye movements are sensitive reflectors of higher cognitive processes and, hence, they are related to central factors. Once the cognitive functions of eye movements are understood, then the relationship between eye movements and dyslexia will become clearer.

RELATIONSHIP BETWEEN EYE MOVEMENTS AND DYSLEXIA

At present, there are at least three different interpretations of the role that eye movements play in dyslexia. One view holds that the dyslexics' erratic eye movements are another reflection of the problems dyslexics experience with reading material (Goldberg and Arnott, 1970; Tinker, 1958). There are no firm data that support this point of view, but its proponents claim that word-recognition, understanding, and comprehension problems force dyslexics to shift their eyes forward and backward across the line. Hence, they exhibit erratic eye movements. Existing data, however, contradict this theory.

If it was true that the dyslexics' erratic eye movements found during reading, were only the result of their reading problems then it would be reasonable to expect that the age-matched retarded readers with equally severe reading problems, would also exhibit erratic eye movements. But the data did not support this hypothesis as the dyslexics had significantly more eye movements than the matched retarded readers, especially in the number of regressions (Pavlidis, 1981b). Additionally, how can this hypothesis explain the dyslexics' erratic eye movement patterns found during non-reading tasks? It can be concluded that although reading problems can negatively affect the dyslexics' eye movement patterns and characteristics, they do not cause them (Lesevre, 1968; Pavlidis, 1985a).

Gilbert (1953), Lesevre (1968), Goldrich and Sedgwick (1982), and Zangwill and Blakemore (1972) among others suggested that at least some dyslexics' erratic eye movements lead to their reading disability. Hence, dyslexia can be sometimes seen as secondary to erratic eye movements. If this hypothesis was true, then how could one explain the language deficits found in dyslexics (Liberman, 1983; Vellutino, 1977)?

Why must it be assumed that eye movements and dyslexia have a cause and effect relationship? They can, instead, be seen as the results of the same or parallel but independent brain malfunctions (Pavlidis, 1985a, 1985c). Such a theory would explain the dyslexics' erratic eye movements found during reading and non-reading tasks, and also their language, attentional, synchronization, and sequential problems.

Neurological evidence is supportive of this view. For instance, Ojemann and his colleagues (Ojemann and Mateer, 1979; Calvin and Ojemann, 1980) during brain surgery asked their adult subjects to name objects, to identify phonemes, and to read. While they were performing these tasks various parts of their brain were stimulated through microelectrodes. If the parts of the brain that controlled these functions were stimulated during the execution of the task their verbal output was disrupted and, thus, the stimulated part of the brain was considered to be involved in the control of the function under examination. Ojemann and his colleagues found that the functions of naming, phoneme identification, and reading were located in the same area of the left hemisphere.

The same subjects were asked to imitate facial expressions of photographs shown separately to them. This motor task was not controlled by these language areas. But, when they were asked to imitate exactly the same facial expressions but in a *rapid sequence*, they found that these motor-sequential actions were controlled by the same areas of the left hemisphere that were involved in the control of reading, phoneme identification, and naming.

These neurological findings are in agreement with the clinical observations and other experimental findings suggesting that dyslexics have problems in sequencing, naming, phoneme identification, and reading. The dyslexics' motor-sequential problems, as reflected in their erratic eye movements, may constitute another manifestation of the malfunction of the same areas of the brain that control sequencing and the language functions involved in reading. The dyslexics' erratic eye movements can be further perceived as being complementary to their language problems, rather than being casually related.

AUTOMATED SEQUENCING AND READING

A well-established relationship also exists between dyslexia and sequential order. This vital component of the reading process is involved from its earliest to its most advanced stages (Vernon, 1977). Dyslexics have been found to have significantly worse performance than matched normal readers in sequential tasks across modalities (Doehring, 1968; Zurif and Carson, 1970; Bakker, 1972; Naidoo, 1972).

By automated sequencing, we refer to the fast sequential skills required for the effective execution of such tasks as blending of letters to create syllables, blending of syllables to make words, and placing words in the correct syntactic order to compose sentences, etc., and to the automated sequential movements of the eyes from one syllable or word to the next.

In his classic paper, Karl Lashley (1951) stated 'temporally integrated actions are especially characteristic of human behavior and contribute as much as does any single factor to the superiority of human intelligence'. The validity and power of this neglected but vital aspect of human cognition has been recognized by the psychological and neurological community. Nevertheless, for a number of reasons research in this area has been rather sparse, with the exception of the area of reading.

Reading is an aspect of language and visuomotor behavior which requires extensive temporal/sequential skills to be effective (Vernon, 1977; Gilbert, 1953). It also represents a sphere of behavior in which the temporal/sequential skills are reflected in, and can be monitored through, eye movement recordings. As previously mentioned, eye movements have proved to be sensitive and objective indicators of the neuropsychological processes subserving the temporal/ sequential and motor components of reading.

Since automated sequencing has been shown to be such a fundamental component of the reading process, and a consistent cross-modal weakness in dyslexics, it is therefore reasonable to expect that dyslexics may also exhibit sequential problems in non-reading tasks that simulate the motor-sequential components of the reading process. Such tasks will be free of the higher level information processing resulting from the comprehension requirements of reading.

ERRATIC EYE MOVEMENTS IN NON-READING TASKS

In an effort to separate the higher information processing requirements from the motor components of reading, Gilbert (1953) asked readers, ranging from best to worst, to: (a) read prose and, (b) to sequentially scan digits spaced across the line from left to right. Gilbert found a substantial correlation between eye movement efficiency while reading prose and while sequentially scanning the digits (Figure 2). The correlation between the average number of regressions per 100 words or digits was particularly high ($r = +0.71$). Gilbert stated: 'there is no overlapping of cases in the extreme groups. For example, there was no instance of a pupil who was very superior in fixation frequency in reading prose and yet proved very inferior in fixation frequency in reading digits.' (1953, p. 203).

Gilbert's findings have been replicated by a number of investigators worldwide (Lesevre, 1964, 1968; Griffin et al., 1974; Goldrich and Sedgwick, 1982). These results have also been replicated in our laboratory. Pavlidis (1985b) carefully matched dyslexics, normal and retarded readers on the basis of the following factors: IQ, age, socioeconomic background, visual and auditory acuity,

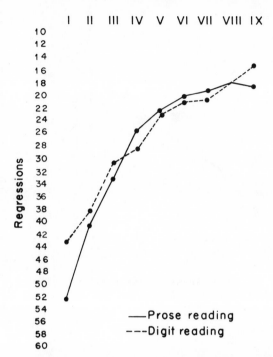

Figure 2. Average number of regressions per 100 words and per 100 digits for the same subjects (from Gilbert, 1953). The high correlation (0.71) is noteworthy.

neurological, psychological, and educational factors, including absenteeism, and school changes. In addition to matched normal readers he also matched dyslexics and retarded readers for reading and chronological ages. It was found that dyslexics made significantly more regressions while sequentially scanning digits than normal and retarded readers (Figure 3).

Almost the same factors that are responsible for the variable results found in the rest of the dyslexia literature are also at work in the various eye movement studies. For instance, some studies (Olson *et al.*, 1983; Stanley *et al.*, 1983; Brown *et al.*, 1983; and Black *et al.*, 1984) have reported different results from the previously mentioned literature on eye movements. These differences can be accounted for by their variable subject selection criteria, experimental designs, stimuli, and data collection and analysis (Pavlidis, 1981a; 1981b; 1983c; 1985c). The importance of subject selection criteria for the results of a study is discussed extensively by Keogh and Babbitt (1986). It is likely that the poor readers of some of those studies were more similar to Pavlidis's retarded readers than to his dyslexic group. If that is the case then the results of those studies are in agreement with Pavlidis's (1981b) results obtained from the retarded readers. The interested reader can find elsewhere details of subject selection criteria and the experimental

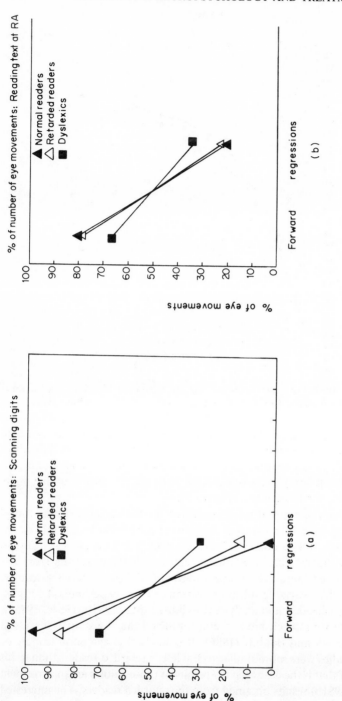

Figure 3. Percentages of forward and regressive eye movements of dyslexics, retarded and normal readers (a) while sequentially scanning the digits, (b) while reading, for comprehension, text at their reading age. (Note similarities with Figure 4, especially for dyslexics.) The similarities in the dyslexics' percentage of regressions while reading and scanning the digits suggest that the causes of the dyslexics' erratic eye movements are independent of reading. In contrast, normal and retarded readers made far fewer regressions while scanning digits than during reading, which suggests that the comprehension requirements and high level information processing of the reading task, as expected, increased their regressions.

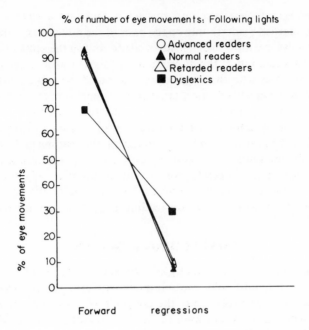

Figure 4. Percentages of forward and regressive eye movements of dyslexics, retarded, normal, and advanced readers while they followed sequentially moving lights. Note the similarity, especially for dyslexics, to when they read text and scanned digits (Figure 3).

procedures used (Pavlidis, 1985b), and a detailed discussion of the factors that may have been responsible for the differing results of those studies (Pavlidis, 1983c; 1985c). It is noteworthy that a number of recent studies indicate that they have replicated his results (Cizek and Jost, 1984; Jerabek, 1984; Mawson, 1982, and personal communication, 1984), including two replications in our laboratory in England and the USA.

In an effort to achieve a higher degree of differentiation between dyslexics and matched controls, Pavlidis (1981a; 1981b) incorporated into the stimulus design tasks that tapped the clinical weaknesses of dyslexics, i.e. attentional and sequential problems coupled with their inability to predict/synchronize their actions with a stimulus and to alternate between mental sets.

The children were asked to fixate at lights that moved sequentially from left to right and right to left across the line. Indeed, the dyslexics made significantly more forward and regressive eye movements than the matched advanced, normal, and retarded readers (Figure 4). There were no significant differences between advanced, normal, and retarded readers in the percentage of their regressions while following the sequentially illuminated lights. However, the difference between dyslexic and non-dyslexic readers in the number and percentage of regressive eye movements was highly significant. Using discriminant analysis the children were reclassified into dyslexics, and non-dyslexics (advanced, normal, and retarded readers) only on the basis of the number and the percentage of their regressive eye movements made while following the sequentially moving lights. The classification of the discriminant analysis was in agreement in 93.2 per cent of the cases with the initial classification of the subject made only on the basis of the original selection criteria (non-including eye movements).

The decreased information processing requirements of the lights task was reflected in the significantly smaller number of regressions made by the non-dyslexic readers during the non-reading task than during the reading task. In contrast, the dyslexics made a similar number of regressions during reading and non-reading tasks, indicating that their erratic eye movements are relatively independent of reading. These findings are important as they can lead to the development of an objective and possibly early non-reading diagnostic test for dyslexia.

CONCLUDING REMARKS

Breakthroughs in the understanding of dyslexia will be facilitated by the use of complete and quantifiable research diagnostic criteria for the selection of dyslexics and their controls. Only the adoption of such criteria will help us understand *who* we study and *what* the characteristics are that distinguish one group from another (Pavlidis, 1983b). For instance, erratic eye movements characterize many dyslexics but not their matched controls.

The use of eye movement records, taken during non-reading tasks, have been shown to be very promising for the diagnosis of dyslexia. The main advantage of a potential eye movement test would be its objectivity, its ease of recording, and its short duration (only a few minutes). The additional bonus of computerized eye movement technology offers an easy and accurate means for the recording and analysis of eye movements by non-experts (e.g. school nurses and special educators). Recent technological advances will lead to a much wider use of eye movements in clinical and educational settings for the diagnosis of neurologically based conditions. The fact that this test is independent of reading leads to the possibility of applying the test even before reading age. Well-controlled developmental studies are needed to determine how early such a test can be applied.

Pertinent to this question are the neuroanatomical findings of Galaburda and Kemper (1979) which suggest that whatever malformations exist in dyslexics' brains, exist even before birth (Geschwind, 1982). It has also been suggested by Geschwind (Chapter 5, this volume) that delayed development of certain parts of the brain at critical periods may reproduce the kind of abnormalities in eye movements which have been found in dyslexics.

These neurological findings are supportive of our view that the dyslexics' erratic eye movements may exist even before reading age and, hence, may provide a useful prognostic test of dyslexia.

Are erratic eye movements the cause, the effect, or a parallel phenomenon of dyslexia? It is not necessary for each of these hypotheses to be either right or wrong, as each of them explains certain clinical symptoms of dyslexia and leaves others unanswered. Hence, each of them may hold true only for one or more subgroups of dyslexics. The hypothesis that explains almost all the clinical and experimental findings of dyslexia is the one that views dyslexia and erratic eye movements as parallel phenomena or the results of the same malfunctioning parts of the brain (Pavlidis, 1985a).

Finding the cause(s) of erratic eye movements will be critical in determining which method of treatment is appropriate or inappropriate for a particular dyslexic. It is not important, however, for the diagnosis of dyslexia whether erratic eye movements represent a trait or a state phenomenon or a biological marker of dyslexia. As long as dyslexia and erratic eye movements coexist, erratic eye movements can be used for the diagnosis of dyslexia.

The early diagnosis or prognosis of dyslexia by erratic eye movements will be beneficial in many ways. It is likely to spare the dyslexics from the secondary emotional problems stemming from their unexpected failure in reading and spelling. Early diagnosis will also help capitalize on the greater plasticity of the younger brain and, hence, even if only the traditional methods of treatment are used they will become more effective.

ACKNOWLEDGEMENTS

I thank the late Professor Norman Geschwind for the constructive suggestions he made during our long conversations on the interpretation of the eye movement data. I also wish to acknowledge research grant CD # 085-D02.0 from Barnes-Hind to the author.

REFERENCES

Bakker, D. J. (1972), *Temporal Order and Disturbed Reading*. Rotterdam, Rotterdam University Press.

Bala, S. P., Cohen, B., Morris, A. G., Atkin, A., Gittelman, R., and Kates, W. (1981), Saccades of hyperactive and normal boys during ocular pursuit. *Developmental Medicine and Child Neurology* 23, 323–336.

Black, J. L., Collins, D. W. K., De Roach, J. N., and Zubrick, S. (1984), A detailed study of sequential saccadic eye movements for normal and poor reading children. *Perceptual and Motor Skills* 51, 423–434.

Brown, B., Haegerstrom-Portnoy, G., Adams, A. J., Yingling, C. D., Galin, D., Herron, J., and Marcus, M. (1983), Predictive eye movements do not discriminate between dyslexic and control children. *Neuropsychologia* 21, 121–128.

Calvin, H., and Ojemann, G. A. (1980), *Inside the Brain*. New York, Mentor.

Ciuffreda, K. J., Bahill, A. T., Kenyon, R. V., and Stark, L. (1976) Eye movements during reading: case reports. *American Journal of Optometry and Physiological Optics* 53, 389–395.

Ciuffreda, K. J., Kenyon, R. V., and Stark, L (1985), Eye movements during reading: further case reports. *American Journal of Optometry and Physiological Optics*, in press.
Cizek, O., and Jost, J. (1984), Eye movements, dyslexia and child development, Prepublication manuscript, Praha, Czechoslovakia.
Coakley, D., and Thomas, J. G. (1977), The ocular microtremor record and the prognosis of the unconscious patient. *Lancet* 1, 512–515.
Critchley, M. (1981), Dyslexia: an overview. In: G. Th. Pavlidis and T. R. Miles (Eds.), *Dyslexia Research and its Application to Education*. Chichester, John Wiley.
Doehring, D. G. (1968), *Patterns of Impairment in Specific Reading Disability*. Bloomington, Indiana, Indiana University Press.
Elterman, R. D., Abel, L. A., Daroff, R. B., Dell'Osso, S. F., and Bornstein, J. L. (1980), Eye movement patterns in dyslexic children. *Journal of Learning Disabilities* 13, 16–21.
Galaburda, A. M., and Kemper, T. L. (1979), Cytoarchitectonic abnormalities in developmental dyslexia: a case study. *Annals of Neurology* 6, 94–100.
Geschwind, N. (1982), Biological foundations of dyslexia. Paper presented at the British Psychological Society's International Conference on Dyslexia. Manchester University, England, March 1–3, 1982.
Geschwind, N. (1986) Dyslexia, Cerebral Dominance, Autoimmunity, and Sex Hormones. In: G. Th. Pavlidis and Fisher, D. F. (Eds.), *Dyslexia: Its Neuropsychology and Treatment*. Chichester, John Wiley.
Gilbert, L. C. (1953), Functional motor efficiency of the eyes and its relation to reading. *University of California Publications in Education* 11, 159–231.
Goldberg, H. K., and Arnott, W. (1970), Ocular motility in learning disabilities. *Journal of Learning Disabilities* 3, 160–162.
Goldrich, S. G., and Sedgwick, H. (1982), An objective comparison of oculomotor functioning in reading disabled and normal children. *American Journal of Optometry and Physiological Optics* 59, 82.
Griffin, D. C., Walton, H. N., and Ives, V. (1974), Saccades as related to reading disorders. *Journal of Learning Disabilities* 7, 310–316.
Holzman, P. S., Levy, D. L., and Proctor, L. R. (1976), Smooth pursuit eye movements, attention, and schizophrenia. *Archives of General Psychiatry* 33, 1415–1420.
Hue, E. B. (1908), *The Psychology and Pedagogy of Reading*. New York, Macmillan.
Javal, Le. (1879), Essai sur la physiologie de la lecture. *Annales d'Occulistique* 82, 242–253.
Jerabek, J. (1984), A contribution to analysis of eye movement disorders in dyslexics. Prepublication manuscript, Praha, Czechoslovakia.
Keogh, B. and Babbitt, B. C. (1986). Sampling issues in Learning Disabilities Research: Markers for the Study of Problems in Mathematics. In. G. Th. Pavlidis and D. F. Fisher (Eds.), *Dyslexia: Its Neuropsychology and Treatment*. Chichester, John Wiley.
Lashley, K. S. (1951), The problems of serial order in behaviour. In: L. A. Jeffress (Ed.), *Cerebral Mechanisms in Behaviour*. New York, John Wiley.
Lesevre, N. (1964), Les mouvemennts oculaires d'exploration: étude electro-oculagraphique comparée d'enfants normaux et dyslexiques. Thèse de 3 cycle (mimeo).
Lesevre, N. (1968), L'organisation du regard chez des enfants d'age scolaire, lecteurs normaux et dyslexiques. *Revue de Neuropsychiatrie des Infant*, 16, 323–349.
Liberman, I. Y. (1983), Linguistic abilities and reading–spelling instruction. Paper presented at the 2nd World Congress on Dyslexia, Halkidiki, Greece, June 27–30, 1983.
Lloyd, P., and Pavlidis, G. Th. (1978), The relationship between child language and eye movements: a developmental study. *Neuroscience Letters Supplement* 1, 248.
Masland, R. L. (1981), Neurological aspects of dyslexia. In: G. Th. Pavlidis and T. R. Miles (Eds.), *Dyslexia Research and its Applications to Education*. Chichester, John Wiley.
Matin, E. (1974), Saccadic suppression: a review and an analysis, *Psychological Bulletin* 81, 899–917.

Mawson, B. (1982), Eye movements and dyslexia. Informal presentation at the British Psychological Society's International Conference on Dyslexia, Manchester University, England, March 1-3, 1982.

Miles, T. R., and Ellis, N. (1981), A lexical encoding deficiency. II: clinical observations. In: G. Th. Pavlidis and T. R. Miles (Eds.), *Dyslexia Research and its Applications to Education*. Chichester, John Wiley.

Naidoo, S. (1972), *Specific Dyslexia*. London, Pitman.

Ojemann, G. and Mateer, K. (1979), Human language cortex: localization of memory, syntax, and sequential motor-phoneme identification systems. *Science* 205, 1401-1403.

Olson, R. K., Kliegl, R., and Davidson, B. J. (1983), Dyslexic and normal readers' eye movements. *Journal of Experimental Psychology*: Human Perception and Performance 9, 816-825.

Pavlidis, G. Th. (1978), The dyslexic's erratic eye movements: case studies. *Dyslexia Review* 1, 22-28.

Pavlidis, G. Th. (1979), How can dyslexia be objectively diagnosed? *Reading* 13, 3-15.

Pavlidis, G. Th. (1981a), Do eye movements hold the key to dyslexia? *Neuropsychologia* 19, 57-64.

Pavlidis, G. Th. (1981b), Sequencing, eye movements and the early objective diagnosis of dyslexia. In: G. Th. Pavlidis, and T. R. Miles, (Eds.), *Dyslexia Research and its Applications to Education*. Chichester, John Wiley.

Pavlidis, G. Th. (1983a), The 'dyslexia syndrome' and its objective diagnosis by erratic eye movements. In: K. Rayner (Ed.), *Eye Movements in Reading: Perceptual and Language Processes*. New York, Academic Press.

Pavlidis, G. Th. (1983b), Research diagnostic criteria for dyslexia: their rationale. Paper presented at the 2nd World Congress on Dyslexia, Halkidiki, Greece, June 27-30.

Pavlidis, G. Th. (1983c), Erratic eye movements in dyslexics: comments and reply to Stanley *et al.*, *British Journal of Psychology*, 74, 189-193.

Pavlidis, G. Th. (1985a), Eye movements in dyslexia: their diagnostic significance. *Journal of Learning Disabilities* 18, 42-50.

Pavlidis, G. Th. (1985b), Eye movement differences between dyslexics, normal and retarded readers while sequentially fixating digits. *American Journal of Optometry and Physiological Optics*, 62, 820-832.

Pavlidis, G. Th. (1985c), Erratic eye movements and dyslexia: factors determining their relationship. *Perceptual and Motor Skills* 60, 319-322.

Pirozzolo, F. J., and Rayner, K. (1978), The neutral control of EM in acquired and developmental reading disorder. In: G. Avakian-Whitaker and H. A. Whitaker (Eds)., *Advances in Neurolinguistics and Psycholinguistics*. New York, Academic Press.

Rubino, C. A., and Minden, H. A. (1973), An analysis of eye movements in children with a reading disability. *Cortex* 9, 217-220.

Schwartz, A. H., Pavlidis, G. Th., Hollander, H. E., and Goldstein, L. (1984), Relation between pursuit eye movements and computerized EEG in schizophrenic in-patients. Paper presented at the Annual Meeting of the American Psychiatric Association, Los Angeles, May, 1984.

Stanley, G., Smith, G. A., and Gowell, E. A. (1983), Eye movements and sequential tracking in dyslexic and control children. *British Journal of Psychology* 74, 181-187.

Taylor, S. E., Franckenpohl, H., and Pette, J. L. (1960), Grade level norms for components of the fundamental reading skills, EDL. *Information Research Bulletin, 3*. Huntington, New York, Educ. Devel. Labs.

Tinker, M. A. (1958), Recent studies of eye movements in reading. *Psychological Bulletin* 55, 215-231.

Vellutino, F. R. (1977), Alternative conceptualizations of dyslexia: evidence in support of a verbal deficit hypothesis. *Harvard Educational Review* 47, 334-354.

Vernon, M. D. (1977), Varieties in deficiency in the reading process. *Harvard Education Review* **47**, 396–410.

Volkman, F. C. (1976), Saccadic suppression. In: R. A. Monty and J. A. Senders (Eds.), *Eye Movements and Psychological Processes*. New Jersey, Lawrence Erlbaum Associates.

Young, L. R., and Sheena, D. (1975), Survey of eye movement recording methods. *Behavioral Research Methods and Instrumentation* **7**, 397–429.

Zangwill, O. L., and Blakemore, C. (1972), Dyslexia: reversal of eye movements during reading. *Neuropsychologia* **10**, 371–373.

Zurif, E. B., and Carson, G. (1970), Dyslexia in relation to cerebral dominance and temporal analysis. *Neuropsychologia* **8**, 351–361.

CHAPTER 9

Eye Movements and the Perceptual Span: Evidence for Dyslexic Typology

KEITH RAYNER
Department of Psychology, University of Massachusetts, Amherst, Massachusetts, USA

There has recently been a great deal of research utilizing eye movement data as dependent variables in studying the reading process. Silent skilled reading is a very private process with few observable indications of what cognitive activities are occurring at a particular point in time. The amount of time that a reader looks at a particular portion of the text has proved to be particularly important in specifying underlying cognitive processes associated with reading (Rayner, 1978; Just and Carpenter, 1980). Given the recent success with respect to investigating perceptual and language processing in reading via eye movement data (see Rayner, 1983a), it is not surprising that investigators interested in reading disability would also be particularly interested in examining eye movement patterns in reading disabled subjects. A number of recent studies have attempted to study the characteristics of eye movement patterns in reading disabled subjects. In this chapter, three basic questions with respect to dyslexia and eye movements will be discussed. They are:

(1) What is different about the pattern of eye movements of normal and dyslexic readers?
(2) Are eye movements the cause of the reading disability or are they a symptom of a more basic underlying problem?
(3) Given that there are differences in eye movement patterns between normals and dyslexics, what relationship may these eye movement patterns have to the perceptual span?

I should also make clear the fact that I will be discussing developmental dyslexia as opposed to acquired dyslexia. With acquired dyslexia, the brain damage that results in reading problems could easily result in abnormalities of the oculomotor system (i.e. damage to the visual cortex or superior colliculus). Patients with lesions in various parts of the brain known to have some relationship to the oculomotor system often, though not always, have reading problems (Pirozzolo and Rayner, 1979). Likewise, patients with low vision due to macular degeneration, optic nerve atrophy, ocular histoplasmosis, diabetic retinopathy, etc., have severe difficulties in reading (Legge *et al.*, 1985; Holcomb and Goodrich, 1976; Goodrich *et al.*, 1977). Often such patients develop foveal scotomas in which central vision is lost. As an experimental simulation of this phenomenon, Rayner and Bertera (1979) created artificial scotomas of the retina by moving a visual mask in perfect synchrony with the reader's eye. Wherever the reader fixated, the mask obliterated the text a given number of character spaces left and right of fixation. One could easily argue that these normal readers were temporarily dyslexic—the reading rate was very slow, they made many fixations, long fixation durations, many regressions, and understood very little of what they read. Studies of acquired dyslexia and visual impairment reveal the importance of various parts of the brain and oculomotor system in reading, but may not shed much light on the mechanisms of developmental dyslexia.

Everyone seems to agree that there are problems associated with categorizing readers as dyslexics (see Vellutino, 1979). There has been considerable controversy over exactly how to define a reader as being dyslexic and a lot of the variability in the results of different studies may be due to that problem. Additionally, it appears somewhat questionable to assume that dyslexics represent a homogeneous group. Recently, a number of researchers (Boder, 1973; Kinsbourne and Warrington, 1963; Mattis, French, and Rapin, 1975; Pirozzolo, 1979) have proposed that dyslexia should be thought of as consisting of heterogenous subgroups. Although the criteria by which different subgroups are defined vary somewhat, the categorization process seems to yield at least two broad groups of dyslexic readers. One group, generally assumed to be considerably more prevalent than the other, consists of readers with a general language deficit. Such dyslexics are referred to as *dysphonetic* by Boder (1973) and *language disorder dyslexics* by Mattis *et al.* (1975). The second group appear to consist of dyslexics with a visual–spatial deficit. They are referred to as *dyseidetic* by Boder (1973), *visual–perceptual dyslexics* by Mattis *et al.*, (1975) and as having *developmental Gerstmann syndrome* by Kinsbourne and Warrington (1963). Additionally, there may be other dyslexics who have mixed patterns having both a language deficit and a visual–spatial deficit. Dyslexics could presumably differ within these subgroups in terms of the severity of the disability. In fact, others have suggested that dyslexia can best be described in terms of a continuum or continuous distributions (Olson *et al.*, 1984). Olson *et al.* (1984) point out that distinct subgroups and continuous distribution views of dyslexia can have quite different implications for the etiology and remediation of reading disability. Clear and distinct subgroups suggest distinct causes for different reading disabilities (such as different training programs, localized brain damage, or gene inheritance patterns). On the other hand, continuous distributions suggest multiple causes. Indeed, reading disability could be thought of as consisting of a number of different continuums on which reading disabled children might differ.

My purpose in this chapter is not to argue for either view as being superior or more appropriate. What is important is that both approaches emphasize that dyslexia is not due to a single underlying cause. Future work will have to determine which approach is more appropriate. My intention in the present chapter is to elucidate some of the recent work relating eye movements and the perceptual span to dyslexia. For expository convenience, I will adopt the convention of referring to subgroups of dyslexic readers. However, it could well turn out that the notion of continuous distributions is equally valid in terms of explanatory power. My impression from examining the eye movement records of dyslexic readers is that there are at least two broad groups of dyslexic readers: one with a general language disorder and one with a visual–spatial disorder. There may also be dyslexic readers with both types of disorders. My observations are due in large part to case studies reported previously by Pirozzolo and Rayner (1978, 1979), Ciuffreda et al., (1976), Zangwill and Blakemore (1972), Pavlidis (1978), and Jones and Stark (1983). One final point to keep in mind is that the dyslexics with a language disorder may outnumber those with a visual–spatial disorder by a factor of more than 10 to 1. Assuming then that at least two broad subgroups of dyslexics exist, let us proceed to the three questions outlined earlier.

EYE MOVEMENT PATTERNS

While reading text, poor readers and dyslexic readers differ from normal readers in that they make more fixations per line, have longer fixation durations, shorter saccade lengths, and a higher frequency of regressions than normals (Elterman et al., 1980; Lefton et al., 1979; Rayner, 1978; Rubino and Minden, 1973; Griffin, et al., 1974). Lefton et al. (1979) also found that normal developmental gains made by children are not shown in the eye movement dynamics of poor readers. That is, normal children tend to show clear developmental trends in that fixation duration decreases, saccade length increases, and the frequency of regressions decrease as children get older and more proficient at the task of reading (Rayner, 1978). Lefton and co-workers found that poor readers showed much less of a developmental trend. In the remainder of this chapter, a general distinction will be made between poor readers and dyslexics in terms of the severity of the disability. Poor readers will be assumed to be those with no gross physical handicaps, who are 1–2 years retarded in reading. The characteristics of poor readers is somewhat muddled with some suggesting that poor reading is due to low intelligence, while others insist that the only interesting poor readers are those with average IQ scores.

Poor reading could also be attributable to motivational and/or socio-economic factors. With adequate instruction, poor readers with average intelligence may improve their reading performance. On the other hand, poor readers with subnormal intelligence may always exhibit reading difficulties. Dyslexic readers, by contrast, do have normal intelligence with no gross emotional or physical handicaps, yet they read two or more years behind expected grade level. Likewise, a number of other factors such as educational history, lack of motivation, absenteeism from school, and frequent school changes presumably cannot account for their reading problems. Unfortunately, it is the case that many of these latter factors are quite subjective and difficult to evaluate.

The dyslexic readers to be described in this section are adults who have extreme difficulties reading. None of the subjective or objective factors listed above can account for their reading problems. The two dyslexic readers whose eye movement characteristics will be described in detail below, for example, were given extensive psychometric test batteries, as well as interviews to consider the subjective factors mentioned above. Both dyslexics had normal IQ scores, with Subject B having a Verbal WAIS score of 97 and a Performance score of 114. Subject C, on the other hand had a Verbal score of 104 and a Performance score of 98 (for details of other psychometric scores, see Pirozzolo, 1979). Table 1 shows representative values for differences in key eye movement measures for normal and dyslexic readers. As seen, when reading text at comparable levels, there are major differences between normal and dyslexic readers. The pattern of eye movements also differs. Table 2 shows two lines of text read by a normal reader (A), and two dyslexic readers. Both dyslexic subjects make many more fixations than the normal subject and, of course, comprehension is markedly poorer in the two dyslexics. What is interesting is a comparison of the pattern of the two dyslexic readers. Subject B can be characterized as having a language processing deficit. Fixations are quite long, there are many regressions and when difficulty is encountered, B resorts to a strategy in which attempts are made to use the context to disambiguate the text. If that fails, every letter may be fixated in an attempt to decode the word. Subjects with language processing

Table 1. Average eye movement measures for normal and dyslexic readers

	Normal	Dyslexic
Average fixation duration	200–250 ms	300–350 ms
Average saccade length	8–9 characters	3–6 characters
Frequency of regressions	10–20%	30–40%

	A	B	C
Average fixation duration	220 ms	310 ms	335 ms
Average saccade length (forward)	9 chars.	5.5 chars.	7 chars.
Average saccade length (regression)	3 chars.	5.5 chars.	8.5 chars.
Frequency of regression	17%	35%	30%

Table 2. Eye movement patterns for a normal (A) and two dyslexic (B and C) readers

As society has become progressively more complex, psychology has

```
 1     2    3      4          5    7   |   8     9
234   310  188    216        242  188  |  177   159
                                  6
                                 144
```

A

assumed an increasingly important role in solving human problems.

```
 11   |    12        13      15   14      16   |   18
244   |   317       229     269  196     277   |  202
      10                                     17
     206                                    144
```

As society has become progressively more complex, psychology has

```
 1    3    2    5 |     6    7    8     9    10  | 15   12 | | 13    14
311  277  115  412|    198  403 266   295  311  |193  317 | |600   312
               4                                  11    18
              222                                 277   206|
                                                       19
                                                      415
```

B

assumed an increasingly important role in solving human problems.

```
 16   |    21   |   22   24  |    25   26   27  | |  28      31  | 32
369   |   302   |  244  310  |   383  119  487  | | 413     277  |366
      17        20           23              29             33
     415       177          288             200|           361
                                             30
                                            117
```

As society has become progressively more complex, psychology has

```
 1   |    2      3    6    7  |  5     9   |   11    10   13 |
282  |   476    322  197  472 |483   177   |  290   268  276 |
     4                           8          12              14
    177                        257         476            399
```

C

assumed an increasingly important role in solving human problems.

```
 19  |    21   22     23   |  18    25   26  |   16   |   15   |
167  |   320  297    302   | 336   256  325  |  259   |  391   |
     20              24             17            27         28
    428             399            323           446        281
```

difficulties like B tend to make short forward saccades and their regressions also tend to be short, often shorter than the forward saccades. Figure 1 shows a strip chart eye movement pattern of each of the three subjects. The normal reader (A) shows a typical 'staircase pattern' in which the eye moves mainly from left to right. By contrast, Subject B shows what can be called a 'partial staircase pattern' in which the movements are from left to right with numerous regressions back over material already traversed. In examining the pattern for Subject C, we can identify what has been referred to as a 'reverse staircase pattern' in which there are clusters of right to left saccades. Also, the amplitude of right to left saccades exceeds that of left to right saccades. Thus, an examination of the pattern of eye movements reveals different characteristics for Subject C than Subject B. Subject C can be characterized as having a visual-spatial processing deficit.

ARE EYE MOVEMENTS THE CAUSE OF DYSLEXIA?

No one would dispute that the eye movements of dyslexics are different from those of normals. The differences in mean values for fixation duration, saccade

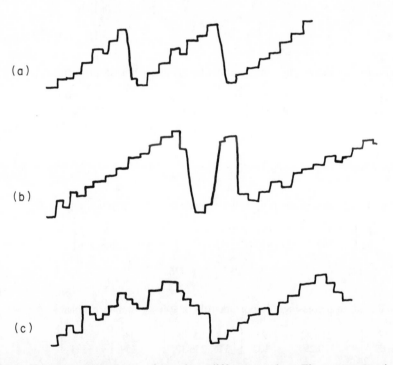

Figure 1. Eye movement patterns from three different readers. The top pattern is for reader A, the middle pattern is for reader B, and the bottom pattern is for reader C.

length, and frequency of regressions have been known for some time. One critical question on which there is controversy concerns the extent to which the eye movements represent the cause of the reading problem, much as in the case of patients with oculomotor problems such as saccade intrusions (Ciuffreda, *et al.*, 1983) or congenital jerk nystagmus (Ciuffreda, 1979). Tinker (1958) argued quite strongly that eye movements were not a cause of reading disability, rather they were a reflection of other underlying problems. The issue, assumed by Tinker to be settled, has been dramatically brought back into the spotlight by some recent work reported by Pavlidis (1981a, 1981b).

Pavlidis presented results which he suggested indicated a central malfunction in dyslexics, namely a sequential disability and/or oculomotor malfunction. He has not been entirely clear as to which of the above factors he believes his results are due to, but others have assumed that his results were support for the notion that faulty eye movements represent the major causative factor in reading disability. Pavlidis quite appropriately noted that any study of dyslexia based on reading experiments alone would be open to the criticism that dyslexics would show different eye movement patterns during reading from normals because they do not read well. However, Pavlidis reasoned, if the cause of dyslexia is constitutional in nature (e.g. is due to a sequential disability or oculomotor malfunction), one would expect that such a disability should manifest itself not only in reading, but also in other tasks in which sequencing and eye movements are important. Pavlidis developed what he has referred to as the 'lights test' in which subjects are asked to continuously fixate on a target that jumps unpredictably (in terms of temporal properties) from left to right or right to left across the screen. This task is actually quite similar to one used by Arnold and Tinker (1939) and more recently by Salthouse and Ellis (1980) and Rayner *et al.* (1983) to study saccadic latency in a task simulating reading, but in which the necessity for verbal encoding is eliminated. Pavlidis tested 12 dyslexic and 12 normal readers in the lights task. His primary finding was that when the target moved from left to right, dyslexic subjects showed significantly more right to left saccades than did the normal readers. Also, when reading text, the dyslexic subjects showed the characteristic reverse staircase pattern described previously. Hence, Pavlidis concluded that the erratic eye movements and reverse staircase pattern often reported in case studies is characteristic of dyslexics. It is also important to note that Pavlidis's results are consistent with data in previous reports by Gilbert (1953); Griffin *et al.* (1974) and Lesevre (1968) and with many case studies mentioned previously in demonstrating erratic eye movements in dyslexic readers. Pavlidis (1983a) has also tested 'backward' readers, those for whom IQ or other factors can be used to account for their poor reading performance. The backward readers did not differ from the controls.

Pavlidis has been criticized by a number of investigators as being vague concerning his definition of dyslexics (1981a). Indeed, the original report is quite sparse on such details[1]. However, elsewhere, Pavlidis (1981b, 1983a) has been more explicit about his criteria in selecting backward and dyslexic readers. However, using variations of Pavlidis's subject selection criteria, stimuli, and experimental procedures (Pavlidis 1983b), three studies have been undertaken (Stanley et al., 1983; Brown et al., 1983; Olson et al., 1983). They did not obtain the same findings reported by Pavlidis. In fact, in none of the three studies was there any indication that the dyslexic subjects differed from the normals in the frequency of regressions during the lights test. Stanley and co-workers further pointed out that they have failed to find differences between their dyslexic and normal readers' eye movement patterns on a visual search task. When asked to read text, the two groups of subjects differed markedly. Adler-Grinberg and Stark (1978) reported similar findings.

What are we to make of the differences between these studies? My own resolution of the discrepancies, biased in part by the fact that I have seen dyslexic readers such as those described by Pavlidis, is that sampling procedures can account for the disagreements. That is, Stanley, Brown, and Olson's samples almost entirely comprise dyslexic readers with a language deficit. On the other hand, Pavlidis may have used a sample comprised primarily of dyslexics with a visual–spatial deficit (see Pollatsek (1983) for similar arguments). Pavlidis's original sample comprised subjects from throughout Great Britain. He is known for specializing in dyslexic subjects with visual problems so it is not surprising that many such subjects would be referred to him. Given that such subjects are considerably rarer than those with a language deficit, it is not surprising that they would not show up in the other studies. In fact, however, one of the 15 dyslexic subjects run by Stanley and co-workers showed a pattern similar to that reported by Pavlidis.

Pavlidis's work is very important because it has focused on certain issues with respect to eye movements and dyslexia. In particular, it emphasizes that dyslexia may be due to different underlying perceptual and cognitive deficits. He may well be quite correct in the implication that dyslexics with a visual–spatial deficit have the more severe form of reading disability. However, it is also the case that there are dyslexic readers who do not exhibit erratic eye movements. Such readers (those with a language deficit who do not have erratic eye movements) may have just as serious a disability as those with a visual–spatial deficit.

Finally, with respect to this issue it is important to point out that when Subject B was presented with text appropriate for his reading level, the eye movement pattern and mean values for the critical eye movement variables were equivalent to children reading at the reading level which was normal for that age (in this case, fifth grade text). On the other hand, when Subject C was presented with age-appropriate text which was rotated 180 degrees, her reading performance (both speed and comprehension) improved dramatically and her eye movement

Table 3. Characteristics of dyslexic sample in the Pavlidis study and three failures to replicate the results

	Pavlidis (1981a)	Pavlidis (1981b)	Stanley et al.	Brown et al.	Olson et al.
Age: $\overline{X}$	Not given	10 yr. 1 mo.	12 yr. 6 mo.	11 yr. 1 mo.	11 yr.
Range	10–16 yr	8-3 to 13-6	11-1 to 13-11	10–12 yr	8-3 to 13-9
IQ: $\overline{X}$	Not given	Not given	113[a]	104[b]	100[c]
Cutoff	Not given (above average)	At least 90	Not given[d]	At least 88	At least 90
Years behind	At least 2 years behind	At least 2 years behind if over 10 and 18 months behind if under 10	2 yr. 10 mo.	2 yr. 6 mo.[e]	1 yr. 8 mo.[f]

[a] Jenkins Non-Verbal IQ Test.
[b] WISC-R.
[c] WISC-R.
[d] The lowest score given for non-verbal is 93 and for verbal is 81.
[e] This value is a composite score based on oral reading and reading comprehension.
[f] The authors note that their dyslexic subjects averaged approximately half of expected grade level on three subscales of the PIAT in comparison to their control subjects.

pattern looked quite normal (staircase pattern), except, of course, the saccades were in a right-to-left direction (see Pirozzolo and Rayner, 1978).

In this section, I have tried to account for the discrepancies in results between data reported by the various investigators. If my analysis is correct, then the discrepancy is due to a subject sampling problem. While I have argued for differences due to different subtypes of dyslexics in a specific task involving sequential eye movements, the problem is really more pervasive and general with respect to research on dyslexia. For almost any type of study done with dyslexics, one can find quite contradictory results leading many not working in the area to be quite skeptical about the research. Let me amplify a bit on this assertion by presenting two examples, one that involves eye movements and one that doesn't.

The type of study that does not involve eye movements is related to hemispheric specialization and dyslexia. Visual half field studies conducted with reading disabled readers have produced quite confusing results. For example, McKeever and Huling (1970; also, McKeever and VanDeventer, 1975) found a right visual field superiority for the recognition of words in poor readers. Olson (1973), however, was unable to find a right visual field superiority for verbal stimuli in disabled readers. Marcel, Katz, and Smith (1974; also Marcel and Rajan, 1975) found a reduced right field superiority in their disabled readers and argued that this represented a linguistic superiority of the disabled readers' right hemispheres rather than a left hemisphere dysfunction. In direct contrast to these results, Yeni-Komshian, Isenberg, and Goldberg (1975) reported that disabled readers have increased right visual field superiorities. The causal relationship between reading disability and hemispheric specialization that has been developed to explain these inconsistent patterns of results has also differed dramatically. How do we account for these differences? There are a number of reasons why the conflicting results might emerge. However, one could conclude that the selection of subjects for entry into the disabled reader group is an important factor that influences group performance data (Pirozzolo, Rayner, and Hynd, 1983).

The second area where there are contradictory results involves dyslexia and saccadic latency. In a task in which stimuli were presented to the left or right of fixation and the subject was instructed to make an eye movement to the stimulus as fast as possible, Lesevre (1966) found that normal readers have a shorter latency to the right. Dyslexic readers, on the other hand, showed no such asymmetry. Dossetor and Papaioannou (1975), however, found quite a different pattern of asymmetry. Reaction times for dyslexics were shorter for movements to the right whereas normals showed shorter reaction times to the left. It should be noted that the reaction times reported for their subjects were very long (400–500 ms) and the target appeared 40 degrees from fixation. Cohen and Ross (1977) found that there were no differences for saccadic latencies to the right or left for either good readers or poor readers in their study of the

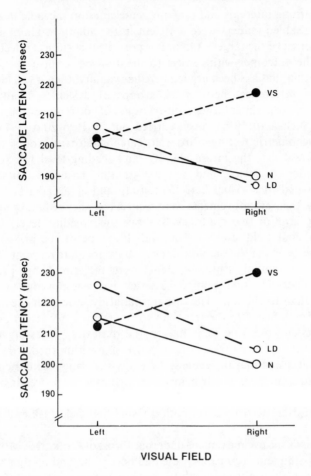

Figure 2. Saccade latencies for normal (N), visual–spatial dyslexics (VS), and language deficit dyslexics (LD). Top panel presents data when three symbols were the target; lower panel presents data when three-letter words were the target. Adapted from Pirozzolo (1979).

Table 4. Mean age, IQ, and reading level for subjects in Pirozzolo's study

	Normal readers	Language deficit dyslexics	Visual–spatial dyslexics
Age	11.0	11.1	11.2
Full-scale IQ	106	103	105
Verbal IQ	106	96	113
Performance IQ	107	113	94
Reading level	5.8	2.9	3.1

effects of warning intervals and target eccentricities on saccadic latencies, but found that disabled readers were deficient in the ability to maintain fixation prior to the onset of the target. Again, it is possible that subject selection effects influenced the outcomes with respect to the dyslexic results.

If the position that has been argued here has validity, then it will be necessary to document differences between subgroups of dyslexics in advance and then look for experimental demonstrations of differences between such subgroups. Such a study has been carried out by Pirozzolo (1979). On the basis of psychometric testing, Pirozzolo categorized two groups of dyslexic readers. Table 4 lists the mean age, IQ, and reading level for 8 normal, 8 language deficit dyslexics, and 8 visual–spatial dyslexics. These subjects then participated in a visual half field study and a saccadic latency study. Additionally, their eye movements were recorded as they read text either below their reading level or two grade levels above their reading level. The results of the visual half field study are beyond the scope of the present chapter. However, the results of the saccadic latency study are quite relevant. The results when words or symbols (three # signs) were the stimuli are presented in Figure 2. The normals and the language deficit dyslexics moved their eyes faster to the right than to the left. The visual–spatial dyslexics, on the other hand moved their eyes faster to the left than to the right. Pirozzolo's explanation of the results suggests that in visual–spatial dyslexics processing within the right hemisphere is more efficient than processing within the left hemisphere. He further suggested that the general difficulty that language deficit dyslexics have is due to some type of left hemisphere disorder for processing language. Be that as it may, Pirozzolo was able to demonstrate differences between two subgroups of dyslexic readers on both a visual half field task and a saccadic latency task.

Table 5 shows the eye movement data that Pirozzolo collected. Most relevant for the discussion and arguments presented here is the finding that the visual–spatial dyslexics showed considerably more return sweep inaccuracies than did the other two groups of subjects.

In short, it appears that there is a group of dyslexic readers that have a tendency to move their eyes to the left in both reading (Pirozzolo and Rayner, 1978; Pavlidis, 1978; Zangwill & Blakemore, 1972) and non-reading tasks (Pavlidis, 1981a). Further, such subjects show shorter eye movement latencies to the left than to the right and have a higher frequency of return sweep inaccuracies (Pirozzolo, 1979). This subgroup of dyslexic readers, called visual–spatial dyslexics here, are proportionally quite smaller than language deficit dyslexics. This latter group of dyslexic readers do not show any form of erratic eye movements. In fact, the eye movements of the language deficit dyslexics are quite normal in non-reading tasks (Stanley et al., 1983a; Brown et al., 1983; Olson et al., 1983; Adler-Grinberg and Stark, 1978). It is only when reading text that their eye movement patterns are abnormal, and such abnormal patterns are a reflection of the difficulty the reader is having processing the language. In the future, more research of the type conducted by Pirozzolo (1979) in which dyslexics are categorized in advance will be necessary to further document the points raised in this chapter. Pirozzolo (1983; Pirozzolo *et al.*, 1983) and others (Boder, 1973; Mattis *et al.*, 1975) have provided categorization schemes for differentiating different subtypes of dyslexic readers.

It should also be noted that other researchers have pointed out qualitative differences in eye movement patterns for disabled readers. Olson *et al.* (1984) identified two reading styles among disabled readers that they referred to as 'plodders' and 'explorers'. The plodders displayed relatively few regressions between words and rarely skipped words on forward movements. They tended to move steadily forward, with more frequent forward saccades within words and to the immediately following word. Explorers, on the other hand, displayed relatively more regressions and word-skipping movements. Olson and co-workers pointed out that the plodders and the explorers might finish reading a given text in the same amount of time, but the patterns of eye movements are markedly different. Olson and co-workers pointed out that the plodder–explorer dimension was normally distributed in their sample and there was no evidence of distinct subgroups. In fact, when they examined the twelve subjects in their sample with the greatest deficit in performance IQ compared to verbal IQ (which Boder and Pirozzolo have suggested as a possible way to identify dyseidetics), they found that these subjects were not different from the rest of the group in their reading

Table 5. Characteristics of subjects' eye movements and fixations during reading in Pirozzolo's study

	Normal readers	Language deficit dyslexics	Visual–spatial dyslexics
Mean number of fixations per line:			
Easy	6.0	5.7	6.3
Difficult	7.8	7.8	7.6
Average fixation duration:			
Easy	252	274	273
Difficult	260	273	274
Mean number of return sweep inaccuracies:			
Easy	0.50	0.75	2.6
Difficult	0.62	0.75	2.75
Mean percentage of regressions:			
Easy	15.1	22.2	22.2
Difficult	21.8	27.7	24.7

patterns. Precisely what to make of this fact is uncertain, since it may be that the severity of the reading disability in Olson's sample may be less extreme than the samples used by those advocating subgroups (which typically include clinically referred children). Nevertheless, the point to be made is that it is clear that different patterns of eye movements emerge among disabled readers that may be indicative of different types of problems associated with processing text.

Finally, this section started with the question concerning the extent to which eye movements are the cause of dyslexia. My conclusion is that for dyslexics with a visual–spatial deficit, the eye movements are a reflection of an underlying spatial processing disorder. For dyslexics with a language deficit, the eye movements reflect the underlying problem with language processing. When reading level appropriate text is presented, the eye movement pattern looks quite normal for that developmental level. Tinker (1946, 1958) reviewed numerous studies in which the eye movements of poor readers were trained so that these subjects would make smooth efficient eye movements. The two assumptions in most of that research were that (1) good readers make smooth efficient eye movements and (2) the problems that poor readers have are due to faulty eye movements. The first assumption, that good readers have smooth efficient eye movements, is quite blatantly incorrect. Good readers are highly variable in how far they move their eyes and in their fixation durations (Rayner, 1978). So it is not surprising that the results of such research endeavors were doomed to failure. In fact, Tinker's summary of the research leads to the conclusion that you can improve the efficiency of poor readers' eye movements, and they will still be poor readers. Hence, while erratic eye movements may well be diagnostic of a group of dyslexic readers (Pavlidis, 1983b), it is most likely futile to think of eye movements as being causative of reading disabilities. Thus I conclude that Tinker was correct in his assessment that eye movements are a reflection of the problems readers have and not the cause of the problem.

THE PERCEPTUAL SPAN AND DYSLEXIA

It is frequently suggested that dyslexics read poorly because their perceptual span is smaller than normal readers (see Pirozzolo (1979) for a review of such suggestions). That is, it is assumed that dyslexics take in less visual information per fixation than do normal readers. Certainly, patients with a loss of vision in the parafovea read quite slowly. In part, the suggestion that dyslexics take in less information per fixation derives from the fact that dyslexics make shorter saccades on average than do normal readers and some techniques used to estimate the perceptual span rely solely on average saccade length (Taylor, 1957). However, while saccade length may bear some relationship to the size of the percetual span, it does not really produce a good estimate of the perceptual span since the average saccade length is at least half the size of the span. Over

Fixation number	Example
1	Xxxxhology means perxxxxxxxx xxxxxxxxx xxxx xxxx xxxxxxx. Xxxx xx x
2	Xxxxxxxxxx xxxxs personality diaxxxxxx xxxx xxxx xxxxxxx. Xxxx xx x
3	Xxxxxxxxxx xxxxx xxxxxxxxxxx xiagnosis from hanx xxxxxxx. Xxxx xx x
4	Xxxxxxxxxx xxxxx xxxxxxxxxxx xxxxxxxxx xxxm hand writing. Xxxx xx x

Figure 3. Example of a moving window with fixation location marked by the dot for four successive fixations. The window is 17 characters around the fixation point.

the past ten years, numerous experiments have been conducted in my laboratory to determine the size of the perceptual span. Subjects are asked to read text presented on a CRT and their eye movements are monitored as they do so. Then display changes contingent upon eye position are made as they read.

As can be seen in Figure 3, our experimental situation creates a 'moving window' of text in which the reader's eye movements determine the location of the window. Wherever the reader looks text is exposed within the window region. The experimenter can vary the size of the window on each fixation, but the subject is always free to look anywhere in the text. Using this technique (see Rayner (1978, 1983a) for reviews), we have been able to reach a number of conclusions about the characteristics of the perceptual span in normal adult readers. We have found that the perceptual span extends from the beginning of the currently fixated word (but no more than 4 letters to the left of fixation) to about 15 characters to the right of fixation. Within the span region, different types of information are acquired. Information useful in identifying words and letters is acquired from a region extending to about 8 characters to the right of fixation. Beyond that region, more gross types of information (such as word length) are acquired and used in guiding the eye movement.

The moving window type of experiment seems ideal to test the notion that dyslexics have smaller perceptual spans than do normals. In fact, such an experiment with reading disabled subjects in the fifth grade has been carried out by Underwood and Zola (1984). If dyslexics have a smaller perceptual span than normals, then they should show the most pronounced deficit since they make shorter saccades. My reading of the Underwood and Zola paper implies that the reading disabled children in the study corresponded to the language deficit subgroup. They had normal IQ (and were matched with the normals) and had no emotional or behavioral problems that could account for their two years below grade level reading performance. Underwood and Zola used a variation of the moving window technique in which all of the letters a certain distance to the left or right of fixation were replaced by other letters on certain fixations. The saccade length data shown in Figure 4 are taken directly from their paper. I have estimated the reading rate for the different conditions and they are also presented in the figure. The striking thing about the figure is that while average saccade length is shorter for the poor readers than the normal readers and while reading rate is also slower (as would be expected), the curves are parallel for both groups suggesting that the effects of changing the letters have exactly the same effect at equal distances from fixation for both groups of subjects. Clearly, more work needs to be done on this issue and perhaps a study of this type with both language deficit and visual–spatial dyslexics would be useful (Rayner, 1983b). But, the results of the Underwood and Zola study

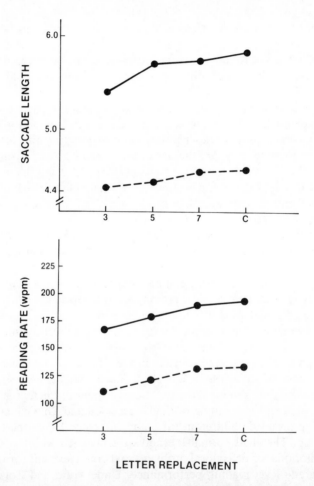

Figure 4. Average saccade length and reading rate for good (solid line) and poor (dashed line) readers in the Underwood and Zola study.

certainly suggest that a small perceptual span is not a major contributing factor in dyslexia. This analysis is also consistent with the conclusion that the pattern of eye movements reflects underlying cognitive or neurological problems and that the eye movements in and of themselves are not the cause of the reading deficiency.

CONCLUSIONS

I have attempted to argue that at least two different subtypes of dyslexics can be identified on the basis of their eye movement patterns while reading text and non-textual material. The language deficit dyslexics have problems processing language. Their speech may show subtle signs of agrammatism (and anomia) and when reading they make many fixations. When they encounter a word which they do not know, they attempt to use context to disambiguate the word. They may then guess what the word is, based on letter cues from the word and context, or they may fixate on each letter in an attempt to sound out the word. When they read reading level appropriate text, their eye movement pattern and characteristics mimic normal children at that age level. When engaged in non-language tasks, their eye movement patterns are indistinguishable from normals. The language deficit group make up the majority of dyslexics. The second group have a visual–spatial disorder. In reading age appropriate text, they frequently exhibit a reverse staircase eye movement pattern. Their regressions tend to be longer than their forward saccades. When presented with reading level appropriate text, the reverse staircase pattern persists. Also in a non-reading task (Pavlidis's lights test) they make many more right-to-left saccades in what Zangwill and Blakemore (1972) referred to as an irrepressible tendency to move to the left. The latency for moving the eye to the left of fixation is also shorter than for moving to the right.

I have further argued that the difference in eye movements between the normal reader and the language deficit dyslexic can be explained in terms of the dyslexic's general difficulty with processing language. In the case of the visual–spatial deficit dyslexic, the difference in eye movements is accounted for on the basis of an underlying spatial orientation problem. Thus, the eye movements are not the cause of dyslexia but reflective of other problems.

Finally, I have argued on the basis of some preliminary data that language deficit dyslexics do not have a smaller perceptual span than normal readers. The fact that they make smaller saccades is not due to them taking in less information per fixation but to the general problem with language as described above. Further research in which dyslexic readers are categorized into subgroups on an *a priori* basis and then presented with eye movement tasks, is needed. If the results of such experimentation were to be successful, it would further document the case for at least two major subgroups of dyslexic readers.

ACKNOWLEDGEMENTS

Preparation of this paper was supported by grant HD12727 from the National Institutes of Health. The author would like to thank Fran Pirozzolo and Richard Olson for their comments on an earlier version of this chapter, and Alexander Pollatsek, Dennis Fisher, and George Pavlidis for discussing their ideas concerning the relationship between eye movements and dyslexia with the author.

NOTES

1. In fairness to Pavlidis, it should be noted that the original paper (1981b) by a more detailed description.

REFERENCES

Adler-Grinberg, D., and Stark, L. (1978), Eye movements, scanpaths, and dyslexia. *American Journal of Optometry and Physiological Optics* 55, 557–570.

Arnold, D., and Tinker, M. A. (1939), The fixational pause of the eyes. *Journal of Experimental Psychology* 25, 271–280.

Boder, E. (1973), Developmental dyslexia: a diagnostic approach based on three atypical reading–spelling patterns. *Developmental Medicine and Child Neurology* 15, 663–687.

Brown, B., Haegerstrom-Portnoy, G., Adams, A. J., Yingling, D. D., Galin, D., Herron, J., and Marcus, M. (1983), Predictive eye movements do not discriminate between dyslexic and control children. *Neuropsychologia* 21, 121–128.

Ciuffreda, K. J. (1979), Jerk nystagmus: some new findings. *American Journal of Optometry and Physiological Optics* 56, 521–530.

Ciuffreda, K. J., Bahill, A. T., Kenyon, R. V., and Stark, L. (1976), Eye movements during reading: case studies. *American Journal of Optometry and Psychological Optics* 53, 389–395.

Ciuffreda, K. J., Kenyon, R. V., and Stark, L. (1983), Saccadic intrusions contributing to reading disability: a case report. *American Journal of Optometry and Physiological Optics* 60, 242–249.

Cohen, M. E., and Ross, L. E. (1977), Saccadic latency in children and adults: effects of warning signal and target eccentricity. *Journal of Experimental Child Psychology* 16, 539–549.

Dossetor, D. R., and Papaioannou, J. (1975), Dyslexia and eye movements. *Language and Speech* 18, 312–317.

Elterman, R. D., Abel, L. A., Daroff, R. B., Dell'Osso, L. F., and Bornstein, J. L. (1980), Eye movement patterns in dyslexic children. *Journal of Learning Disabilities* 13, 16–21.

Gilbert, L. C. (1953), Functional motor efficiency of the eyes and its relation to reading. *University of California Publications in Education* 11, 159–231.

Goodrich, G. L., Mehr, E. B., Quillman, R. D., Shaw, H. K., and Wiley, J. K. (1977), Training and practice effects in performance with low-vision aids: a preliminary study. *American Journal of Optometry and Physiological Optics*, 54, 312–318.

Griffin, D. C., Walton, H. N., and Ives, V. (1974). Saccades as related to reading disability. *Journal of Learning Disabilities* 7, 310–316.

Holcomb, J. G., and Goodrich, G. L. (1976), Eccentric viewing training. *Journal of the American Optometric Society* **47**, 1438–1443.

Jones, A., and Stark, L. (1983), Abnormal patterns of normal eye movements in specific dyslexia. In: K. Rayner (Ed.), *Eye Movements in Reading: Perceptual and Language Processes*. New York, Academic Press.

Just, M. A., and Carpenter, P. A. (1980), A theory of reading: from eye fixations to comprehension. *Psychological Review* **87**, 329–354.

Kinsbourne, M., and Warrington, E. K. (1963), Developmental factors in reading and writing backwardness. *British Journal of Psychology* **54**, 145–156.

Lefton, L. A., Nagle, R. J., Johnson, G., and Fisher, D. F. (1979), Eye movement dynamics of good and poor readers: then and now. *Journal of Reading Behavior* **11**, 319–328.

Legge, G. E., Rubin, G. S., Pelli, D. G., and Schleske, M. M. (1985), Psychophysics of reading, II: Low vision. *Vision Research*, **25**, 253–266.

Lesevre, N. (1966), Les mouvements oculaires d'exploration. *ICAA Word Blind Bulletin* **4**, 15–24.

Lesevre, N. (1968), L'organisation du regard chez infants d'age scolaire, lecteurs, normaux et dyslexiques. *Revue de neuropsychiatrie infantile* **16**, 323–349.

Marcel, T., Katz, L., and Smith, M. (1974). Laterality and reading proficiency. *Neuropsychologia* **12**, 131–139.

Marcel, T., and Rajan, P. (1975), Lateral specialization of words and faces in good and poor readers. *Neuropsychologia* **13**, 489–497.

Mattis, S., French, J., and Rapin, E. (1975), Dyslexia in children and young adults: three independent neuropsychological syndromes. *Developmental Medicine and Child Neurology* **17**, 150–163.

McKeever, W., and Huling, M. D. (1970), Lateral dominance in tachistoscopic word recognition of children at two levels of ability. *Quarterly Journal of Experimental Psychology* **22**, 600–604.

McKeever, W. and VanDeventer, A. D. (1975), Dyslexic adolescents: evidence of impaired visual and auditory language processing associated with normal lateralization and visual responsivity. *Cortex* **11**, 361–378.

Olson, M. E. (1973), Laterality differences in tachistoscopic word recognition in normal and delayed readers in elementary school. *Neuropsychologia* **11**, 343–350.

Olson, R. K., Kliegl, R., and Davidson, B. J. (1983), Dyslexic and normal readers' eye movements. *Journal of Experimental Psychology: Human Perception and Performance* **9**, 816–825.

Olson, R. K., Kliegl, R., Davidson, B. J., and Foltz, G. (1984), Individual and developmental differences in reading. In: T. G. Waller (Ed.), *Reading Research: Advances in Theory and Practice*. New York, Academic Press.

Pavlidis, G. T. (1978), The dyslexic's erratic eye movements: case studies. *Dyslexia Review* **1**, 22–28.

Pavlidis, G. T. (1981a), Do eye movements hold the key to dyslexia? *Neuropsychologia* **19**, 57–64.

Pavlidis, G. T. (1981b), Sequencing, eye movements, and the early objective diagnosis of dyslexia. In: G. T. Pavlidis and T. R. Miles (Eds.) *Dyslexia Research and its Applications to Education*. Chichester, J. Wiley.

Pavlidis, G. T. (1983a), The 'dyslexia syndrome' and its objective diagnosis by erratic eye movements. In: K. Rayner (Ed.) *Eye Movements in Reading: Perceptual and Language Processes*. New York, Academic Press.

Pavlidis, G. T. (1983b), Erratic sequential eye movements in dyslexics: comments and reply to Stanley *et al. British Journal of Psychology* **74**, 189–193.

Pirozzolo, F. J. (1979), *The Neuropsychology of Developmental Reading Disorders.* New York, Praeger.

Pirozzolo, F. J. (1983), Eye movements and reading disability. In: K. Rayner (Ed.), *Eye Movements in Reading: Perceptual and Language Processes.* New York, Academic Press.

Pirozzolo, F. J., and Rayner, K. (1978), Disorders of oculomotor scanning and graphic orientation in developmental Gerstmann syndrome. *Brain and Language* 5, 119–126.

Pirozzolo, F. J., and Rayner, K. (1979), The neutral control of eye movements in acquired and developmental reading disorders. In: H. A. Whitaker and H. A. Whitaker (Eds.), *Studies in Neurolinguistics*, Vol. 4. New York, Academic Press.

Pirozzolo, F. J., Rayner, K., and Hynd, G. W. (1983), The measurement of hemispheric asymmetries in children with developmental reading disabilities. In: J. B. Hellige (Ed.)., *Cerebral Hemispheric Asymmetry: Method, Theory, and Application.* New York, Praegar.

Pollatsek, A. (1983), What can eye movements tell us about dyslexia? In: K. Rayner (Ed.), *Eye Movements in Reading: Perceptual and Language Processes.* New York, Academic Press.

Rayner, K. (1978), Eye movements in reading and information processing. *Psychological Bulletin* **85**, 618–660.

Rayner, K. (1983a), *Eye Movements in Reading: Perceptual and Language Process.* New York, Academic Press.

Rayner, K. (1983b), Eye movements, perceptual span, and reading disability. *Annals of Dyslexia* 33, 163–173.

Rayner, K., and Bertera, J. H. (1979), Reading without a fovea. *Science* **206**, 468–469.

Rayner, K., Slowiaczek, M. L., Clifton, C., and Bentera, J. H. (1983), Latency of sequential eye movements: implications for reading. *Journal of Experimental Psychology: Human Perception and Performance*, **9**, 912–922.

Rubino, C. A., and Minden, H. A. (1973), An analysis of eye-movements in children with a reading disability. *Cortex* **9**, 217–220.

Salthouse, T. A., and Ellis, C. L. (1980), Determinants of eye fixation duration. *American Journal of Psychology* **93**, 207–234.

Stanley, G., Smith, G. A., and Howell, E. A. (1983), Eye-movements and sequential tracking in dyslexic and control children. *British Journal of Psychology* **74**, 181–187.

Taylor, E. A. (1957), The spans: perception, apprehension, and recognition. *American Journal of Ophthalmology*, **44**, 501–507.

Tinker, M. A. (1946), The study of eye movements in reading. *Psychological Bulletin* **43**, 93–120.

Tinker, M. A. (1958), Recent studies of eye movements in reading. *Psychological Bulletin* **55**, 215–231.

Underwood, R., and Zola, D. (1986), The span of letter recognition of good and poor readers. *Reading Research Quarterly.*

Vellutino, F. R. (1979), *Dyslexia: Theory and Research.* Cambridge, Mass., MIT Press.

Yeni-Komshian, G., Isenberg, D., and Goldberg, H. (1975), Cerebral dominance and reading disability: left visual field deficit in poor readers. *Neuropsychologia* **13**, 83–94.

Zangwill, O. L., and Blakemore, C. (1972), Dyslexia: reversal of eye movements during reading. *Neuropsychologia* **10**, 371–373.

CHAPTER 10

The Role of Language Awareness in Reading Proficiency

CHE KAN LEONG
Department for the Education of Exceptional Children, University of Saskatchewan, Saskatoon, Saskatchewan S7N 0W0, Canada.

It is appropriate in the land of Hippocrates and Aristotle that we have come together from diverse disciplines — neurology, experimental and child psychology, psycholinguistics, and education — to discuss issues of dyslexia. For Hippocrates, diseases and higher cortical functions are constrained by natural laws. For Aristotle, the faculties of sensing, perceiving, cognizing, and memorizing follow some form of information-processing. So, going back two millennia, ancient Greek scholars were well aware of brain–behavior relationship, even though explanations could be sought in the temples of the gods!

The multi-faceted approach is needed in understanding dyslexia which, simply put, deals with difficulties in language — language heard, spoken, written, and internalized. For the purpose of this chapter, I will focus on reading difficulties and disabilities within the language continuum, particularly language awareness.

OVERVIEW OF LANGUAGE AWARENESS

The subject of language awareness has occupied much of the attention of linguists, psycholinguists, experimental and child psychologists, and educators. Noam Chomsky (1972, p. 115), for example, conceives of such awareness as referring to the language user having internalized a system of rules in relation to their phonetic and semantic representations. Compare this with Cazden's (1974, p. 29) explanation: 'Metalinguistic awareness, the ability to make language forms opaque and attend to them in and for themselves, is a special kind of language performance, one which makes special cognitive demands, and seems to be less easily and less universally acquired than the language performance of speaking and listening . . .'. It is clear from even these short references that Chomsky conceives of language awareness as abstract, idealized systems while Cazden, and many others, conceive of it in more pragmatic terms.

These two different but related aspects of language awareness from the psycholinguistic and cognitive aspects are best represented by the work of Mattingly (1972, 1984) and such major works as the Nijmegen Max-Planck psycholinguistic project on the child's conception of language (Sinclair, Jarvella, and Levelt, 1978). Mattingly draws attention to the relationship between the primary activities of speaking and listening and the secondary activities of reading and writing. He and his colleagues at the Haskins Laboratories have shown that speech cues and print materials carry different levels of linguistic information. The language cues for speaking–listening are largely phonetic; the writing–reading cues involve the more abstract phonological coding. Specifically, the speaker must produce a phonetic representation (perceived pronunciation) of a sentence with a semantic representation. The listener must synthesize a sentence which matches a particular phonetic representation and recovers the semantic representation. The reader must know the rules of the phonological, graphological, syntactic, and semantic cues to produce, construct, and reconstruct what is contained on the printed page. Mattingly suggested that reading be regarded as 'a deliberately acquired, language-based skill, dependent upon the speaker–hearer's awareness of certain aspects of primary linguistic activity. By virtue of this linguistic awareness, written text initiates the synthetic linguistic processes common to both reading and speech, enabling the reader to get the writer's message and so to recognize what has been written' (Mattingly, 1972, p. 145).

In his 1984 paper Mattingly refined and elaborated on his earlier concepts of linguistic awareness. He now suggests that linguistic awareness is a matter of access to 'knowledge of the grammatical structure of sentences' (p. 9). Further, reading is just as natural an activity as listening and speaking, albeit more 'linguistic' than these two primary activities. Basing his linguistic and psycholinguistic assumptions largely on Noam Chomsky's transformational generative grammar, Mattingly suggests that the speaker–hearer's grammatical knowledge is also tacit knowledge but is accessible in the same way that the speaker–hearer has intuition about grammaticality. Following Chomsky's competence and performance distinction, Mattingly stresses that grammatical knowledge is intuitive knowledge and hence accessible while strategies to use such knowledge (strategies such as speech perception, parsing mechanisms) are inaccessible empirically, if not linguistically.

To answer the question of how the intuitive grammatical knowledge or listening and speaking are related to reading acquisition, Mattingly discusses the role of the 'practical orthography'. Such an orthography is not phonetic but is based on semantic representation of sentences, and that lexical items are transcribed morphemically as a morpheme carries both semantic and phonological values. It therefore follows that the language-learner/reader has to exploit the morphophonemic representations in practical orthographies which presuppose the learner's/reader's access to such representations. There is both theoretical and empirical evidence to support the claim that an alphabetic writing system such as English can be coded, or represented in memory, both phonologically and semantically just as a morphemic writing system such as Chinese can be accessed through phonological coding. Downing and Leong (1982, Chapters 9 and 10) have critically reviewed theoretical and empirical works on phonological coding and visual coding of accessing English words and have drawn attention to the parallel-coding, multiple-paths approach. The reader has the option of sometimes using the one route, sometimes the other, depending on his/her skill as a reader, task demand, and purposes of reading.

The Mattingly view of language awareness may be compared with the more cognitive-developmental approach of explaining language as a skill, as a conscious repairing. Thus language awareness is explained by the Nijmegen project group (Sinclair, Jarvella, and Levelt, 1978) as 'meta-cognition', 'reflective abilities', 'general development of consciousness and self-consciousness', and 'objects of reflection' over and above language as a formal system. One participant, Read (1978), a linguist, brings language awareness directly into the realm of reading:

> The performances of adapting, manipulating, segmenting, correcting, and judging language seem to play an important role in at least three processes: learning to read and write, learning a non-native language, and responding to social expectations. In short, they have a great deal to do with using language effectively under varied circumstances. Whether they are conscious or can easily be brought to consciousness appears to be of secondary importance. (Read, 1978, p. 66).

From the cognitive-developmental perspective, 'becoming aware' is interpreted as 'becoming aware' of the *how*, and eventually the *why* of certain actions and their interactions. Becoming aware should also refer to the process of monitoring, control, and repair. Clark (1978, p. 34) summarized different types of metalinguistic awareness. They include: (a) monitoring one's ongoing utterances, (b) checking the result of an utterance, (c) testing for reality, (d) deliberately trying to learn, (e) predicting the consequences of using inflections, words, phrases, or sentences and (f) reflecting on the product of an utterance. As an example, monitoring of language refers to practising sounds, adjusting speech to different groups, ages, and status; and 'checking the result of an utterance' includes such activities as commenting on others' utterances and correcting the utterances of others. Under (f) 'reflecting on the product of an utterance' we will include disambiguation of ambiguous sentences, understanding of jokes, riddles and humours, and explaining anomalous sentences. An example of such reflection is the joke: ' "Why can't you starve in the desert?" "Because of the sand which is [sandwiches] there" '. There is a developmental trend in the various kinds of metalinguistic awareness discussed by Clark with the last two-named 'predicting' and 'reflecting' being the later emerging.

The view of language awareness as relating to the monitoring, control, and repair of, and generally reflection on, language may seem far removed from the rule-governed, logical, and mentalistic position of Chomsky. Yet the apparent distinction between the internalized mentalistic concept of language as structure of the mind and the communicative competence of language use is not as rigid as is usually claimed. Chomsky agrees, at least in part, that understanding of syntax also entails understanding the communicative use of language. He does state, however, that the contribution of 'pragmatic considerations' to language is not at all clear for the simple reason that the wider realm of 'semantic representation', is not as yet well understood. His assertion that he can use language in the strictest sense with no intention of communication, except communication with himself, is best interpreted as inner speech or internalized thought with rules corresponding to grammatical categories. It is likely that Chomsky's communication with himself represents a form of decentration in the Piagetian sense with full recognition not only of contexts but of intentions. Thus, it is the formal linguistic system that determines mental operations and such operations are triggered off and elaborated on through social interactions. Seen in this way, it is possible to reconcile the essentially Chomskyan viewpoint as propounded by Mattingly and the pragmatic approach of the Nijmegen group.

LANGUAGE AWARENESS AND READING—SOME EVIDENCE

Integrating and extending the theoretical and experimental works discussed in the foregoing and also studies on language awareness in different countries (Canada, England, New Zealand, Spain, Sweden, USA, Switzerland, USSR), Downing and Leong (1982) suggest that there are two main strands in relating language awareness to reading. These strands are: the need to understand the purposes of reading and the importance of understanding the internal structure (e.g. meaning of a phoneme, a word, a sentence) of language. Both concepts have generated testable hypotheses and have been found to underpin learning to read.

Language Segmentation

Working within the above framework and especially drawing on the research programmes of Liberman and her associates (Liberman *et al.*, 1977), I have attempted to provide some empirical evidence on the way in which language awareness affects reading acquisition. In several experiments, Leong and Haines (1978) studied beginning readers' analysis of words and sentences. We examined the performance of grades 1, 2, and 3 children in segmenting syllables into phonemes, words into syllables, concepts of the number and order of sounds within a spoken pattern and the children's ability to repeat sentences of different complexities (e.g. 'A little girl by the pond was watching some ducks' contrasted with 'The not very well painted toys want painting during holidays'). The overall poorer performance of the children in phoneme segmentation was accentuated with the addition of a test tapping auditory conceptualization of both the number and order of speech patterns. Further, children across the grades found high complexity sentences more difficult to repeat accurately than low complexity sentences with almost parallel relative facility grade for grade. These results can be interpreted in relation to the philosopher Polanyi's (1964) discussion of maxims, or rules of art: 'Maxims cannot be understood, still less applied by anyone not already possessing a good practical knowledge of the art . . . there exists rules which are useful only within the operation of our personal knowledge' (p. 31). He distinguishes between two kinds of skilled performance: subsidiary and focal. For many children, their awareness of words and sentences is at the subsidiary level. Their acquisition of verbal skills is facilitated if their understanding is brought to the focal level. The reflection on and manipulation of words and sentences, which can be taught in the form of word games and play activities, will go some way towards helping the child in the learning to read process.

Cognitive Processing and Language Awareness

In another study, Leong and Sheh (1982) used multivariate techniques to tease out the relationship between cognitive processing, language awareness and reading (word recognition) in grades 2 and 4 children. Very briefly, cognitive processing is predicated on the Russian neuropsychologist Luria's (1973) simultaneous and successive modes of information processing while language awareness to the understanding of implicit phonological rules (e.g. flexibility and interchangeability of phonemes to make new words), appreciation of ambiguities (lexical, surface, and deep structures), of riddles and jokes and judgment of well-formed and ill-formed sentences. In Luria's terms, simultaneous synthesis (primarily spatial, groups) and successive synthesis (primarily temporally organized series) are the two main forms of integrative activity and these syntheses operate at the perceptual, memory, and conceptual levels. In my ongoing factor analytic work (Leong, 1976, 1976–1977, 1980) these two modes of information processing have consistently distinguished between dyslexics and their controls and skilled and less skilled readers. In the Leong and Sheh study we obtained factor scores from the simultaneous and successive components for the unselected grade 2 and grade 4 children. On the basis of these factor scores, scores in the different language awareness tasks and a word recognition test, analyses proceeded in two directions. In one, we hypothesized that those children who were high on both the simultaneous and successive dimensions would also perform better on language awareness tasks and on reading and that there would be a main effect for grade. This hypothesis was upheld. The second direction is a more fundamental one. By using path analysis we hoped to make more explicit the theoretical framework. In other words, by analyzing the different components of cognitive processing, language awareness and reading we can at least determine the direct and indirect effects on reading. In a larger study involving 120 children (Leong, 1984) path analysis results showed much greater direct effect from language awareness on reading than antecedent cognitive processing. Thus, knowing *about* language as well as knowing language is central to reading acquisition.

Appreciation of Ambiguities and Reading

Unselected Readers

To explore further the role of language awareness, or more specifically the comprehension of ambiguities, in reading, a study involving grades 3, 4, 5 and 6 children was conducted by Leong (1982b). The sample consisted of 24 children in each of these grades with a total of 96 children. The broad question was how well would grade 3 to grade 6 children comprehend verbal ambiguities and whether or not 'skilled readers' and 'less skilled readers' could be differentiated with ambiguity tasks. The main instrument used was an 18-item ambiguity task designed and pretested by the author. There are three components with six items each: one component assesses the comprehension of *lexical ambiguity* (e.g. 'The investor's money earned interest'. 'Why did the farmer name his hog ink? Because he kept running out of the pen.'); the next component taps *surface structure ambiguity* (e.g. 'The foreman (boss) fired the worker with little care') and the third assesses *deep structure ambiguity* (e.g. 'The duck is ready to eat'). The approach used was quasi-experimental and quasi-interviewing. Each child was seen in his/her school by the author or the research assistant. Each child was presented verbally twice with a panel of ambiguous sentence or sentences and was also shown simultaneously the printed version of the panel with the sentence(s) lettered in Helvetica 20 point lettering on a 21 × 14 cm card. This simultaneous presentation of the stimuli in both the spoken and the written forms should not penalize the 'less skilled' readers. With surface structure ambiguities, special care was taken to balance juncture and intonation patterns (e.g. 'They fed her/dog biscuits' counterbalanced with 'They fed her dog/biscuits'). Through a series of interlocking probes the child was asked for the meaning or meanings of each panel.

   This approach was an adaptation of the 'clinical method' of Piaget. In his [translated] words:

The clinical examination is . . . experimental in the sense that the practitioner sets himself a problem, makes hypotheses, adapts the conditions to them and finally controls each hypothesis by testing it against reactions he stimulates in conversation. But the clinical examination is also dependent on direct observation, in the sense that a good practitioner lets himself be led, though always in control, and takes account of the whole of the mental context. (Piaget, 1963, p. 8)

Following this dictum there are several main criteria used in assessing the clinical interview. The child must: (a) make a 'correct' or best judgment to show the appreciation of ambiguities, (b) clearly and logically explain that judgment (the meanings of the ambiguities) and (c) successfully resist a verbal counter-suggestion, if needed for clarification. This quasi-experimental and quasi-interviewing approach gets around the all or none kind of answer, avoids predetermined adult standards of correctness and enables the child to provide his/her answers. Thus, there is a much richer source of information on how the child reasons and comes to grips with a set of hypotheses.

In the present study with the 96 children in grades 3, 4, 5 and 6 they were first administered The Word Reading Test of the British Ability Scales (BAS) (Elliott, Murray, and Pearson, 1978) to determine their reading level. The British Ability Scales were used because of the painstaking research underpinning the standardization of the Scales and because of the Piagetian approach and the robustness of the Rasch model in item calibration. All the tests or subtests provide different scores (ability scores, T scores, and percentiles) and make adjustments for differential chronological ages of the subjects. On the basis of the BAS Word Reading the 24 children in each grade were dichotomized into 'skilled' and 'less skilled' readers at or near the sixtieth percentile. This dichotomy provided subgroups of 12 skilled readers and 12 less skilled readers for each grade. The Sentential Ambiguity task was administered to each child in the way described in the preceding paragraphs and scored according to the criteria outlined. A 2 (reading) $\times$ 4 (grades) ANOVA showed significant main effects for skilled/less skilled readers ($F(1, 88) = 38.77$, $p < 0.001$) and for grades ($F(3, 88) = 34.36$, $p < 0.001$). There was no reading by grade interaction effect. Newman–Keuls multiple comparisons further showed that all pairwise comparisons (with the exception of the grade 5 and grade 6 comparison) were significantly different at the 0.01 level. The results show that the skilled and less skilled readers are clearly differentiated, that they follow a similar pattern and that there is a monotonic increase in the performance in ambiguity tasks from grade 3 to at least the grade 5 level. That grade 5 and grade 6 are not differentiated could be attributed to the need for a more discriminating task at these levels; although there is no evidence for the ubiquitous 'ceiling' and 'floor' effects for a task spanning four grades with mean ages ranging from 106.67 months (for the 24 children in grade 3) to 143.67 months (for the 24 children in grade 6).

While the statistical findings are of interest, it is equally revealing, if not more so, in examining the verbatim records of the children's responses. It is clear that not a few children do not understand the subtleties of such constructions as 'They are (flying planes)', '(They are flying) planes'. Many children spoke of people piloting, 'driving' (sic) planes and almost none of flying as contrasted with stationary planes. This and similar response patterns are analogous to the findings of the Leong and Sheh (1982) study. There, it was found that children reason from 'human sense', as Donaldson (1978) so aptly put it. As an example, when children were asked in the Leong and Sheh study, 'Is it OK to say Joe [the child's name] loves Joe?', many grade 4 children simply laughed and insisted that the sentence was not OK because 'You must say "Dad loves mom"'. The intent of this item, which formed part of a large item pool tapping the appreciation of incongruities, was to assess understanding of the *reflexive form*. The sentence is admissible if and only if Joe$_1$ is not the same as Joe$_2$; otherwise the reflexive 'himself' must be used. To be able to resolve this item and to resolve incongruities, the child must go 'beyond the bounds of human sense' (Donaldson, 1978, p. 82). Donaldson goes on to emphasize: 'In order to handle the world with maximum competence it is necessary to consider the *structure* of things. It is necessary to become skilled in manipulating *systems* and in abstracting forms and patterns' (Donaldson, 1978, p. 82). This is another way of stating that learners must systematize their knowledge to unify different facts into a higher-order structure; they must generate hypotheses and test these and they must make knowledge more explicit and hence more accessible. This is also the essence of the statement in the earlier section that reading is part of knowing and that teaching reading is teaching or helping learning through reading.

While the study with the 96 children has shown the contribution of understanding of ambiguities to reading in skilled and less skilled readers, there are many more questions that need to be answered. For example, what are the other areas of ambiguities and incongruities that form the larger aspect of language awareness? How well does the appreciation or comprehension of ambiguities contribute to reading? What are the mutually facilitating effects of disambiguation of ambiguities on reading and the other way round? These and other aspects will need to be examined.

Poor Readers

To further examine some of the above questions, Leong (1982b), Leong and Carrier (in press) conducted three experiments with carefully selected samples of 'poor' readers (a 'younger' sample consisting of 15 grade 5 poor readers nominated by their teachers and an 'older' sample consisting of 15 grade 6 poor readers similarly nominated). Each of these experimental groups was compared with two control groups: a Chronological Age (CA) Control group of 15 children from the same rooms as the poor readers but reading at an 'average' or 'above average' level; a Reading Age (RA) Control group of another 15 children from grades 3 and 4 respectively, who were regarded as reading at about the same level as that of the younger sample or older sample poor readers respectively. There was thus a group of 45 readers in the younger sample with three subgroups: Experimental, CA Control, and RA Control with 15 children each and another 45 readers in the older sample similarly constituted with three subgroups. A total of 90 children was studied in depth in quasi-experimental and quasi-interviewing situations.

The use of two control groups is not often found in the learning or reading disabilities literature. The rationale for this design with two control groups is as follows. If disabled readers differ from their CA controls but not from their RA controls, then an impairment is shown but such an impairment is no greater than would be predicted on the hypothesis that the child has not developed much of the language awareness experience which would normally be acquired by readers of that age. It is only when disabled readers perform less well than both their CA controls and their RA controls can we conclude that the tasks under investigation do make a difference in reading.

The aim of the three experiments was to study the effect of three different kinds of ambiguity materials on reading. These materials were: *ambiguity in pictorial materials* as typically found in cartoons; *sentential ambiguity* with lexical, surface, and deep structure ambiguities (this being a refinement of the task used in the 1982b Leong study with 96 children as discussed earlier); and *ambiguity in paragraphs or short stories*. As with previous studies, each of the 90 children in the several schools was interviewed individually and asked to explain the ambiguities. Again, scoring took into account the differential qualities of the responses in disambiguating the ambiguities and detecting the incongruities.

The results of the three experiments can be summarized as follows. First, The Word Reading Test of the British Ability Scales established within limits of probability the equivalency of the reading performance of the Experimental and Reading Age Control groups for each of the younger and older samples and that teachers were generally quite accurate in identifying their 'poor' readers, 'average', and 'good' readers. Next, to guard against the possible effect of differential general ability on reading and language awareness, the short form of the British Ability Scales consisting of speed of Information Processing, Matrices, Similarities, and Recall of Digits was administered. It was indeed found that the RA Control group for each of the younger and older samples was significantly higher in general ability than their corresponding Experimental and CA Control groups. It was likely that for children in grades 3 and 4 to be reading about one grade above their respective levels they would also be more 'intelligent'. It should be noted here that no assumption is made as to 'cause' and 'effect'. While 'intelligence' affects reading, it is also possible that reading 'causes' general ability. In any case, the differential general ability between the RA Control and the other two groups for each sample could be accommodated statistically. This adjustment was made with the analyses of covariance (ANCOVA) with 'IQ' from the British Ability Scales as the covariate in the various analyses.

The disambiguation of ambiguities in cartoons and in sentences and the recall of short stories with incongruous elements (sentences) was analyzed in a series of two (sample) × three (reading groups) analyses of variance (ANOVA) followed by ANCOVA to make adjustments for possible effects of differential general ability. The results are:

(a) For *pictorial ambiguity* through the use of cartoons there was a significant main effect for the Experimental, CA Control, and RA Control groups ($F(2, 84) = 8.670$, $p < 0.001$) while there was no difference between the younger and older samples, nor was there any interaction effect. Newman–Keuls multiple comparisons showed that the poor readers performed significantly worse than their CA controls but were comparable to their RA controls. This finding was also verified in the two-way ANCOVA with general ability as the covariate. There is thus evidence, though it is not very strong, that poor readers lag behind in detecting, appreciating, and explaining ambiguities embedded in cartoons and the accompanying short captions.

(b) For *sentential ambiguity* the Experimental group in each of the younger and older samples generally performed much more poorly than the controls in each of the three types of verbal ambiguities: lexical, surface, and deep structures. In *lexical ambiguity* there were significant main effects for samples ($F(1, 84) = 4.609$, $p < 0.05$) and for reading groups ($F(2, 84) = 9.845$, $p < 0.001$). There was no interaction effect. Newman–Keuls multiple comparisons showed that the poor readers performed significantly worse than their CA controls but were comparable to their RA controls. The findings of the ANOVA were verified in the two-way ANCOVA with general ability as the covariate.

In *surface structure ambiguity* there were significant main effects for the younger and older samples ($F(1, 84) = 7.485$, $p < 0.01$) and for reading groups ($F(2, 84) = 6.886$, $p < 0.01$). There was no sample × reading group interaction. These findings were supported in a two-way ANCOVA with general ability as the covariate. Newman–Keuls multiple comparisons showed that the poor readers performed significantly less well than their CA controls but not their RA controls.

In *deep structure ambiguity* there were significant main effects for the younger and older samples ($F(1, 84) = 4.639$, $p < 0.05$) and for reading groups ($F(2, 84) = 12.459$, $p < 0.001$). There was no sample × reading group interaction. The results were verified in a two-way ANCOVA when adjustment was made for initial differences in general ability. Newman–Keuls multiple comparisons showed that the poor readers performed significantly worse than *both* their CA controls and RA controls. Thus it would appear that of the three main kinds of sentential ambiguities: lexical, surface structure, and deep structure, it was deep structure

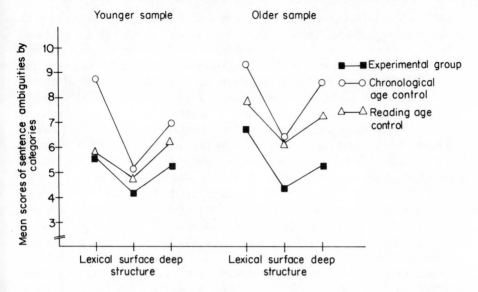

Figure 1. Poor readers' comprehension of lexical, surface structure, and deep structure ambiguities.

ambiguity that led to much more difficulties in readers. This aspect will be elaborated on in subsequent sections.

The comparative performance in lexical, surface structure and deep structure ambiguities by the Experimental group and the two control groups in the younger and older samples is illustrated in Figure 1.

(c) For the *recall of ideas* in short stories with incongruous elements the main effect for reading groups was significant ($F(2, 84) = 6.255$, $p < 0.01$) while the effect for sample was not significant. There was also no reading group × sample interaction. The time it took the children to read the passages and to detect the incongruous elements (sentences) was also examined, but the results were not significant. This was likely due to the more involved nature of the stories or paragraphs in order to avoid the 'ceiling' effect for the older children and the 'floor' effect for the younger ones and also to the confounding of the time needed to read the passages alone and to detect the ambiguous or incongruous sentences. As it was, the recall of main ideas provided a reasonable estimate of one aspect of awareness of the subtleties of language.

Taken together, the Leong and Haines (1978) study, the Leong and Sheh (1982), Leong (1984) projects, the 1982b Leong study, and the Leong and Carrier (in press) investigation all point to the role of language awareness tasks in reading and provide empirical evidence to support this claim. These results with unselected readers in grades 1, 2, and 3 (Leong and Haines, 1978), in grades 2 and 4 (Leong and Sheh,

1982; Leong, 1984), in grades 3, 4, 5, and 6 (Leong, 1982b), and with poor readers in grades 5 and 6 (Leong and Carrier, in press) have highlighted the contribution to reading of knowledge of 'language registers' (ability to segment words into syllables and syllables into phonemes) and the understanding of ambiguities and incongruities. A question about possible cause and effect may well be asked. While the studies cited were not addressed to the question of whether or not language awareness 'causes' reading or vice versa, there is nevertheless tangible evidence that language awareness tasks have a potent, direct effect on reading. Part of this evidence is derived from the use of stepwise multiple regression analysis and path analysis to analyze cognitive processing and language awareness in relation to reading. In the study with 120 children cognitive processing affects reading through its relationship with language awareness as shown by the indirect path coefficients in the region of 0.30 while language awareness has a much greater direct effect as shown by the path coefficient of 0.74 (Leong, 1984). In an elegant study using path analysis Lundberg, Olofsson, and Wall (1980) demonstrated that metalinguistic tasks including segmentation and synthesis of words given to preschoolers, predicted with a high degree of accuracy reading and spelling achievement of these children in first and second grades. Lundberg (1982) further suggested that the development of metalinguistic skills over early schools presents an approach to studying dyslexia, especially that subgroup of dyslexics with verbal deficits. Collaborative evidence of the role of phonological awareness in reading comes from Bradley (1980) and Bradley and Bryant (1983) who have shown that backward readers are markedly insensitive to rhymes and alliterations. In a recent study involving 164 ten-year-old children Leong, Cheng, Lundberg, Olofsson and Mulcahy (1985) have found from maximum likelihood analyses that language awareness as latent domain subserved by ambiguities and anomalies as manifest variables has considerable direct effect on reading proficiency.

PRACTICAL IMPLICATIONS FOR READING AND READING DIFFICULTIES

Reading as a Skill

In their book on the psychology of reading Downing and Leong (1982) emphasize reading as a skill — an organized, coordinated chain of complex intentional actions. As a highly complex pattern behavior, reading as a skill includes these main characteristics: (1) smooth performance, (2) integration of subskills, (3) timing, proper pacing and flexibility, (4) anticipation of future events, (5) automaticity beyond mere accuracy so as to free readers' attention for other subskills, (6) consciousness of the reading activities and their functions, (7) ability to react to both internal and external cues such as feedbacks and to modify these cues, (8) utilization of increasingly larger perceptual units as reading skill develops. For each of these main characteristics there is considerable support from the psychological literature to point to the application in reading.

In general, there are at least three phases of skill development: the *cognitive, mastering,* and *automaticity* phases (see Downing and Leong, 1982, Chapters 2 and 3). During the initial cognitive phase learners must find out what to do in unfamiliar situations. They must master both the purposes and the processes of their activities. Consider beginning readers or those children with reading difficulties. Quite often, the purposes (there are many purposes for reading) of reading are not made clear to them. Nor are the coding processes. By the latter is meant the way spoken and written language is used to communicate meaning. Very early on, children read about such terms as 'sentences', 'words', 'syllables', 'consonants', 'vowels' when these concepts mean very little to them. I am reminded of the anecdote in Donaldson (1978) when a preschooler Laurie came home the first day from school very disappointed. She was told by the teacher '. . . to sit there for the *present*, and sit there she did without getting a present (gift)!

What Donaldson in her powerful book *Children's Minds* emphasizes, just as Downing and Leong do in their treatise, is that given a proper setting with a language that makes 'human sense' even young children can perform tasks often thought to be beyond them. To do this, schools need to encourage children to develop their reflective skills in the early years, to guide children to come to grips with a set of options when unknowns are encountered. Above all, teachers need to stand back to see issues from the children's viewpoints and to be able to decenter in guiding their language growth and development.

Knowing Words and Sounds—Phonemic Awareness

There is evidence (for example, Leong and Haines, 1978) that children's reflection on the components of words (syllables and phonemes), on the grammatical structures of sentences, facilitates the reading process. For beginning readers and readers with difficulties they need instruction to codify their spoken language and to understand the spatial–temporal correspondence of symbols and sounds and the internal representation. Some readers acquire this knowledge fairly easily and in a relatively short time; while others need a great deal of teaching to go from the cognitive phase to the mastering phase to attain automaticity.

There are teaching programs which help train phonemic awareness subskills. These programs include: Lindamood and Lindamood (1969), Rosner (1975), Wallach and Wallach (1976), and Williams (1979, 1980), among others. A useful review of phonemic awareness training with suggestions on the 'what' and 'how' to teach these tasks is provided by Lewkowicz (1980). In general, these teaching programs owe much of their theoretical underpinning to the work of Elkonin (1963, 1973) on teaching beginning reading to Russian children. Elkonin emphasizes the creation and re-creation of the sound form of the word from its graphic representation, and spells out ways of representing concretely 'sound structure of spoken words'. He is careful in emphasizing that the aim is 'not the symbolizing of separate sounds, but their separation and modeling as a succession' (Elkonin, 1973, p. 563). Moreover, this aim is to show not only the basic sound units of language but also how language is constructed from the orthographic and phonologic components. Similar line of reasoning can be found in the writing of Samuel Orton (1937). From his clinical experience with developmental dyslexics, Orton suggested: 'It is this process of synthesizing the word as a spoken unit from its component sounds that often makes much more difficulty for the strephosymbolic child than do the static reversals and letter confusions' (Orton, 1937, p. 162). Orton advocated the training for the simultaneous association of visual, auditory, and kinesthetic language stimuli and the multi-sensory approach to remediating dyslexics is exemplified in the Orton-Gillingham approach (see Gillingham and Stillman, 1960).

The phonemic awareness tasks outlined in the different teaching programs parallel detailed studies of children's speech plays in the child language literature. Weir (1962), for example, recorded 'language in the crib'. The Opies (Opie and Opie, 1959) have provided many examples of nursery rhymes and 'topsy-turvies' that children invent and use. The Russian writer Kornei Chukovsky (1963) has documented children's delight in sounds with 'topsy-turvey meanings'. He points out that while many children's rhymes are the results of games, 'topsy turvies [pereviortyshi] are a game in themselves' (p. 98). It is not so much the 'gameful' aspect that the child seeks but the opaqueness of the topsy-turvey in sounds and words when the real juxtaposition is transparent to him or her. This mental play is an indication of the child exercising his/her newly acquired language skill and of varying this knowledge. What characterizes children's speech plays as following certain morphophonemic patterns such as the use of alliterations, rhymes, and Pig Latin takes on a slightly different course with older individuals. These older children delight in the kind of language play with fairly intact phonological and syntactic rules but rather meaningless items or pseudo-lexemes (the kind of 'frumious Bandersnatch' Jabberwocky of Lewis Carroll).

Knowing about Rules of Grammar

The early study of Gleitman, Gleitman, and Shipley (1972) alerted us to children's sensitivity to syntactic and semantic rules in the grammar of the language. There is evidence that children progress from lexical to surface and deep structures in their understanding of verbal ambiguities and that detection of surface and deep structure ambiguities appears rather late in development (Kessel, 1970; Shultz and Pilon, 1973). Indeed, Carol Chomsky (1969) shows that active syntactic acquisition takes place to the age of ten and beyond and that the order and rate of acquisition vary widely amongst individuals.

It was after these and other works that the Leong and Sheh (1982) and Leong and Carrier (in press) studies were patterned. Our statistical findings generally uphold the claim of the progression in comprehension from surface to deep structure ambiguities, at least with children. Our qualitative analyses of the protocols from the readers of varying proficiency highlight the need to understand *speech acts*. This refers to treating language not so much as a rule-bound formalized system, but more in relation to the speaker, the listener and context. This pragmatic approach to discourse comprehension is predicated on certain conversational postulates including the speaker's intention in uttering a particular sentence, the 'world knowledge' that both speaker and listener bring to bear on the speech act and the total situation. There are, of course, differences between speech acts and reading. These differences pertain to the nature of the oral/aural and written channels, the physical separation in space and time between the reader and the writer as contrasted with the speaker/listener dyad and certain pragmatic rule differences between oral and written discourse. Still, the shared linguistic context in reading and 'auding' is both referential and metalingual. It is referential in that the context tells the reader/listener something. It is metalingual in that the language code and its internal representation must be made explicit.

Directly in the realm of reading, Pearson and Johnson (1978) in their very informative work on reading comprehension discuss nine proposition-level comprehension tasks. These tasks are: (1) paraphrase, (2) association, (3) main ideas or details, (4) comparison, (5) figurative language, (6) ambiguous statements, (7) causal relations, (8) sequence, and (9) anaphoras or pronominalization. In addition to these nine main tasks, Pearson and Johnson further suggest that readers should separate fact from fiction, evaluate bias, analyze the author's craft, use imageries while reading, distinguish reality from fantasy, and know the literacy form of writing (e.g. setting, theme, plot, characterization, and resolution). Inherent in all the above tasks is the need to make inferences which underpin much of comprehending. We may note the role of figurative language (e.g. metaphors) and ambiguities in the propositional levels of the Pearson and Johnson schema. We should also note that in the field of reading disabilities reading comprehension has been sorely neglected. In a review of research and theories in learning disabilities Leong (1982a) emphasizes the role of language awareness and training of learning strategies. He states:

> Learning to learn over and above learning content areas must be integrative (bringing together inter-related concepts), inferential (going beyond the information given), and performance-oriented (applicable to different situations). The many facets of training in prose learning include training in the use of mental imagery, self-questioning and monitoring, reorganization of incoming materials, elaboration training to link new with old knowledge; building of networks of important concepts (nodes) and learning their interrelationships. Training strategies must be specified in detail and should not simply rely on the inductive power of learning disabled or reading disabled children as they are less inner-directed. The training

pace must be specified and moderated. Feedback to and motivation of the learners are important considerations. As well, long-term effects of strategy learning must be assessed. (p. 12)

The above view is reiterated at some length as it represents the way the present author views as important in developing reading proficiency. To help poor readers and dyslexics, language including reading must be treated as a flexible and not so much a rigid, formalized system; and learning to learn is important. These children in turn must be encouraged to adapt, correct, judge, reflect on incongruities, almost savoring them.

SUMMARY

In this chapter, the role of language awareness in reading proficiency is sketched and several studies pertaining to language segmentation, the appreciation of ambiguities, in unselected readers and poor readers are discussed. Empirical findings show that the understanding of ambiguities, of incongruities as presented in pictorial and verbal materials, does have a direct effect on reading. Development of language awareness at the lexical, phonological, and syntactic/semantic levels helps children to read effectively and efficiently.

ACKNOWLEDGEMENTS

Studies reported in this chapter were supported in part by the University of Saskatchewan President's Humanities and Social Sciences Research Fund and grants from the Saskatchewan School Trustees Association and the Orton Dyslexia Society.

I gratefully acknowledge interactions at various times with Lynette Bradley of Oxford University, Isabelle Liberman of the University of Connecticut and the Haskins Laboratories, and Ingvar Lundberg of the University of Umeå. Any shortcomings are necessarily my own.

REFERENCES

Bradley, L. (1980), *Assessing Reading Difficulties: A Diagnostic and Remedial Approach.* London, Macmillan.
Bradley, L., and Bryant, P. E. (1983), Categorizing sounds and learning to read—a causal connection. *Nature* **301** (5899), 419–420.
Cazden, C. (1974), Metalinguistic awareness: one dimension of language experience. *The Urban Review* **7**, 28–39.
Chomsky, C. (1969), *The Acquisition of Syntax in Children from Five to Ten.* Cambridge, MA, MIT Press.
Chomsky, N. (1972), *Language and Mind*, enlarged edition. New York, Harcourt, Brace & World.
Chukovsky, K. (1963), *From Two to Five.* Berkeley, University of California Press.

Clark, E. V. (1978), Awareness of language: some evidence from what children say and do. In: A. Sinclair, R. J. Jarvella, and W. J. M. Levelt (Eds.), *The Child's Conception of Language*. New York, Springer-Verlag, pp. 17–43.
Donaldson, M. (1978), *Children's Minds*. Glasgow, Fontana/Collins.
Downing, J., and Leong, C. K. (1982), *Psychology of Reading*. New York, Macmillan.
Elkonin, D. B. (1963), The psychology of mastering the elements of reading. In: B. Simon and J. Simon (Eds.), *Educational Psychology in the U.S.S.R.* London, Routledge & Kegan Paul, pp. 165–179.
Elkonin, D. B. (1973), U.S.S.R. In: J. Downing (Ed.), *Comparative Reading*. New York, Macmillan, pp. 551–579.
Elliott, C. D., Murray, D. J., and Pearson, L. S. (1978), *British Ability Scales: Manual 3: Directions for Administration and Scoring* and *Manual 4: Tables of Abilities and Norms*. Windsor, Berks, NFER.
Gillingham, A., and Stillman, B. W. (1960), *Remedial Training for Children with Specific Disability in Reading, Spelling and Penmanship* (6th edn). Cambridge, MA, Educators Publishing Service.
Gleitman, L. R., Gleitman, H., and Shipley, E. F. (1972), The emergence of the child as grammarian. *Cognition* 1, 137–164.
Kessel, F. S. (1970), The role of syntax in children's comprehension from age six to twelve. *Monographs of the Society for Research in Child Development* 35 (6, Serial no. 139).
Leong, C. K. (1976), Lateralization in severly disabled readers in relation to functional cerebral development and synthesis of information. In: R. M. Knights and D. J. Bakker (Eds.), *The Neuropsychology of Learning Disorders: Theoretical Approaches.* Baltimore, University Park Press, pp. 221–231.
Leong, C. K. (1976–1977), Spatial–temporal information-processing in children with specific reading disability. *Reading Research Quarterly* 12, 204–215.
Leong, C. K. (1980), Cognitive patterns of 'retarded' and below-average readers. *Contemporary Educational Psychology* 5, 101–117.
Leong, C. K. (1982a), Promising areas of research into learning disabilities with emphasis on reading disabilities. In: J. P. Das, R. Mulcahy, and A. E. Wall (Eds.), *Theory and Research in Learning Disability*. New York, Plenum, pp. 3–26.
Leong, C. K. (1982b), *Language Awareness in Readers*. (Research Rep.) Saskatchewan, Canada, Saskatchewan School Trustees Association.
Leong, C. K. (1984), Cognitive processing, language awareness and reading in grade 2 and grade 4 children. *Contemporary Education Psychology*. 9, 369–383.
Leong, C. K., and Carrier, C. (in press), Readers' comprehension of ambiguous sentences. *Scientia Paedagogica Experimentalis*.
Leong, C. K., Cheng, S. C., Lundberg, I. Olofsson, A., and Mulcahy, R. (1985). *The Effects of Cognitive Processing, Language Access on Academic Performance — Linear Structural Equation Modelling*. Manuscript submitted for publication.
Leong, C. K., and Haines, C. F. (1978), Beginning readers' analysis of words and sentences. *Journal of Reading Behavior* 10, 393–407.
Leong, C. K., and Sheh, S. (1982), Knowing about language — some evidence from readers. *Annals of Dyslexia* 32, 149–161.
Lewkowicz, N. K. (1980), Phonemic awareness training: what to teach and how to teach it. *Journal of Educational Psychology* 72, 686–700.
Liberman, I., Shankweiler, D., Liberman, A. M., Fowler, C., and Fischer, F. W. (1977), Phonetic segmentation and recoding in the beginning reader. In: A. S. Reber and D. L. Scarborough (Eds.), *Toward a Psychology of Reading*. NJ, Erlbaum, pp. 207–225.
Lindamood, C. H., and Lindamood, P. C. (1969), *Auditory Discrimination in Depth*. Boston, MA, Teaching Resources.

Lundberg, I. (1982), Linguistic awareness as related to dyslexia. In: Y. Zotterman (Ed.), *Dyslexia: Neuronal, Cognitive and Linguistic Aspects*. New York, Pergamon, pp. 141–153.

Lundberg, I., Olofsson, Å., and Wall, S. (1980), Reading and spelling skills in the first school years predicted from phonemic awareness skills in kindergarten. *Scandinavian Journal of Psychology* **21**, 159–173.

Luria, A. R. (1973), *The Working Brain: An Introduction to Neuropsychology*. London, Penguin.

Mattingly, I. G. (1972), Reading, the linguistic process, and linguistic awareness. In: J. F. Kavanagh and I. G. Mattingly (Eds.), *Language by Ear and by Eye: The Relationship between Speech and Reading*. Cambridge, MA, MIT Press. pp. 133–147.

Mattingly, I. G. (1984), Reading, linguistic awareness, and language acquisition. In: J. Downing and R. Valtin (Eds.), *Language Awareness and Learning to Read*. New York, Springer-Verlag. pp. 9–25.

Opie, I., and Opie, P. (1959), *The Lore and Language of School Children*. Oxford, Oxford University Press.

Orton, S. T. (1937), *Reading, Writing, and Speech Problems in Children*. New York, Norton.

Pearson, P. D., and Johnson, D. D. (1978), *Teaching Reading Comprehension*. New York, Holt, Rinehart & Winston.

Piaget, J. (1963), *The Child's Conception of the World*. Paterson, NJ, Littlefield, Adams.

Polanyi, M. (1964), *Personal Knowledge: Towards a Post-critical Philosophy*. New York, Harper & Row.

Read, C. (1978), Children's awareness of language, with emphasis on sound systems. In: A. Sinclair, R. J. Jarvella, and W. J. M. Levelt (Eds.), *The Child's Conception of Language*. New York, Springer-Verlag, pp. 65–82.

Rosner, J. (1975), *Helping Children Overcome Learning Difficulties*. New York, Walker.

Shultz, T. R., and Pilon, R. (1973), Development of the ability to detect linguistic ambiguity. *Child Development* **44**, 728–733.

Sinclair, A., Jarvella, R. J., and Levelt, W. J. M. (Eds.) (1978), *The Child's Conception of Language*. New York, Springer-Verlag.

Wallach, M. A., and Wallach, L. (1976), *Teaching all Children to Read*. Chicago, University of Chicago Press.

Weir, R. H. (1962), *Language in the Crib*. The Hague, Mouton.

Williams, J. P. (1979), The ABD's of reading: a program for the learning disabled. In: L. B. Resnick and P. A. Weaver (Eds.), *Theory and Practice of Early Reading*, Vol. 3. Hillsdale, NJ, Erlbaum, pp. 179–195.

Williams, J. P. (1980), Teaching decoding with an emphasis on phoneme analysis and phoneme blending. *Journal of Educational Psychology* **72**, 1–15.

CHAPTER 11

On the Persistence of Dyslexic Difficulties into Adulthood

T. R. MILES
Department of Psychology, University College of North Wales, Bangor, Gwynedd LL57 2DG, UK

INTRODUCTION

There are many reports in the literature which suggest that adolescent and adult dyslexics do not simply outgrow their problems despite the many respects in which they can make progress. Thus Stone (1980) claims that 'even under ideal conditions . . . problems remain for some' (p. 79), while Critchley (1970) cites, among other case studies, that of a young woman who 'can read traffic signs in the street, and . . . can follow T.V. and the cinema—except foreign films where she cannot fathom the English sub-titles because they are exposed for too short a period of time' (p. 114). He also mentions the case of 'a brilliant violinist [who] was considerably handicapped at the Royal College because of her persistent inability to read musical notation' (p. 114). Even Rawson (1978), while emphasizing that for many of the boys whom she studied 'advice to keep the educational and occupational sights very modest would have been inappropriate' (p. 82), does not dispute that some 'have been slowed in their progress' (p. 109), and cites, among other cases, a highly successful medical student 'whose extreme childhood dyslexia left him with residuals such as "rather slow reading speed" and continued "very poor spelling" (his own 1965 appraisal)' (p. 91). Slowness at reading among dyslexic undergraduates has also been reported by Ellis and Miles (1978), and also slowness at recognizing visually presented digits (Miles and Wheeler, 1977; Ellis and Miles, 1977), while Miles (1983) has shown that when asked to recall auditorily presented digits dyslexic adolescents, aged 16 to 18, were only marginally more successful than dyslexic children of a much younger age. Stirling and Miles (1984) have presented evidence showing a relative lack of oral fluency even among those dyslexic adolescents who had been receiving special help with reading and spelling.

149

The main purpose of the present chapter is to investigate further whether the difficulties of the dyslexic person do indeed persist into adulthood, and, if so, in what form. The exact procedure has been guided by the model offered by Ellis and Miles (1981). These authors cite evidence suggesting that there are no major differences between dyslexic and non-dyslexic persons in respect of the VIS (visual information store), the mechanisms for visual coding, or the semantic system. The important differences arise, so they claim, when symbolic material has to be identified and named; and they argue that the reading and spelling difficulties of the dyslexic person should be seen as examples of this wider limitation.

Now if it were simply the case that those with reading and spelling problems are able to improve their performance in varying degrees and that there is no evidence among adults for any 'wider limitation' such as they postulate, then the concept of dyslexia—in so far as it implies such a limitation—would not be supported. To put the matter another way, if a number of allegedly dyslexic adults performed no differently from suitably matched controls on tasks which were believed to present difficulty to the dyslexic, this would cast doubt on the legitimacy of the classification into dyslexic and non-dyslexic. In contrast, if differences were found, then to that extent the attempt to challenge the legitimacy of the distinction would have been unsuccessful. The three following experiments were based on the supposition that the distinction between 'dyslexic' and 'non-dyslexic' is a valid one and were designed to test whether the lexical system of a dyslexic adult ever achieves full normality.

SELECTION OF SUBJECTS

It was important in the context of the present research to investigate only those dyslexic subjects who had achieved some measure of academic success. Otherwise any figures suggesting that they were slower 'information-processers' than some of the controls could have been interpreted in terms of a general all-round intellectual weakness rather than in terms of a specific deficiency. It was decided, therefore, not to include anyone in either the dyslexic or the control group unless he or she had qualified for the tertiary stage of education, i.e. had reached a high enough level of academic attainment to have qualified for either university or technical college.

The following further selection criteria were adopted: (i) all subjects had to be native English speakers; (ii) all had to be within the normal age-range for students, which for this purpose was taken to be between ages 17 and 26, and (iii) all had to be free of any gross physical handicap. In addition those in the dyslexic group had to satisfy the criteria for inclusion in 'Group I' as set out by Miles (1983). Full details of the diagnostic procedures will not be repeated here; but, in brief, what is claimed is that assessment yielded 'a "pool" of 223 subjects who could be regarded as pure or typical cases of dyslexia' (p. 26). All the present subjects had been assessed, either by the present writer or one of his colleagues, at the Dyslexia Unit, University College of North Wales, Bangor, and none has been included who would not have qualified for membership of the same 'pool'. The criteria are, of course, both multiple and disjunctive. This means that the reasons for diagnosing subject A as dyslexic need not be precisely the same as those for diagnosing subject B, and positive diagnosis is not made without sufficient accumulation of positive signs. These signs are now widely known (compare Newton and Thomson, 1976; Critchley and Critchley, 1978). They include not only a history of lateness in learning to read but persistent difficulty with spelling, a variety of difficulties with ordering and sequencing, and an incongruous discrepancy between intelligence level on the one hand and performance at written work on the other.

Exact matching of dyslexic and control subjects in respect of 'IQ' was not attempted. This was because any intelligence test necessarily taps a variety of different skills, of which some will almost certainly present distinctive difficulty to a dyslexic person (for evidence on this point see Spache, 1976 and Rugel, 1974, and for further discussion see Miles and Ellis, 1981). It follows that the notion of an exact or 'true' IQ makes little sense in the case of a dyslexic person (if, indeed, it makes sense in the case of any person). For present purposes the criterion of whether the subject had qualified for the tertiary stage of education was a more appropriate way of ensuring that those of limited intellectual ability were excluded.

Apart from having to satisfy this requirement the control subjects were selected largely on grounds of availability. All the subjects in both groups were volunteers. Five dyslexic subjects took part in both experiment 2 and experiment 3; otherwise no subject took part in more than one of the experiments.

EXPERIMENT 1.   EFFECTS OF PRACTICE

Background

That the reading and spelling of dyslexic children will improve as a result of suitable practice and training is not in doubt (Hornsby and Miles, 1980). In the case of memory for digits, however, it is not clear whether the typical dyslexic weakness is something which can be overcome. It has in fact been argued by Ellis and Miles (1978) that the dyslexic person is distinctive not because he is a 'slow processer' as such but because he *remains* a slow processer when those without his limitation have learned to speed up. If this is right one might expect to be able to demonstrate a gradual decrease in processing time on the part of a non-dyslexic person during the time when initially unfamiliar material was becoming familiar. A convenient example of unfamiliar material would be the letters of an alphabet other than the English one; and for the present experiment it was possible to secure the cooperation of a student who was learning Russian but who was not yet very far advanced. It was also possible to enlist the help of two other subjects, one of them dyslexic, who were willing, over a 28-day period, to try to find out if their ability to process familiar material could be improved by practice.

The experiment was designed to investigate four questions, viz. (i) Is there evidence that *any* adult subject (whether dyslexic or not) can improve his processing speed with practice when digits are presented visually?, (ii) Does the improvement 'hold up' with other types of stimulus? (iii) Can the processing speed of a dyslexic person be brought up, with practice, to that of a non-dyslexic person?, and (iv) How does his performance compare with that of a non-dyslexic native English person who is given similar practice with letters of the Russian alphabet?

Subjects, Apparatus, and Method

Three subjects took part in the experiment, one of whom had been diagnosed as dyslexic in accordance with the criteria specified above. Of the two non-dyslexic subjects one had recently started a degree in Russian and therefore had some limited familiarity with the letters of the Russian alphabet.

The apparatus was a two-field tachistoscope supplied by Electronic Developments. The viewing distance was 490 mm from the subject's eyes, the illumination at the eye being about 3.125 lux.

The stimuli were of three different types, viz. numerals, letters of the English alphabet, and, in the case of the one subject, letters of the Russian alphabet. Six letters or numerals were exposed at each presentation, the sequences being randomly generated except that no individual letter or numeral was permitted to occur more than once per card. Since Russian letters were unobtainable in Letraset all stimuli were painted by hand with a black felt pen, the background being a white card measuring 220 by 200 mm. The letters used were lower case, and they and the digits were 10 mm high. No mask was used, but a cross was exposed in the other field of the tachistoscope 1 second before the letters or numerals were presented. The experimenter was present throughout the sessions and between each trial she adjusted the timer (where necessary) and changed the stimulus card.

Eight practice trials were given. The subject was told: 'I am now going to show you six letters (numbers, Russian letters). After the sequence has gone off the screen I want you to tell me what they are'. The experimenter noted the exposure-time and recorded whether or not the response was correct.

Each session involved either ascending or descending exposure-times. In the 'ascending' condition, if there were two consecutive failures at a given exposure-time the exposure-time was increased by 50 ms (or 10 ms in the case of times below 100 ms). This procedure was repeated until the subject responded correctly on both trials. In the 'descending' condition, whenever the subject was successful on both trials the exposure-time was decreased by 50 ms (or 10 ms in the case of times below 100 ms) until the subject responded incorrectly on both trials. 'Ascending' and 'descending' conditions were used on alternate days over a period of 28 days. 'Information processing time' (IPT) was reckoned as the mid-point between two consecutively correct and two consecutively incorrect trials.

Results and Discussion

There were in fact systematically lower IPTs in the 'ascending' condition than there were in the 'descending' condition. This finding, however, will not be discussed here. The important data are those given in Table 1 which show, for each subject and with each type of stimulus, the initial IPT and the IPT after 28 days. From this table it can be seen: (i) that all three subjects improved their performance with practice, (ii) that the improvement occurred whatever the nature of the stimulus (digit, English letter, Russian letter), (iii) that the IPT of the dyslexic subject remained well below that of the other two subjects (he did in fact achieve an IPT of 475 ms on five occasions between days 12 and 20 but was never below 525 ms otherwise), and (iv) that the subject who was exposed to the Russian letters was slower than the dyslexic subject at the outset but by day 28 had achieved an IPT of 150 ms. Despite the relative unfamiliarity of the Russian material this subject had thus achieved a processing time which was considerably faster than that achieved by the dyslexic subject in processing symbols to which he had been regularly exposed over many years. The idea of a constitutionally caused limitation seems the most likely explanation; or, at the very least, it seems that even after considerable practice a dyslexic person does not learn to process this kind of material as fast as a non-dyslexic person.

Table 1. Changes in information-processing times (ms) between day 1 and day 28

| | English letters | | Numerals | | Russian letters | |
	Day 1	Day 28	Day 1	Day 28	Day 1	Day 28
Subject 1	725	10	675	7.5	1600	150
Subject 2	775	7.5	550	7.5	–	
Subject 3 (dyslexic)	1500	525	1100	525	–	

EXPERIMENT 2.   THE 'HENRY' TASKS: A PILOT STUDY

Introduction

Although this experiment was carried out simply as a pilot study and is incomplete as it stands, some results emerged which support the central thesis of this paper and are therefore worth quoting.

The purpose behind the 'Henry' tasks was to carry out a variant of the clinical procedures described in item 1 of the Bangor Dyslexia Test (Miles, 1982) under timed conditions. This item consists of a series of tests in which the subject, seated opposite the tester, is required to respond to instructions such as 'Touch my right hand with your left hand'.

In the present experiment, in place of the tester a human figure ('Henry') was made to appear on the VDU of an Apple II microcomputer and the subjects were required to direct an arrow so that it pointed to Henry's ear, hand, or foot (see below for further details). This procedure made it possible to determine whether dyslexic subjects made more errors and/or took more time than controls in carrying out this task.

Subjects, Apparatus, and Method

Twelve dyslexic and twelve non-dyslexic subjects took part in this experiment. In each group six were male and six female. The apparatus was an Apple II microcomputer to which were connected two paddles. These were placed between the subject and the VDU, one by his right hand, one by his left. Their function was to control an arrow which could be moved to different positions on the VDU.

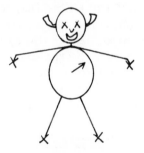

Figure 1.

A figure ('Henry') was made to appear on the VDU, with distinctive ears, arms, and legs (see Figure 1). Instructions, which were given either visually on the VDU or auditorily on tape, were of the form 'With the paddle on your right (left) point to my right (left) ear (hand, foot)'. In the visual condition the instructions

with the paddle   point to Henry's
on your   . . . .
. . . . .

were present throughout. Timing started when the rest of the instructions appeared (as indicated by the dots) and finished when the subject pressed a button attached to the paddle. In the auditory condition timing started when the voice first said the word 'right' or 'left' ('with the paddle on your right/left . . .') and finished in the same way as in the visual condition. A print-out gave the required response, the given response, the execution time in centiseconds, and the number of errors.

On their arrival in the laboratory the purpose of the experiment was explained to the subjects. Half of those in the dyslexic group started with the auditory condition and half with the visual condition, and similarly with the non-dyslexic group. In each condition there were eight questions, such as 'With the paddle on your left point to Henry's right foot'. Each condition was repeated five times; this gave 40 readings in all, of which the first eight were treated as practice trials.

Results and Discussion

Table 2(a) shows the numbers of dyslexic and control subjects who made a specified number of errors. This table makes clear that even for dyslexic subjects an almost error-free performance is possible; and it is worth noting that of the 36 errors made by the dyslexic subjects 20 were contributed by three individuals. One of the control subjects was error-free but most of the subjects in both groups made occasional errors.

Table 2(a). Numbers of dyslexic and control subjects who made a specified number of left–right errors

No. of errors	Frequencies Dyslexic subjects	Control subjects
0	—	1
1	5	5
2	2	2
3	1	2
4	1	1
5	1	1
6	1	—
7	—	—
8	—	—
9	1	—

Table 2(b). Mean times in seconds taken by dyslexic and control subjects in the visual and auditory conditions

	Visual condition	Auditory condition
Dyslexic subjects	5.74	5.85
Control subjects	3.96	5.02
	$U = 5.5$	$U = 26.0$
	$p < 0.001$	$p < 0.01$

The response times, however, tell a very different story. This can be seen from Table 2(b). In both the visual and the auditory conditions the dyslexic subjects were taking longer. In the visual condition the lowest time for a dyslexic subject was 4.56 s, only three of the twelve non-dyslexic subjects taking more time than this. In the auditory condition one dyslexic subject achieved 4.67 s (at a cost of four errors), which was faster than all but two of the non-dyslexic subjects; otherwise the lowest time for a dyslexic subject was 5.21 s, only two of the twelve non-dyslexic subjects taking more time than this. There is thus a consistent tendency over both conditions for the dyslexic subjects to need longer time for correct responding.

Overall it seems fair to conclude that for *some* of the time *some* adult dyslexic subjects can be as fast or as accurate at processing symbolic material as suitably matched controls but that they continue to be at risk; it is not the case that earlier difficulties simply disappear.

These results as they stand are not sufficient to show that the 'left–right' requirement in the Henry tasks is the decisive factor which accounts for the difference between dyslexic and control subjects. In view of the findings of experiment 3 (see below) and the findings reported by Miles (1983, Chapter 10), the conclusion is a likely one; but before the claim can be regarded as conclusively established it would be necessary to run a similar experiment with stimuli other than 'left' and 'right' and compare the differences. The differences between results in the auditory and in the visual condition should also be treated with caution pending further experimentation. From the point of view of the present paper what is important is that the dyslexic subjects were slower overall. Whatever the precise nature of the processing tasks involved there is clear evidence of persisting difficulties.

EXPERIMENT 3. VISUAL AND SEMANTIC INFORMATION

Background

The ability to match a visual display against a verbal description of that display has been extensively investigated by Chase and Clark (1971, 1972) and by Clark and Chase (1972, 1974). In a typical experiment the subjects were presented with a display such as the following:

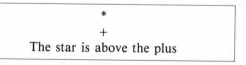

They were then timed on their ability to say whether the sentence (semantic information) did or did not match the display (visual information). Both affirmative and negative sentences were used, and each sentence contained either the word 'above' or the word 'below'.

In the present experiment, in view of what was known about the special difficulties of dyslexic subjects, it was decided to introduce the left–right dimension, with the above–below dimension as a control to it, and examine whether comparison of visual and semantic information took longer when 'left' and 'right' were involved than it did when 'above' and 'below' were involved. Moreover, since there is a documented case of a dyslexic young man aged 18 muddling 'b' and 'd' in the year of his entrance to university (Miles, 1983, pp. 101 and 194), it was decided to examine whether a choice between 'b' and 'd' took longer time than a choice between a star and a plus. At the same time it seemed appropriate to check whether any similar problems existed with B and D (upper case letters) and with the auditorily confusable letters, 'f' and 's'.

Subjects, Apparatus, and Method

The apparatus was an Apple II microcomputer which was programmed to record the time taken for each decision. The subjects were selected in accordance with the criteria given above, ten being dyslexic and fifteen non-dyslexic. Of the dyslexic subjects five were male and five female; of the control group seven were male and eight female.

Since it seemed unsafe to have fewer than four exposures in each condition and since it was thought undesirable to have sessions involving more than 128 exposures, it was decided not to include the affirmative/negative dimension. Indeed, in view of the adequacy of the 'semantic system' in dyslexic persons (Ellis and Miles, 1981), there was no particular reason for thinking that the presence or absence of the word 'not' would distinctively affect dyslexic subjects. The two 'directions' used were above/below and left/right, and the four stimulus pairs were b/d, f/s, B/D, and */ + . There were thus 32 different combinations, each of the eight stimuli being combined with 'above', 'below', 'left', and 'right'. With four exposures in each condition this gave a total of 128 exposures in all. The subjects were instructed to sit so that they could immediately press one or another key on the Apple keyboard, viz. the key marked 'Y' in order to respond 'yes' and the key marked 'N' in order to respond 'no'. The VDU was immediately above the keyboard. The experimenter was present throughout.

Below is a typical presentation (to which the correct answer is 'N').

b   d
The b is to the right of the d

Five practice trials were written into the program, with the opportunity to take them over again if the subject so wished. The presentations were in random order, with the constraint that the same presentation should not appear twice consecutively. The items on which the subject made errors were presented again at the end, if necessary more than once, until response-times had been obtained for all 128 exposures.

Results and Discussion

The first requirement was to check whether, overall, the dyslexic subjects were taking longer over the various tasks than the control subjects. The mean reaction times in each condition and overall are set out in Tables 3(a), 3(b), and 3(c). From simple inspection it is plain that there were differences between dyslexic and control subjects in all four directions and with all four types of stimulus.

Table 3(a). Mean reaction time in seconds for dyslexic and control subjects in the four different directions

	Dyslexic	Control
Above	3.619	2.007
Below	3.624	2.125
Right	5.245	2.377
Left	5.450	2.405
Overall mean	4.497	2.228

Table 3(b). Mean reaction time in seconds for dyslexic and control subjects in response to the four different types of stimulus

	Dyslexic	Control
* +	3.882	2.129
b d	5.984	2.473
B D	4.186	2.118
f s	3.936	2.193
Overall mean	4.497	2.228

Table 3(c). Mean reaction time in seconds in the 'yes' and condition and in the 'no' condition

Correct answer 'yes'	:	3.002
Correct answer 'no'	:	3.270

Table 3(d). Analysis of variance (extracts only)

		df	F	p
D	Direction (left/right; above/below)	3	79.65	<0.001
S	Stimulus (b/d; f/s; B/D; */+)	3	56.25	<0.001
A	Answer (yes, no)	1	43.68	<0.001
G	Group (dyslexic, non-dyslexic)	1	23.63	<0.001
D×S		9	0.99	ns
D×A		3	1.81	ns
S×A		3	0.93	ns
D×G		3	15.41	<0.001
S×G		3	20.58	<0.001
A×G		1	0.79	ns
D×A×G		3	1.51	ns
S×A×G		3	0.39	ns

In order to examine matters in further detail a six-factor ANOVA was carried out (four directions × four stimuli × two answers × two groups with ten Group One subjects and fifteen Group Two subjects nested within groups × four observations within each cell). Because of the greater scatter of scores in the dyslexic group a $\log_{10}$ transformation was used, and it was decided in advance to treat the results as statistically significant only if there was significance at the 1 per cent level in the case of both transformed and non-transformed data. Extracts from the ANOVA are set out in Table 3(d). This table shows that there were significant differences (i) between the four different directions (above, below, left, right), (ii) between the four pairs of stimuli (*/+, b/d, B/D, f/s), (iii) between the two answers (yes, no), and (iv) between the two groups (dyslexic and non-dyslexic). It also shows significant group × direction and group × stimulus interactions, which implies that among the stimuli and among the directions there were at least some which presented extra difficulty to the dyslexic subjects as compared with the controls. In contrast there was no additional difficulty for the dyslexic subjects in responding 'no' as opposed to 'yes'.

In the case of the data in Table 3(a), use of the Tukey test showed that a difference between means of 0.228 would be needed for significance at the 5 per cent level. It follows that overall there is no significant difference between the 'above' and 'below' conditions or between the 'left' and 'right' conditions but that for both groups the left–right dimension requires longer than the above–below dimension. Clark (1970) has argued that 'above' can be expected to take shorter time than 'below' but this claim was not borne out in the present study.

With regard to Table 3(b), a similar Tukey test showed that for both groups there was a significantly longer reaction time to the b/d stimuli than to any of the other pairs. In the case of the dyslexic group B/D took significantly longer than */+ but in neither group were there any other significant differences.

As predicted by Clark and Chase (1972) responses of 'no' tended to require longer time than responses of 'yes' (see Table 3(c)) but the dyslexic group were not differentially slower.

The main findings, therefore, were:

(i) In every condition the dyslexic subjects were slower than the control subjects.

(ii) Longer time was needed by both groups in the case of left/right than in the case of above/below, this task being differentially harder for dyslexic subjects.

(iii) Longer time was needed by both groups in the case of b/d than in the case of the other pairs, this task being differentially harder for the dyslexic subjects.

(iv) 'No' answers took longer than 'yes' answers but the dyslexic subjects had no distinctive difficulty in this respect.

These results are compatible with the hypothesis of a lexical encoding deficiency (Ellis and Miles, 1981). Since all the stimuli were symbolic, a longer response-time in all conditions is predicted by the hypothesis, but since answers of 'yes' and 'no' involve the semantic system ('processing for meaning') rather than the lexical system the non-significant answer × group interaction is quite expected.

It is of interest that even in the case of the control subjects both b/d and left/right produced some small degree of extra difficulty. This seems to be an example of a more general phenomenon, viz. that symbolic processing tasks which are *particularly* difficult for a dyslexic person are likely to present *some degree* of difficulty to the non-dyslexic person. For example, if a lecture is delivered in so incoherent a fashion that note-taking is difficult for most students, then dyslexic students can be expected to find the task virtually impossible.

The results do not rule out the possibility of a serial ordering deficiency in dyslexia or even a deficiency in terms of inter-sensory integration (for a detailed review of such theories see Vellutino, 1979). Nor do they rule out Orton's (1937) theory of non-elision of engrams, since slight tendencies towards non-elision could quite well exist in non-dyslexic subjects. It should be noted, however, that confusion between mirror images appears to be a widespread phenomenon among living organisms and is known to occur in birds and monkeys (Brown and Ettlinger, 1983). A possible hypothesis, therefore, is that mirror-image confusions and the weakness of the lexical system of a dyslexic person are, at bottom, quite different phenomena but that when a dyslexic person is confronted with stimuli which are mirror images he is less able than the non-dyslexic person to help himself out by means of labelling.

As for the extra difficulties experienced by the non-dyslexic subjects in the case of tasks involving 'left' and 'right', the explanation could be the same as that put forward by Miles and Ellis (1981) to explain the difficulties of dyslexic subjects, viz. that *left* and *right* fluctuate in their 'referents' in a way in which *up* and *down* do not; thus 'up' remains 'up' and 'down' remains 'down' whichever way one is facing, but if one turns round one has to change one's account of what is on the left and what is on the right. There seems no reason why a similar difficulty in milder form should not also occur in non-dyslexic persons, and the present results suggest that in fact it does.

No attempt will be made in this paper to discuss individual differences between subjects, but it is perhaps worth recording that only one out of the ten dyslexic subjects consistently achieved response-times of under 4 s, while fourteen out of the fifteen control subjects invariably did so. One dyslexic subject had a median response-time of 23 s in the 'left–yes–b/d' condition and twelve other median response-times of over 10 s. The longest median response-time for a control subject was 5 s, and fewer than 8 per cent of the median response-times in the control group were over 3 s.

CONCLUSIONS

On the basis of these three experiments there can be no doubt at all that dyslexic difficulties sometimes persist into adulthood. This claim can be regarded as firmly established.

Now all three experiments called for the processing of symbolic material: in experiment 1 the subjects were required to recall tachistoscopically presented letters and digits; in experiment 2 they had to read or listen to heard or written instructions involving left and right and respond accordingly, while in experiment 3 visual-non-symbolic and visual-symbolic information had to be compared. The results are therefore compatible with the idea (Miles and Ellis, 1981) that developmental dyslexia should not be thought of simply as difficulty with reading or even as difficulty with spelling, but that the reading and spelling problems of a dyslexic person are part of a wider disability which shows itself whenever symbolic material has to be identified and named. At the very least one should treat with caution the view that when the reading and spelling of a dyslexic person have reached an adequate level no other problems remain.

It should be added that over the three experiments eighteen dyslexic subjects were involved (one in experiment 1, twelve in experiment 2, and an additional five in experiment 3), along with twenty-four non-dyslexic subjects (two in experiment 1, twelve in experiment 2, and ten in experiment 3). The massive difference in experiment 1 between the dyslexic subject and the other two subjects is plain on inspection, while in experiments 2 and 3 there is one comparison between dyslexic and control subjects which gives a confidence level of $p < 0.01$ (that in the 'talking Henry' condition), while all others give a confidence level of $p < 0.001$ (see Tables 2(b) and 3(d)). Since there are massive differences one can have increased confidence in the generality of the findings. The notion of a 'population' of adult dyslexic subjects may well turn out to be one in which the boundaries are not clearly defined, but predictions about the difficulties to be expected in typical cases can be made with a high degree of confidence.

Finally, experiments such as those reported in this paper start with the assumption that a distinction can usefully be drawn between those who are dyslexic and those who are not. This seems to be what is at issue when there is argument as to whether 'something called dyslexia exists' or whether one should 'believe in' dyslexia. If under controlled conditions allegedly 'dyslexic' persons regularly performed no differently from anyone else, then, as was suggested in the Introduction, the distinction between 'dyslexic' and 'non-dyslexic' would become progressively more uncomfortable. If, on the other hand, highly significant differences are sometimes found — differences, that is, other than the trivial one that some people are better readers and spellers than others — then to that extent the distinction resists refutation and therefore holds up. The present experiments were concerned with a specific prediction, viz. that if people are classified into dyslexic and non-dyslexic some of those in the former group will continue to be slow in processing symbolic information despite academic success in other ways. This prediction is a 'risky' one in Popper's sense (see Popper, 1963, p. 36), since negative results could not easily have been explained away. Only a long series of similar results could show that the usefulness of the concept of dyslexia is decisively established, but one can argue from the present experiments that yet another attempt to 'refute' its value has been unsuccessful.

ACKNOWLEDGEMENTS

I should like to emphasize the extent to which this paper was a team effort. The data for experiment 1 were collected by Laura Ritchie, with the help of Helen Ritchie, Simon Bush, and Rebecca Mousley. The data for experiment 2 were collected by Stephanie Christie and the data for experiment 3 by Joyce McCulloch who was also responsible for the analysis of variance. Dr Nick Ellis has given a large amount of help on both the theoretical and technical aspects of the research, and I am grateful to Patrick Miles, my son, for writing the programs for the Apple II microcomputer which were used in experiments 2 and 3. Details of these programs are available on request.

REFERENCES

Brown, J. V., and Ettlinger, G. (1983), Intermanual transfer of mirror-image discrimination by monkeys. *Quart. J. Exp. Psychol.* **35B**, 2, 119–124.
Chase, W. G., and Clark, H. H. (1971), Semantics in the perception of verticality. *Brit. J. Psychol.* **62**, 311–326.

Chase, W. G., and Clark, H. H. (1972), Mental operations in the comparison of sentences against pictures. In Gregg, L. (Ed.), *Cognition in Learning and Memory*. New York, John Wiley.
Clark, H. H. (1970), Comprehending comparatives. In: G. B. Flores D'Arcais and W. J. M. Levelt (Eds.), *Advances in Psycholinguistics*. Amsterdam, North Holland Press.
Clark, H. H., and Chase, W. G. (1972), On the process of comparing sentences against pictures. *Cog. Psych.* **3**, 472–517.
Clark, H. H., and Chase, W. G. (1974), Perceptual coding strategies in the formation and verification of descriptions. *Memory and Cognition* **2**, 101–111.
Critchley, M. (1970), *The Dyslexic Child*. London, Heinemann Medical Books.
Critchley, M., and Critchley, E. A. (1978), *Dyslexia Defined*. London, Heinemann Medical Books.
Ellis, N. C., and Miles, T. R. (1977), Dyslexia as a limitation in the ability to process information. *Bull. Orton Soc.* **27**, 72–81.
Ellis, N. C., and Miles, T. R. (1978), Visual information processing as a determinant of reading speed. *J. Reading Res.* **1**, 2, 108–120.
Ellis, N. C., and Miles, T. R. (1981), A lexical encoding deficiency I. In: G. Th. Pavlidis and T. R. Miles (Eds.), *Dyslexia Research and its Applications to Education*. Chichester, John Wiley.
Hornsby, B., and Miles, T. R. (1980), The effects of a dyslexia-centred teaching programme. *Brit. J. Educ. Psychol.* **50**, 236–242.
Miles, T. R. (1982), *The Bangor Dyslexia Test*. Wisbech, Cambs., Learning Development Aids.
Miles, T. R. (1983), *Dyslexia: The Pattern of Difficulties*. St. Albans, Granada Press. Also Springfield, Illinois, Charles C. Thomas.
Miles, T. R., and Ellis, N. C. (1981), A lexical encoding deficiency II. In: G. Th. Pavlidis and T. R. Miles (Eds.), *Dyslexia Research and its Applications to Education*. Chichester, John Wiley.
Miles, T. R., and Wheeler, T. J. (1977), Responses of dyslexic and non-dyslexic subjects to tachistoscopically presented digits. *IRCS Med. Sci.* **5**, 149.
Newton, M., and Thomson, M. (1976), *The Aston Index: a Classroom Test for Screening and Diagnosis of Language Difficulties*. Wisbech, Cambs., Learning Development Aids.
Orton, S. T. (1937), *Reading, Writing, and Speech Problems in Children*. London, Chapman & Hall.
Popper, K. (1963), *Conjectures and Refutations*. London, Routledge & Kegan Paul.
Rawson, M. B. (1978), *Developmental Language Disability. Adult Accomplishments of Dyslexic Boys*. Cambridge, Mass., Educators Publishing Service Inc.
Rugel, R. P. (1974), W.I.S.C. sub-test scores of disabled readers. *J. Learning Disabilities* **7**, 48–55.
Spache, G. D. (1976), *Investigating the Issues of Reading Disabilities*. Boston, Allyn & Bacon.
Stirling, E. G., and Miles, T. R. (1984), Naming ability and oral fluency in dyslexic adolescents. Paper delivered at Chatauqua Academy, Baltimore.
Stone, C. A. (1980), Adolescent cognitive development: implications for learning disabilities. *Bull. Orton Soc.* **30**, 79–93.
Vellutino, F. R. (1979), *Dyslexia: Theory and Research*. Cambridge, Mass., MIT Press.

CHAPTER 12

Models of Dyslexia and its Subtypes

MARCEL KINSBOURNE
Eunice Kennedy Shriver Center, 200 Trapelo Road, Waltham, MA 02254, USA

Two contrasting models have been applied to dyslexia, each of which subdivides further. One view regards dyslexia as a *unitary disorder*. Dyslexics differ from nonspecifically retarded readers both in the cause of their reading difficulty and in its observable characteristics. This includes the 'medical' or 'disease' model of dyslexia. Some proponents of this view construe the disorder *narrowly* as 'pure'. It specifically implicates a critical mental operation involved only in learning to read and write. Others refer it more *broadly* to cognitive processes which, in addition to being essential for reading and writing, also participate in other measurable activities. A contrasting view regards dyslexia as a syndrome that comprises *heterogeneous* disorders. This view divides into discontinuity theory and continuity theory. The *discontinuity* model of the dyslexia syndrome incorporates a finite number of discrete disorders or dyslexia subtypes, the sum total of which accounts for the general problem of dyslexia. According to *continuity* theory, dyslexic children differ in degree only from normal readers. In such a child, one or more of the many mental operations involved in learning to read or write is underdeveloped and the patterns of underdevelopment varies from child to child. This individual difference approach regards dyslexic children as diverse in the locus of their difficulty, but does not admit of discrete subtypes.

The narrow unitary theory of pure dyslexia was the one put forward by Hinshelwood (1900) and other proponents of the concept of pure or specific 'word blindness'. It reflected the then current preoccupation with functional localization in the brain, and an uncritical equating of mental operation as subserved by brain with real life activity (such as reading). Though it is largely disregarded nowadays, the present state of knowledge does not permit its exclusion in a modified form. In some children who experience profound difficulty in learning to read and write, neuropsychological and psychometric measures reveal little or no cognitive inadequacy of a type that could plausibly be involved in explaining the reading problem. Although by exclusion, some

165

would be inclined then to hypothesize motivational difficulties, these also are not apparent. It remains possible that there exists a mental operation that is 'performance-limiting' for reading and spelling. When this is impaired, children find it difficult to learn to read and spell, but experience undue difficulty on no other task.

The broad version of the unitary hypothesis has held sway more than any other idea: dyslexia is unitary, but based on a more general processing difficulty. The problem was often assumed to be visuospatial or visuodirectional (cf. Orton, 1937; Hermann and Norrie, 1958). More recently, the emphasis within this theory has radically shifted toward incriminating a general language difficulty (Vellutino, 1979). This viewpoint regards linguistic factors (verbal coding, mastering the phonological structure of the language) as the crucial stumbling block for these children. Other associated test-elicited deficiencies are dismissed as coincidental and not critical for reading progress. Other unitary approaches incriminate auditory processing (Tallal and Piercy, 1973), temporal ordering (Bakker, 1970), or sequential eye movement (Pavlidis, 1981) as explanatory principles.

Subtype theory, the discontinuity variant of the diversity theory of dyslexia, was launched by Kinsbourne and Warrington (1963). They demonstrated two developmental neuropsychological syndromes in children referred for reading backwardness. In some children language disorder was the limiting factor. These children, usually male, were slow to develop language and relatively inferior on the verbal as compared to performance subscale of the Wechsler Intelligence Scale for Children (WISC). They also had a subtle impairment of verbal comprehension, as measured by the Token Test. Their spelling errors predominantly involved choosing wrong letters, namely ones that lacked even phonetic correspondence to the sound of the word. In a contrasting syndrome no evidence of a central language disorder was present. The 'Gerstmann' subtype showed a performance deficit on the WISC, notably involving the block design and object assembly subtests. It also featured a problem in arithmetic, both on the WISC and on academic achievement test (in contrast to the language type in which the difficulties were limited to reading and writing *per se*). Failure on test of finger order sense demonstrated a difficulty in identifying body parts based on their sequential position as opposed to their individual forms. Right–left discrimination difficulties again exemplified difficulty in making distinctions based on relative position. The children had more difficulty spelling than reading, and made letter order errors. That is, after choosing correct letters, they would put a letter in too soon, too late, or reverse the position of two letters. In arithmetic, the significance of the digit was compromised, in terms of its spatial relationship to other digits on the same line ('place value'). That is, they would mistake 56 for 65 and showed particular difficulty in arithmetic computations in which numbers have to be carried from column to column. The syndrome was construed as a sequential processing problem (analogous to the Gerstmann syndrome of acquired left posterior parietal damage) and not specifically affecting or limited to verbal material. Indeed, sequences of words or speech sounds seem to be established by a separate processor or in some way that bypasses the impaired process in the sequential difficulty of the Gerstmann type. More recently, Pirozzolo (1979) has discovered that the children also have difficulty in left-to-right sequential eye movement and with the return sweep from the right end of one line to the left beginning of the one beneath. In contrast to normal children, their eye movement reaction time to laterally displaced words is faster leftward than to the right.

Kinsbourne and Warrington (1963) chose clear-cut instances of these two problems from a much larger group of children referred for backward reading. They did not claim to be able to subdivide all backward readers into either one (or a combination of) these two categories. They left open (1) whether other subtypes also await discovery and (2) whether these extreme cases represent specific subtypes or the extremes of continua of individual variation in the development of the relevant underlying mental processes.

The dichotomizing approach was further developed by Boder (1973). She devised ways of detecting a selective propensity of children to misapply phonic analysis (dysphonetic errors) or whole word pattern identification (dyseidetic errors) to reading. The dysphonetic classification corresponded to the language based subtype of Kinsbourne and Warrington. The dyseidetic one, however, departed from the Gerstmann type, and referred back instead to Myklebust's (1965) notion of a 'visual' weakness on the part of some backward readers. This subgrouping lent itself to later attempts to subgroup dyslexia into types due to relative weakness either of the right or the left hemisphere, whereas the language and Gerstmann subtypes were both based on analogies with adult left hemisphere syndromes.

The possibility of subtyping of dyslexia was rediscovered by Mattis, French, and Rapin (1975). They described a language , a visual–spatial and a grapho-motor–dysarticulatory subtype. They introduced an interesting further control. They reasoned that to demonstrate the validity of attributing a reading disability to the associated finding of a neuropsychological deficit on test performance it is necessary to show that any child who has that finding on tests also must have trouble learning to read. They included a brain-damaged but not reading handicapped control group and excluded from consideration those test performances on which that subgroup also did poorly. They argued that if one could do badly on a test and still learn to read, than the ability underlying that test performance could not be considered crucial for reading. On this basis, apparently, they excluded the Gerstmann syndrome from consideration, at least as tested by their methodologies. This refinement addresses a crucial issue in subtyping: the evaluation of the negative instance. Whereas Mattis and co-workers' classification has had wide currency, the issue of the brain-damaged but reading control has escaped attention. Subsequent investigators have not checked the concatenations of test results by which they have characterized the dyslectic subtypes for validity. The methodology may, however, be questioned. The number of patterns of neuropsychological profiles excluded from consideration because they do occur in normally reading children could simply be a function of how many tests are given to how many children. If one kept on testing children who can read but are otherwise neuropsychologically handicapped, one might well find that virtually every possible combination of test results accompanies tolerable reading development *in some cases*. Of course, one could then argue that the children who were able to learn to read in spite of neuropsychological deficits that 'should' have stopped them, were doing so by some alternative or unusual route, or after intensive practice to overcome their disability.

Mattis *et al.* (1975) added a third subtype, which, however, hardly meets the usual criteria for dyslexia. These children have articulatory and graphomotor deficits: that is, they had trouble in oral reading (but not silent) and script (but not spelling). Based on their three subtypes, they claimed to be able to account for every child in their sample. They did so by using generous criteria for identifying deficient test performance (including even performance only one standard deviation below the mean). Although on empirical grounds this appears to have worked, it certainly makes one doubtful that the subgroups are valid. In a subsequent publication, Mattis (1978) confirmed the subgroups, added a 'temporal sequencing disability' group, but this time did find some children whose reading problem was not accounted for (Denckla, 1977).

The main subsequent departure from the clinical approach to subtyping consisted of its rejection for an empirical one. Briefly, it was argued that a less *post hoc* and a more objective procedure would be to administer an extensive neuropsychological test battery to an adequate sample of reading retarded children and then, by statistical means, determine what neuropsychological pattern or patterns of findings characterized most members of the group. The technique applied most appropriately to this end is cluster analysis. This statistical approach determines how subjects cluster in terms of the dependent variables. Doehring and Hoshko (1977), Petrauskas and Rourke (1979) and Satz and Morris (1981) have applied cluster analytic techniques to substantial samples of reading retarded children. Each emerge with a substantial number of clusters of backward readers.

These sets of cluster are superficially in some agreement in that they all include one or more language-based clusters. Some also include a visuospatial cluster, suggestive either of a sequential or of a right hemisphere pattern perception deficit. However, in detail, the clusters do not superimpose. We should note that cluster analytic technique is capable of determining which clusters exist on the assumption that some do. But it would derive clusters even from a random data set (Satz and Morris, 1981). The technique is not capable of disconfirming the hypothesis that clusters do not exist, or of ruling out that the form of the data is continuous variation along multiple dimensions of performance (i.e. individual difference model). Thus, two further tests need to be applied to the cluster: one is, do they make neuropsychological sense? That is, do the clusters really characterize mental operations plausibly deficient in reading (Lyon *et al.*, 1981) but preserved among similarly tested children who read normally? The second test is the extent to which the clusters replicate (see Doehring's work; Fisk and Rourke, 1979; Lyon *et al.*, 1981). At this time the empirical derivation of clusters cannot carry conviction alone but should be bolstered by ancillary findings.

The individual differences approach is exemplified by the work of Olson *et al.* (1984). They determine continuous variation on a variety of plausibly reading-relevant parameters and attribute reading problems to the child's situation at particular intersects of performance on multiple relevant dimensions. This approach conforms to the informal belief of many educators that academic difficulties are multifactorial.

It is evident that each of the four major approaches to the understanding of dyslexia has something to commend it, and no one of them is consensually superior to the rest. It thus behooves us to look for supporting evidence from outside children's reading and neuropsychological test performance. The most obvious of these is: which of these approaches yields the most helpful information remediating the dyslexic? This question cannot yet be answered. Recommendations based on neuropsychological assessment are broad and often idiosyncratic. It is not clear that any of the above-mentioned approaches generates better individualized educational programs than the others, or indeed that they are superior to those formed in the absence of the type of analysis we have been discussing.

Given the legitimate uncertainties about the appropriate model for dyslexia, as derived from corollary test performance, interest is renewed in the search for brain-based correlates (or, as it is fashionable to call them, biological markers). Does some bodily or brain-based attribute reliably pick out a particular subtype of dyslexia from the rest (or even dyslexia as such from nonspecific reading disorders)? Among possible biological markers, none that are metabolic have been proposed. The recent claim for an abnormality of the short limb of chromosome 15 in certain pedigrees with cases of dyslexia is worth noting (Kimberling *et al.*, 1983). We also note that a selective language-based reading disability is prevalent among children with 47XXY karyotype (Bender *et al.*, in press) and that Friedrich *et al.* (1982) found this syndrome, or translocation, in 8 of 92 language-delayed children. For the rest, we shall focus on proceeds of the extended neurological and of the neuropsychological examination.

The various approaches to dyslexia that have been considered leave their brain basis unspecified. A performance deficit can derive from selective brain damage or maldevelopment. It can arise from problems of local neuronal circuitry that currently defy detection. It can result from deviant brain organization, rendering certain processes vulnerable to cross-talk interference. Or it can result from defective or deviant patterns of task-related selective cerebral activation. Any of these concepts could be applied to any of the cited views of the nature of dyslexia. Indeed, where a heterogeneity hypothesis is adopted, multiple factors could be invoked — e.g. activation deficiency for one subtype, structural damage for another.

The most direct evidence for the brain basis of dyslexia would accrue from examination at autopsy of relevant portions of brain. This was recently accomplished in one case by Galaburda and Kemper (1979), who reported evidence of neuronal developmental abnormality in the language area of the left hemisphere. Two more such cases have reportedly since been studied (Kemper, 1984). If this type of finding were to characterize many of the children diagnosed as dyslexics, and shown to be absent in normal readers, then this would revolutionize our concept of that disorder (and also give evidence for a prevalence of developmentally based cerebral neuropathology far greater than currently suspected). However, more normal control autopsy data is needed to confirm that the 'abnormalities' are not within the range of normal variation. Pending confirmation of the Galaburda and Kemper findings, we proceed to consider alternative techniques that might indirectly contribute to the choice between models. These are neurophysiological and radiological methodologies of recent devising.

The use of EEG in dyslexia has not given demonstrably useful information. However, brain electrical activity mapping (BEAM) has been presented as identifying areas of cerebral cortex significantly different with respect to electrophysiological dependent variables in dyslexics than control groups (Duffy et al., 1980a, 1980b). Although these might represent structural differences (in the left hemisphere language area and in both supplementary motor cortices), by their nature the dependent variables are not capable of distinguishing structurally abnormal from functionally deviantly utilized brain. We cannot tell from the data thus far whether the abnormalities represent brain-based differences in how the two groups of children approach tasks or even what they are thinking or feeling about during the test situation. These are not insoluble problems. Indeed, a fuller presentation of data already acquired might resolve them. They have not yet been solved, however.

Neuroradiological methods displaying anatomy are generally not subject to such reservations as they assess structure not function. One study using computerized tomography has claimed a substantial incidence of left lateral ventricular dilatation in a dyslexic group (Hier et al., 1978), but another study has failed to replicate this finding (Haslam et al., 1981). We should note that children come to CT-scan for clinical cause, and scanned dyslexics are far from being a random or representative sample of the dyslexic population. Given that developmental abnormality is suspected and left-handedness is supposed to be a risk factor for dyslexia, it becomes interesting to determine whether 'reversed asymmetry', namely, a reversal of the usual right anterior and left posterior predominance in brain size (LeMay, 1977), characterizes a substantial number of dyslexics. A preliminary report suggests that this may be so (Hier *et al.* 1978). Neuroradiological examination of function (positron emission tomography, regional cerebral blood flow estimation) might prove capable of identifying abnormal patterns of brain use in dyslexia, but they have not yet been applied to children. For this population, the methodology of nuclear magnetic resonance, which is free of radiation hazard, is more promising. For purposes of revealing brain function rather than structure (and for use in children), however, this method is still in the development phase. In summary, neuroradiological investigations open interesting leads, but do not yet settle the issues under discussion.

The left-handedness associated with reading failures (Zangwill, 1960) attracts much current interest. The pioneering finding of an association of immune disorders, left-handedness and dyslexia, is discussed by Geschwind elsewhere in this volume. We have findings supporting the existence of this phenomenon, and extending the relationship to families which include left-handers (Kinsbourne, 1986). Whether familial sinistrality indexes a *specific* subgroup of dyslexics or whether the association with left-handedness contributes a general risk factor for cognitive deficit is unclear.

A possible association between left-handedness and a dyslexia subtype has recently been expored by Satz and his colleagues. They have applied to the problem the concept of pathological left-handedness (Satz, 1972). This proposes that a subset of left-handers represents genotypic dextrals who have assumed left-hand preference on account of minor early left hemisphere damage involving areas of right-hand motor control. This hypothesized damage could also be responsible for left hemisphere malfunction involving the cognitive underpinning of language and learning ability. They have compiled some intriguing case study material which could be interpreted as relating the developmental Gerstmann syndrome to this particular pathogenesis. Kinsbourne and Warrington (1963) had been struck by the profusion of minor neurological abnormalities in the Gerstmann cases, in contrast to their absence in the language subtype. Satz and his colleagues have explored the possibility that mild but measurable underdevelopment of right-sided body parts (hands and feet) identify pathological left-handedness (Satz *et al.*, submitted). Bishop (1984) identifies clumsiness of the non-preferred hand as indicating pathological handedness.

The pathological left-handedness syndrome is one of a number of constructs relating at least some subset of dyslexia to an impairment of left hemisphere function. In general, neuropsychological testing that treats these children as a single group finds left rather than right hemisphere disability. Thus, Gordon, using a battery of tests validated on patients with lateralized structural brain damage, found his dyslexic group to be relatively deficient on tests that in the clinical context detect damage of the left hemisphere. He even found evidence that dyslexic children were superior on right hemisphere tests (Gordon, 1983). Whether this apparent trade-off will have to be considered in any valid model of the dyslexic disorder, or whether it represents the results of sampling bias, remains to be determined.

A non-invasive and widely applicable methodology for determining a hemispheric basis for dyslexia involves the use of laterality tests. In most cases, they have been applied to unselected groups of dyslexic children. In some cases, the subtype distinction was incorporated in the design.

Laterality testing demonstrates whether one hemisphere is more active than the other during the performance of the laterality task. Hemisphere specialization provides the structural basis for the effect. Its mechanism involves selective activation of the hemisphere that subserves the problem solving mode chosen by the subject. The activated hemisphere is a more efficient processor, bestowing a processing advantage on input from the contralateral side of space (Kinsbourne and Hiscock, 1983). Thus, in a normally functioning right-hander, hemifield viewing and dichotic listening for verbal material yield a right-sided superiority. For certain nonverbal materials, the superiority is left-sided.

A number of studies have shown no deviation from the normally expected laterality pattern in samples of reading-disabled children. Some studies have found lack of right-side advantage for verbal material. A few have found the opposite: an enhanced right-sided advantage (Satz, 1976). The deviant patterns found in these studies will be considered with reference to the possible models for the dyslexic disability.

(1) The left hemisphere is structurally inadequate.
(2) Language is not lateralized, but bisymetrically distributed between the hemispheres.
(3) Language is right lateralized.
(4) Language is left lateralized, but overlapped by bilateral spatial functions.
(5) Language is right lateralized and overlapped by spatial functions.

To these structural lateralization variants, we add selective activation variants.

(6) Selective activation of the left hemisphere in task-related circumstances is inadequate.
(7) Selective activation appropriate to the left hemisphere spreads bilaterally.
(8) Selective activation is anomalously diverted to the right side.

Variant 1 currently relies largely on the work of Geschwind and collaborators. Variant 2 was hypothesized by Orton and supported by Lenneberg's (1967) notion of progressive lateralization: the bisymmetric language state in this theory represents a developmental immaturity. Variant 3 is the situation found in some left-handers. Variant 4 and 5 represent hemisphere 'crowding' hypotheses as suggested by Levy (1969) and Witelson (1977). The activation models are based on the attentional model of laterality effects (Kinsbourne, 1970, 1975), adapted by Kinsbourne (1980) to explain laterality findings and ease of recovery of language function in non right-handers with cerebral lesions.

As we already remarked, model 1 is feasible but requires further documentation. Model 2 loses appeal in view of the refutation of the progressive lateralization hypothesis in favor of invariant lateralization (Kinsbourne and Hiscock, 1977, 1983). Some findings do show a failure of laterality effects for verbal material to arise, consistent with this model, but also consistent with model 7. Variant 3 lacks support. Variants 6, 7, and 8 are alternative to structural hypotheses in explaining the diminution of lateral asymmetries for verbal material found in some studies of dyslexic children and more consistently where there is frank development language delay.

In two studies, laterality tests were analyzed with respect to subtype. In one, the expected lack of right-sided advantage for verbal material was found in the language subtype, but the usual right-sided advantages prevailed in the sequential (Gerstmann) subtype (Pirozzolo, 1979). As the verbal test taps the verbal deficiency in the language subtype, the lack of asymmetry is not unexpected. In the Gerstmann type, specifically linguistic processes are unaffected (Kinsbourne and Warrington, 1964). The sequential ordering difficulty obtains both verbal and non-verbal information. Thus a verbal dichotic test would not be expected to yield abnormal results.

Dalby and Gibson (1981) classified their sample of backward readers into dysphonetic, dyseidetic, and nonspecific. Respectively, these yielded no perceptual asymmetry, asymmetry only for spatial tests, and asymmetry only for verbal tests. Malatesha and Aaron (1982) found the expected asymmetry for dyseidetics but none for dysphonetics. Bakker and his colleagues (Bakker, 1979; Bakker et al., 1980) interpreted their laterality findings as indicating two subtypes, involving right and left hemisphere deficiencies respectively. Diverse as these findings are, there is a common thread of *lack of right-sided advantage for verbal material* in these dyslexics with evidence of language disorder. This is consistent with the findings of no asymmetry for verbal processing by children with frank language disorder (Rosenblum and Dorman, 1978).

The alternative approach to the hemisphere basis of dyslexia is to determine any deviation in cognitive style. Some evidence for a tendency toward a nonverbal (right hemisphere) style in reading disabled children has been found (Caplan and Kinsbourne, 1981; Oexle and Zenhausern, 1981). In the former study, the stylistic deviation was found in the presence of normal laterality on dichotic listening tests.

In summary, the laterality data so far do not resolve the choice between the alternative models for the brain basis of dyslexia. The data that exist are consistent with underutilization of the left hemisphere in some cases but it is unclear whether this is based on defective structure or insufficient use of intact structure. In other cases, the laterality evidence for general hemispheric abnormality of use is absent, suggesting a more limited dysfunction not involving the whole hemisphere.

The choice of model for the brain basis of dyslexia could have some impact on the resolution of another basic question: does the dyslexic function in a manner qualitatively or only quantitatively different from normal? The quantitative alternative can be subdivided into two further hypotheses: the dyslexic functions like an equal age normal who is not trying hard (cf. the underactivation models) or like a younger normal child (underdevelopment models). Early attempts to identify diagnostic error types in reading and writing (Orton, 1937; Critchley, 1970) have not found support. The most recent claim for a qualitative difference is by Boder and Jarrico (1982), who hold spelling to be disproportionately disadvantaged in both their subtypes of dyslexia. But even an imbalance theory such as that of Boder and Jarrico (1982) can be reduced to a quantitative formulation in terms of weakness in an individual cognitive system with compensatory readjustment. A selective cognitive weakness, such as in phonologial analysis, might leave the child with an imbalance between that and other systems, causing changes in strategy leading to outcomes not found normally at any stage of development. But the nature of the change *within* the affected cognitive system could conform to one of the quantitative models. So we ask, does the affected system operate immaturely or weakly? *Weak* performance could be simulated by a normal learner of reading who is paying limited attention, perhaps because he is time-sharing this performance with another one. Thus weak or unstable left hemisphere activation might render the learner vulnerable to frequent changes in mental set, deviating from the task at hand to other types of data processing, that are the responsibility of better-activated parts of brain. Gordon's report of dyslexic children's superiority on right hemisphere tasks could be explained in this way, as could the above-mentioned preliminary findings of a relatively nonverbal cognitive style in dyslexic children. Immature performance would call for different types of observation altogether. The delays (and presumed immature) reader should set about the task of learning to read under the handicap of the same constraints that would limit a much younger normal child's efforts to learn the same skill. What, then, characterizes the learning performance of a young child who is not yet 'ready' to learn to read? We cannot answer this question directly, as it has not been addressed in this way. But we can describe principles of mental maturation, and conclude from these what type of observations future research into this issue would attempt to make.

NORMAL MENTAL DEVELOPMENT

Among the momentous changes humans experience in the first five years of their life, none is as dramatic as their acquisition of mental skills. From a helpless organism lacking flexibility of mental resource, there emerges an individual so mentally skilled that many child developmentalists lose interest in changes still to occur before brain maturation is complete. Yet, the principles that control the nature of that development in the major domains of perception, language, memory, reasoning, and skill are parsimonious and have much in common.

If the human mind contains 'modules' that serve distinct special purposes (such as the ones listed), we must admit that they are organized in similar ways.

The newborn child's sensory equipment falls little short of complete development. Within a few months, color vision will develop and depth perception parallel that of the adult. Visual acuity and the extent of the visual fields are already fully elaborated at birth. In the acoustic domain, the newborn is still more advanced, not only in pure tone acuity, but also in discriminating speech sounds. Only the less crucial ability to localize sound sources awaits further development. Although his musculature is small, the newborn already commands a full repertoire of muscles. Thus, we cannot explain the newborn's gross limitation of behavioral control at the sensory motor level.

What develops in mental development? Not sensory receptors nor control over individual muscles; rather, the ability to use the sensory motor equipment to adaptive purpose; advance not in seeing but in purposeful listening; advance in the finer differentiation of movement and flexible combination of movement patterns, rather than in the ability to move at all.

Newborn perception is tied to salient input—vivid colors and interesting shapes, such as faces. When it would be more useful to detach attention and take note of less salient aspects of the environment, then this the infant cannot do. His perceptual controls are preprogrammed to give priority to certain aspects of the environment, when present. Only when vivid and salient impressions are absent can the infant reveal his impressively wide range of perceptual skills.

In movement, the infant is similarly constrained. He has available basic coordinated movements patterns (synergisms), which are adaptively useful— sucking, swallowing, breathing, coughing, startle, and sidewards orienting. To use implicated muscles individually or in alternative combination is beyond the infant's ability.

The growing child becomes more able to distribute his attention flexibly, in response to the situation, rather than in hardwired stereotyped fashion. Nevertheless, preschoolers still are attentionally unskilled (not through want of practice, but for lack of the appropriately differentiated neuronal substrate). They survey displays incompletely, redundantly, and unsystematically. Only part of the display is inspected; that is, the child may inspect several times without gaining further information. The next time he may scan from quite a different direction. This deficiency handicaps the child's acquisition of knowledge that depends not on a single distinctive stimulus, but upon a pattern or set of relationships. In the auditory realm, the child, very capable of discriminating words, or isolated speech sounds, cannot analyze them into their constituent speech sounds (until the age of 7 in most children).

In the course of motor development, the child becomes able to override primitive synergisms and to move one joint without also moving several others. The grip is an example. At first, all five fingers flex together. At around 8 months comes the inferior palmar grasp: the thumb is opposed to the four fingers. Only at age 1 year does the child use pincer grip—opposing index and thumb selectively. This is accomplished by simultaneously inhibiting the associated synergic flexion of the three unwanted fingers. Synergisms continue to fragment well beyond the preschool years. They become fewer and less overt, at least through the first decade. They never disappear completely. Rather, the mature nervous system holds them in inhibitory abeyance, permitting them expression only at extremes of muscular exertion.

The same principles characterize the development of language in the preschool child. Speech initially amounts to naming that at which the child looks and points. Over time, the child can name without pointing, increase the number of words in his utterance, use increasingly complex syntactical forms, and use words as labels for present and remembered experience. By the end of the preschool period, he has only begun to use words in support of creative thinking.

Development in the function of memory depends on the above changes. We remember that to which we attend, and the more efficient and relevant the pattern of attention, the more likely is the experience subsequently to return to mind. When verbal labeling becomes available, this also serves as a 'retrieval cue', further facilitating not only the coding of information but also its recollection. The ability to remember episodes from previous experience is not present from the start, but develops to the extent permitted by the differentation of perceptual and linguistic skills.

Finally, in reasoning, the same organization of development obtains. Given problems, initially children are tied to the first solution that comes to mind, whether it is right or wrong, that is, the most obvious or salient solution. As mental maturation progresses, it is possible for a child to inhibit an obvious but incorrect response, and instead to entertain decreasingly probable solutions which, however, might be more apt. This ability to withhold familiar and attempt unfamiliar responses becomes progressively more possible through childhood (and is the quality which, when most developed, best characterizes the individual with brilliance).

When children experience developmental delay in any of the major domains of mental growth, the form that that deficiency takes can generally be predicted from a knowledge of principles of normal mental development. Within the realm of his impairment, the child functions like a younger normal child.

REMEDIAL IMPLICATIONS OF PRINCIPLES
OF MENTAL DEVELOPMENT

Basing our perception of learning disability on a developmental model, we assume that the patients may be experiencing limitations in learning comparable to those experienced by younger normal children (Kinsbourne, 1973). Our procedure should take this into account, as follows:

(1) Instruction is individual, to maintain the child's attention.
(2) Potentially distracting stimulation is limited.
(3) Learning materials are graduated in difficulty.
(4) Learning materials contain no irrelevant features or decorations.
(5) At each level of difficulty, the skill is learned to the point of fluency before the next level is attempted.
(6) Within each level, additional units of information are phased in one by one. No new item is added unless response to existing items is totally correct.
(7) Length of instruction is determined by needs of child, not of administrative (as long as gains are made, no longer than attention is maintained).
(8) Learning is as 'nearly errorless' as possible. If the child makes an erroneous response, the form of questioning is changed lest the mistake become habitual
(9) Reinforcement is immediate and tangible.

An expanded account of these principles is to be found in Kinsbourne & Caplan, (1979).

REMEDIAL IMPLICATIONS OF
UNDERACTIVATION MODEL

Based on the notion that the child finds it hard to maintain verbal (left hemispheric) mental set, remediation can address both the child's shifting attention by behavioural means, and the selective hemisphere activation mechanisms themselves.

(1) Individual instruction can add external sources of activation to supplement those generated by the child. The teacher continually orients the child to the type of thinking called for by the task. Programmed instruction could serve the same purpose. Each item of information is 'overlearned' to the point of automaticity (at which categorical mental sets are no longer necessary for fluent performance).

(2) Some peripheral maneuvers hold promise of bolstering selective hemisphere activation. These are 'priming' manipulations such as contralateral head and eye turning (Lempert and Kinsbourne, 1982) or contralateral visual (Bakker and Vinke, 1985) or monaural (Bakker, 1979) stimulation. It is not currently clear how to vary the balance of hemispheric activation chemically. However, if reports of lateralization of catecholamine neurotransmitters that subserve left as compared to right hemisphere activation (Oke et al., 1978) are confirmed then a drug with sufficiently selective catecholaminergic properties could conceivably be used to help activate a flagging lateralized cognitive system.

The stage seems set for the systematic study of remedial techniques based on models of dyslexia that reflect what is known about brain function *today*.

REFERENCES

Bakker, D. J. (1970), Temporal order perception and reading retardation. In: Bakker, D. J., and Satz, P. (Eds.). *Specific reading Disability—Advances in theory and method*, Amsterdam, Rotterdam University Press.

Bakker, D. J. (1979), Hemispheric differences and reading strategies: two dyslexias? *Bulletin of the Orton Society* **29**, 84–100.

Bakker, D. J., Litcht, R., Kok, A., and Bouma, A. (1980), Cortical responses to word reading by right- and left-eared normal and reading-disturbed children. *Journal of Clinical Neuropsychology* **2**, 1–12.

Bakker, D. J. and Vinke, (1985), Effects of hemisphere-specific stimulation on brain activity and reading in dyslexia. *Journal of Experimental and Clinical Neuropsychology.* **5**, 505–525.

Bender, B., Fry, E., Pennington, B., Puck, M., Salbenblatt, J., and Robinson, A. (1983), Speech and language development in 41 children with sex chromosome anomalies. *Pediatrics* **71**, 262–267.

Bishop, D. M. V. (1984) Using non-preferred hand skill to investigate pathological left-handedness in an unselected population. *Developmental Medicine and Child Neurology*, **26**, 214–226.

Boder, E. (1973) Developmental dyslexia: A diagnostic approach based on three atypical reading–spelling patterns. *Developmental Medicine and Child Neurology*, **15**, 663–687.

Boder, E., and Jarrico, S. (1982), *The Boder Test of Reading–Spelling Patterns*. New York, Grune & Stratton.

Caplan, B., and Kinsbourne, M. (1981), Cerebral lateralization, preferred cognitive mode, and reading ability in normal children. *Brain and Language*, **14**, 349–370.

Critchley, M. (1970), *The Dyslexic Child*. London, Heinemann.

Dalby, J. T., and Gibson, D. (1981), Functional cerebral lateralization in subtypes of disabled readers. *Brain and Language*, **14**, 34–48.

Denckla, M. B. (1977), Minimal brain dysfunction and dyslexia: beyond diagnosis by exclusion. In: Blaw, M. E., Rapin, I., and Kinsbourne, M. (Eds.), *Topics in Child Neurology*. New York, Spectrum Publications.

Doehring, D. G., and Hoshko, I. M. (1977), Classification of reading problems by the Q-technique of factor analysis. *Cortex* **13**, 281–294.

Duffy, F., Denckla, M., Bartels, P., Sandini, G., and Kiessling, A. (1980a), Dyslexia: Regional differences in brain electrical activity by topographic mapping. *Annals of Neurology* **7**, 5, 412–419.

Duffy, F., Denckla, M., Bartels, P., Sandini, G., and Kiessling, A. (1980b), Dyslexia: Automated diagnosis by computerized classification of brain electrical activity. *Annals of Neurology* **7**, 421–428.

Fisk, J. L., and Rourke, B. P. (1979), Identification of subtypes of learning disabled children at three age levels: a neuropsychological, multivariate approach. *Journal of Clinical Neuropsychology* **2**, 23–37.

Friedrich, U., Dalby, M., Staehelin-Jensen, T., and Bruun-Petersen, G. (1982), Chromosomal studies of children with developmental language retardation. *Developmental Medicine and Child Neurology* **24**, 645–652.

Galaburda, A. M., and Kemper, T. L. (1979), Cytoarchitectonic abnormalities in developmental dyslexia: a case study. *Annals of Neurology* **6**, 94–100.

Gordon, H. W. (1983), The learning disabled are cognitively right. In: M. Kinsbourne (Ed.), *Topics in Learning Disabilities*, Vol. 3. pp. 48–65. London,

Haslam, R. H., Dalby, J. T., Johns, R. D., and Rademaker, A. W. Cerebral asymmetry in developmental dyslexia. *Archives of Neurology* **38**, 679–682.

Hermann, K., and Norrie, E. (1958), Is congenital word blindness a hereditary type Gerstmann syndrome? *Psychiatrica et Neurologia* **1136**, 59–73.

Hier, D., LeMay, M., Rosenberger, P., and Perlo, V. P. (1978), Developmental dyslexia: evidence of a subgroup with a reversal of cerebral asymmetry. *Archives of Neurology* **35**, 90–92.

Hinshelwood, J. (1900), *Letter-word and Mind Blindness*. London, H. K. Lewis.

Kemper, T. L. Asymmetrical lesions in dyslexia. In: Geschwind, N. and Galaburda, A. M. (Eds.) *Cerebral Dominance*, Cambridge, Mass, Harvard University Press.

Kimberling, W. J., Pennington, B. F., and Lubs, H. A. (1983), Specific reading disability: identification of an inherited form through linkage analysis. *Science*, **219**, 1345–1347.

Kinsbourne, M. (1970), The cerebral basis of lateral asymmetries in attention. In: Sanders, A. F. (Ed.), *Attention and Performance*, Vol. 3. Amsterdam, North Holland.

Kinsbourne, M. (1973), Minimal brain dysfunction as a neurodevelopmental lag. *Annals of the New York Academy of Sciences* **205**, 263–273.

Kinsbourne, M. (1975), The mechanism of hemispheric control of the lateral gradient of attention. In: Rabbitt, P. M. A. and Dornic, S. (Eds.), *Attention and Performance*, Vol. 5. London, Academic Press.

Kinsbourne, M. (1980), A model for the ontogeny of cerebral organization in non-righthanders. In: Herron, J. (Ed.), *Neuropsychology of Left Handedness*. New York, Academic Press.

Kinsbourne, M. (1986), Relationship between left-handedness and diseases of the immune system. Paper to the annual meeting of the International Neuropsychological Society, Denver, Colorado.

Kinsbourne, M., and Caplan, P. (1979), Children's learning and attention problems. Boston, Little, Brown.

Kinsbourne, M., and Hiscock, M. (1977), Does cerebral dominance develop? In: S. J. Segalowitz and F. A. Gruber (Eds.), *Language Development and Neurological Theory*, New York, Academic Press.

Kinsbourne, M., and Hiscock, M. (1983) Functional lateralization of the brain: implications for normal and deviant development. In: Mussen, P., Haith, M., and Campos, J. (Eds.), *Handbook of Child Psychology*, 4th edn, Vol. 2, Ch. 4. New York, Wiley.

Kinsbourne, M., and Warrington, E. (1963), Developmental factors in reading and writing backwardness. *British Journal of Psychology* **54**, 145–156.

Kinsbourne, M., and Warrington, E. (1964), Disorders of spelling. *Journal of Neurology, Neurosurgery and Psychiatry* **27**, 224–228.

LeMay, M. (1977), Asymmetries of the skull and handedness: phrenology revisited. *Journal of Neurological Science* **32**, 243–253.

Lempert, H., and Kinsbourne, M. Effects of laterality of orientation on verbal memory. *Neuropsychologia* **20**, 211–214.

Lenneberg, E. H. (1967), *Biological Foundations of Language*. New York, Wiley.

Levy, J. (1969), Possible basis for the evolution of lateral specialization of the human brain. *Nature* **224**, 614–615.

Lyon, G. R., and Watson, B. (1981), Empirically derived subgroups of learning disabled readers. *Journal of Learning Disabilities* **14**, 256–261.

Lyon, G. R., Reitta, S., Watson, B., Porch, B., and Rhodes, J. (1981). Selected linguistic and perceptual abilities of empirically derived subgroups of learning disabled readers. *Journal of School Psychology*, **19**, 152–166.

Malatesha, R. N., and Aaron, P. G. (Eds.) (1982), *Reading Disorders: Varieties and Treatments*. New York, Academic Press.

Mattis, S. (1978), Dyslexia syndromes: a working hypothesis that works. In: Benton, A. L., and Pearl, D. (Eds.), *Dyslexia–An Appraisal of Current Knowledge*. New York, Oxford University Press.

Mattis, S., French, J., and Rapin, E. (1975), Dyslexia in children and young adults: three independent neuropsychological syndromes. *Developmental Medicine and Child Neurology* **17**, 150–163.

Myklebust, H. (1965), *Development and Disorders of Written Language*. Vol. 1. *Picture Story Language Test*. New York, Grune & Stratton.

Oexle, J. E., and Zenhausern, R. (1981), Differential hemispheric activation in good and poor readers. *International Journal of Neuroscience* **15**, 31–36.

Olson, R. K. Kliegl, R., Davidson, B. J., and Foltz, G. (submitted), Individual and developmental differences in reading disability. In: Waller, T. G. (Ed.), *Reading Research: Advances in Theory and Practice*. Academic Press.

Oke, A., Keller, R., Mefford, I., and Adams, R. N. (1978), Lateralization of norepinephrine in human thalamus. *Science* **200**, 1411–1413.

Orton, S. T. (1937), *Reading, Writing and Speech Problems in Children*. New York, Norton.

Pavlidis, G. Th. (1981), Do eye movements hold the key to dyslexia? *Neuropsychologia* **19**, 57–64.

Petrauskas, R. J., and Rourke, B. P. (1979), Identification of subtypes of retarded readers: a neuropsychological, multivariate approach. *Journal of Clinical Neuropsychology* **1**, 17–37.

Pirozzolo, F. J. (1979), *The Neuropsychology of Developmental Reading Disorders*. New York, Praeger.

Pirozzolo, F. J., and Rayner, K. (1980), Disorders of oculomotor scanning and graphic orientation in developmental Gerstmann syndrome, *Brain and Language* **5**, 119–126.

Rosenblum, D. R., and Dorman, M. F. (1978), Hemisphere specialization for speech perception in language deficient kindergarden children. *Brain and Language* **6**, 378–389.

Satz, P. (1972), Pathological left-handedness: An explanatory model, *Cortex*, **8**, 121–135.

Satz, P. (1976), Cerebral dominance and reading disability: an old problem revisited. In: Knights, R. M., and Bakker, D. J. (Eds.), *The Neuropsychology of Learning Disorders*. Baltimore, University Park Press.

Satz, P., and Morris, R. (1981), Learning disability subtypes: a review. In: Pirozzolo, F. J., and Wittrock M. C. (Eds.), *Neuropsychological and cognitive processes in reading*. New York, Academic Press.

Satz, P., Orsini, D., Saslow, E., and Henry, K. (submitted), The pathological left-handedness syndrome.

Tallal, P., and Piercy, M. (1973), Defects of nonverbal auditory perception in children with developmental aphasia. *Nature* **241**, 468–469.

Vellutino, F. R. (1979), *Dyslexia, Theory and Research*. Cambridge, Mass., MIT Press.

Witelson, S. E. (1977), Developmental dyslexia: two right hemispheres and none left. *Science*, **195**, 300–311.

Zangwill, O. (1960), *Cerebral Dominance and its Relation to Psychological Function*. London, Oliver & Boyd.

CHAPTER 13

Analysis of Subtypes of Specific Reading Disability: Genetic and Cluster Analytic Approaches

SHELLEY D. SMITH,[1] DAVID E. GOLDGAR,[1] BRUCE F. PENNINGTON,[2]
WILLIAM J. KIMBERLING,[1] and HERBERT A. LUBS[3]
[1]*Boys Town National Institute, Omaha, NE, USA*
[2]*University of Colorado Health Sciences Center, Denver, CO, USA*
[3]*University of Miami, Miami, FL, USA*

The understanding of specific reading disability has been hindered most by the lack of firm diagnostic criteria. There have been numerous definitions, particularly of the term dyslexia, which reflect the changing ideas about the underlying mechanism, and the different definitions each suggest different means of diagnosis. With uncertainty as to what the disorder is and who actually has it, it is not surprising that there have been conflicting views of what the characteristics and causes are. The most significant development in this field, as reviewed by Doehring *et al.* (1981), has been the recognition that reading disability is a heterogeneous disorder. Thus, the early conceptions of a unitary disorder with a laundry list of possible characteristics had been rejected, and the whole idea of a specific reading disability was in danger of being tossed out as well, until it was recognized that a complex process could be expected to be subject to many different types of interruptions. Since children with different types of reading disability may be expected to perform differently on a given measure, studies comparing 'good' and 'poor' readers, particularly with small sample sizes, were apt to be inconsistent, if not fruitless.

The problem now has become how to separate the subtypes of reading disability, so that homogeneous groups with the same characteristics can be studied and the underlying mechanisms and etiologies can be discovered. Subtyping has been done in three basic ways: intuitively, clinically, and statistically. Intuitive approaches have analysed the reading process for potential points of breakdown, and then looked for the types of disabled readers that should result. Examples of this are the auditory and visual types of Ingram *et al.* (1970) and Johnson and Myklebust (1964), and in the development of the left hemisphere strategy vs. right hemisphere strategy subtypes defined by Bakker *et al.* (1976).

In the clinical approach, subtypes have been grouped by examination of performance on a given test or battery of tests. One of the first to do this was Boder (1970, 1973) who grouped disabled readers according to their pattern of spelling errors. Mattis *et al.* (1975) distinguished three types of disabled readers based on neuropsychological characteristics, and there have been many other such subtyping systems (see Doehring *et al.*, 1981). Finally, several studies have used statistical methods rather than clinical judgement to group disabled readers by performance on any number and type of tests. Methods such as cluster analysis or the Q-technique of factor analysis define subgroups that are mathematically the most homogeneous (Doehring and Hoshko, 1977; Satz and Morris, 1981; Lyon *et al.*, 1982; Watson *et al.*, 1983). All of these methods have certain problems. The intuitive and clinical methods are dependent upon the underlying hypotheses and biases of the investigator. The statistical methods will create subgroups out of any data set, so the subgroups must be validated as being consistent and distinct (see Watson *et al.*, 1983), and caution must be used in presuming underlying biological or etiological differences between subgroups. With any of these approaches, a further problem has been the inability to compare studies to see if some may be describing different aspects of the same subgroups.

Genetic studies of reading disability have essentially paralleled the development of the field as a whole. In the early 1900s it was recognized that dyslexia was sometimes familial, and a positive family history was considered one of the many possible characteristics on the laundry list of possible findings. Although several case reports and a few studies supported autosomal dominant inheritance (Hallgren, 1950; Drew, 1956; Brewer, 1963; Zahalkova *et al.*, 1972), this clearly did not explain all cases, and familial occurrence could also be explained by environmental transmission. More recent family studies have supported the idea of genetic heterogeneity in specific reading disability, meaning that among the possible causes of reading disability are genetic types with different modes of inheritance. Finucci *et al.* (1976), examined individual family histories of disabled readers and found that they were not consistent with any one mode of inheritance. Lewitter *et al.* (1980) utilized statistical methods to find evidence of dominant and recessive subtypes, and DeFries and Decker (1982) described further statistical results consistent with a major (dominant) gene in some families. The task remains to validate these findings and to see if subgroups defined by mode of inheritance have consistent and distinguishing characteristics. Presumably, if a test is measuring an attribute that is directly related to a given genetic etiology, all individuals with the same genetic make-up should have the same findings on that test. On measures that are farther removed from the basic defect, however, performance between individuals may be quite different, owing to modification by environment or other genes.

There have been various ways to examine the genetic contributions to learning abilities. The first studies examined within-family correlations on cognitive measures, including those involved in reading (Foch *et al.*, 1977). While this information is important in establishing a potential genetic influence, this methodology does not define a mode or modes of inheritance or subgroups. Later studies developed subgrouping systems, and then looked for genetic factors. Decker and DeFries (1981) described four subgroups of disabled readers based on the values of three factors derived from a large battery of tests, and then looked for familial consistency of subtype classification. One subtype did show more of a tendency for consistency of subtype classification among siblings. Omenn and Weber (1978) also found familial consistency for type of spelling error (phonetic vs. dysphonetic) and Finucci (1978) reported familial consistency for the proportion of dysphonetic spelling errors.

Another approach would be to identify subgroups on the basis of genetic characteristics and then see which measures show consistency within the genetic subgroups. This is analogous to the cognitive studies of children with sex chromosome aneuploidy, in which the phenotype for the different karyotypes is being determined (Robinson *et al.*, 1979). In the case of reading disability, this could be done by defining a population with a given mode of inheritance. However, since a pattern of transmission in a family could occur by coincidence or environmental transmission, an additional criterion is needed to insure that the families identified actually manifest a genetic influence. As an example of this, our own studies have utilized the technique of linkage analysis to identify an autosomal dominant gene with an influence on reading disability.

Two genes are said to be linked when they are located close together on a chromosome such that recombination between them is decreased. In contrast, unlinked gene loci (either on different chromosomes or far apart on the same chromosome) show free recombination, that is, maternally and paternally derived genes are equally likely to be transmitted to the next generation. Mendel's experiments with peas were the first to demonstrate the free recombination of unlinked traits, where the traits 'wrinkled vs. smooth' seeds were compared with 'yellow vs. green' seed color. A cross of plants with wrinkled/green seeds with those with smooth/yellow seeds resulted in equal combinations of the four types of seeds; the two parental types and the two recombinant types, wrinkled/yellow and smooth/green. If the loci had been linked, there would be an overabundance of the parental types at the expense of recombinant types. Linkage, then, is detected by looking at the distribution of traits among offspring from a given mating. The likelihood that the resultant offspring could be produced by chance is compared with the likelihood that the distribution could be produced by linkage at several distances. The log of these odds is taken and the resultant 'lod scores' are computed. A lod score of at least 3.0 (odds 1000:1 favoring linkage) are required before linkage can be accepted, and then it must be replicated by a separate study. A lod score of −2.0 (100:1 against linkage) refutes the hypothesis of linkage.

If two genes are found to be linked, the inference may be made that they are on the same chromosome. (Alternative explanations such as association and disequilibrium must be ruled out.) In this way, if a disorder is found to be linked to a known genetic trait, the disorder may be presumed to be influenced by a gene linked to the known trait. Further, if a group of different families show different linkage results, such as some families showing linkage of the disorder to a given gene, and other families showing non-linkage with that gene or linkage of the disorder to a different gene, genetic heterogeneity can be detected (that is, that two separate genes or mechanisms can produce the same phenotype) (Morton, 1956).

Linkage studies are generally performed by comparing the inheritance of the disorder in question to the inheritance patterns of a variety of known genetic traits, termed markers. If the gene influencing the disorder is located close to the gene for one of the marker traits, a positive linkage will result. The more marker genes that are available, scattered throughout the chromosomes, the more likely the possibility will be that one of them will happen to be linked to the disorder.

For this study, the linkage studies were performed between specific reading disability and a battery of known genetic traits. For the corresponding phenotype analysis, the participating family members were also given a battery of achievement and neuropsychological tests to see if there was consistency of subtype within and between families. Subtypes were defined in three different ways: on the basis of spelling errors, using an adaptation of the criteria of Boder (1973) and newly developed criteria (Pennington et al., 1983); using neuropsychological tests to replicate the work of Mattis et al. (1975) and Mattis (1978); and using cluster analysis.

The ascertainment and diagnosis of subjects in these studies has been reported elsewhere (Smith et al., 1983a, 1983b) but will be reviewed here for clarity.

Families were solicited from parents' groups and special schools for the learning disabled, and through referral from educators and other professionals. They had to fit the following criteria: a history of specific reading disability in three generations of one side of a family in an autosomal dominant pattern; Verbal or Performance IQ on Weschler or equivalent test of at least 90 for all members; native English-speaking; and both biological parents and at least two children over age 7 had to be available for study.

The criteria of apparent autosomal dominant transmission was used because such families would be the only ones in which linkage, if present, could be found. This would not constitute a bias towards finding linkage, since the families were not selected with knowledge of the segregation of any of the genetic markers used in the linkage analysis. The IQ and ethnic criteria, along with the later testing criteria, were used to insure that the family members actually manifested a specific reading disability, without other possible causes. This is not to say that reading disability cannot co-exist with other factors such as low SES, bilingualism, or decreased IQ; however, for this study, we wished to maximize the probability that the cause of RD in these families was genetic.

If the family history met these criteria, all family members were asked to take a series of achievement tests which included the Peabody Individual Achievement Tests (PIAT) (Dunn and Markwardt, 1970), the Gray Oral Reading Test (Robinson, 1963), and the spelling subtest of the Wide Range Achievement Test (Jastak and Jastak, 1970), and the Colorado Perceptual Speed Test (Foch et al., 1977). Diagnosis of reading disability was dependent upon two criteria: testing results and historical information. For children, diagnosis as affected required a history of reading disability from the time reading was introduced and performance on the Gray Oral Reading Test at least two years below the mean grade level of the PIAT Mathematics and General Information scores. Similar criteria were used for adults; however, if an adult gave a history of early and persistent difficulty learning to read, but passed the tests, the possibility of compensation for an earlier ability was considered. In that case, the adult had to have an affected child and sibling or parent who could be documented to be affected. The compensated adult would then be an 'obligate carrier' of the putative gene.

If, after testing, family members could be classified as affected or unaffected and the pattern of transmission followed that of an autosomal dominant trait, the family was included in the linkage analysis and subtyping studies. Since the subtyping constituted a second phase of the study, not all families who were involved in the linkage analysis took the second battery of tests.

Linkage analysis involved the drawing of about 30 ml of blood from each participating family member. Twenty-one genotyping markers (blood and enzyme types) and Q- and C-band chromosomal heteromorphisms were determined. The inheritance of these markers was compared with the transmission of reading disability using the linkage program LIPED (Ott, 1974).

A total of 80 individuals from 9 families were included in the linkage analysis, and a maximum lod score of 3.241 at 13 per cent recombination was obtained with heteromorphisms of chromosome 15 (Smith et al., 1983a, 1983b). The heteromorphisms in this case were variations in fluorescent intensity of the short arm and satellite regions of chromosome 15 as seen with Q-banding, or variations in the size of the centromeric and short arm heterochromatin as seen with C-banding. These are presumed to be normal variations without clinical significance, and different families had different fluorescent or C-band variations segregating with the reading disability. That is, there was no relationship between level of fluorescence and reading disability *between* families. Thus, the

Table 1. Neuropsychological test battery

Mattis System
  Language Disorder
    Boston Naming Test (E. Kaplan, H. Goodglass, S. Weintraub)
    Spreen–Benton Token Test
    Spreen–Benton Sentence Repetition Test
    Goldman–Fristoe–Woodcock Test of Auditory Discrimination
  Articulation and Graphomotor Dyscoordination
    Goldman–Fristoe–Woodcock Sound Blending Test
    Graphomotor Test (Mattis et al., 1975)
    Grooved Pegboard (Lafayette Instruments)
    Verbal and Nonverbal Oral Expression (H. Goodglass, E. Kaplan)
  Visuo-spatial Perceptual Disorder
    Raven's Progressive Matrices (adapted by Institute for Behavior Genetics, University of Colorado)
    Primary Mental Abilities Test of Spatial Rotation
  Weschler Adult Intelligence Scale (WAIS) or Weschler Intelligence Scale for Children-Revised (WISC-R)

Boder (1973) System
  Denver Reading and Spelling Test (B. Camp, L. McCabe)

---

heteromorphisms themselves are not causal or diagnostic of reading disability. Rather, the results suggest that a gene with a major influence on specific reading disability is located close to the variable region. Since the short arm of chromosome 15 is primarily involved in nucleolar organization, it is most likely that such a gene would be located on the proximal long arm.

The tests given for the analysis of subtypes were the Denver Reading and Spelling Test (DRST) (Camp and McCabe, unpublished), which was designed to replicate the classification system of Boder (1973), and adaptations of the neuropsychological tests given by Mattis et al. (1975, Table 1). On the basis of the neuropsychological tests, each subject was classified as showing the Language Disorder, Articulatory and Graphomotor Dyscoordination Disorder, Visuo-spatial Perceptual Disorder, Temporal Sequencing Disorder, or as Normal according to the criteria outlined in Mattis et al. (1975) and Mattis (1978). The DRST involved the oral reading of selected lists of 20 words at each grade level until a criterion of approximately 10 words missed was reached. The same 20 words were then dictated for spelling, and errors were scored as phonetic or non-phonetic by specific rules. Based on these scores, the individual's spelling pattern was classified as dysphonetic, dyseidetic, or normal.

Results of the Mattis and Boder subtyping systems have been reported elsewhere (Smith et al., 1983b; Pennington et al., 1983) and will be summarized here.

In all, 74 subjects from 12 families took the battery of tests for the classification study, although not all had complete tests. There were 46 affecteds and 27 unaffecteds, and one individual could not be diagnosed. The first phase involved the classification of subjects into one of the four Mattis *et al.* subtypes. Only 43 affecteds and 26 unaffecteds had sufficient data for classification. Of these, only 9 individuals were classified into any of the categories. Eight affected children fit the Language Disorder subtype, and one unaffected man fit the Articulatory and Graphomotor Dyscoordination subtype. The remaining subjects all had normal profiles.

Because of the wide age range in the study (7–69, mean 28.50), a more relaxed set of criteria were developed to classify individual profiles as 'suggestive' of a given subtype. Six more affecteds were classified as 'suggestive' of the Language Disorder; this included three adults and three children. One affected adult, one affected child, and one unaffected individual were classified as 'suggestive' of the Articulatory and Graphomotor Dyscoordination Disorder. Four affected children, one affected adult, and five unaffected individuals were suggestive of the Visual–spatial Perceptual Disorder. None of the subjects were classified in, nor were they suggestive of the Temporal Sequencing Disorder. The primary result of the relaxed criteria, then, was to ascertain additional affecteds in the Language Disorder subtype, which was not seen in any of the unaffecteds. For the other subtypes, affecteds and unaffecteds were fairly equally represented, implying that these findings were not related to reading disability.

Analysis of variance was performed on each test individually, comparing affecteds and unaffecteds with age and intelligence as covariates. Only three tests showed significant differences: the Boston Naming test, Auditory Discrimination in Noise, and the Digit Span subtest of the WISC-R or WAIS. To investigate if a more subtle cognitive profile existed which could differentiate the two groups, stepwise discriminant analysis was performed (Nie *et al.*, 1975) using only the neuropsychological variables. Using the variables Auditory Discrimination in Noise, Digit Span, Block Design, Picture Arrangement, Grooved Pegboard (non-dominant hand), and Object Assembly, this procedure correctly classified 78.1 per cent of the 65 individuals with sufficient data, with five false positives and 9 false negatives.

The DRST criteria resulted in the classification of 20 affecteds and 2 unaffecteds as dyseidetic. All other subjects were classified as normal.

The results of the attempted replication of the subtyping system of Mattis *et al.* (1975) have suggested either that the system was not appropriate for this population, or that the replication was inadequate. As reviewed by Pennington *et al.* (1983), the Boder (1973) system as assessed by the DRST also failed to classify many of the disabled readers, even when a subset with a valid test (e.g. no ceiling effect) was used. It may be that the theoretical basis of 'auditory' vs. 'visual' spelling errors (Boder, 1973) over-generalizes the complexity of the spelling problems in this population. When Pennington *et al.* (1983) classified spelling errors on the WRAT spelling test according to systems which took into account orthographic rules and strategies, and statistical analyses rather than clinical judgement were used to group subjects, the discrimination between affecteds and unaffecteds was much improved.

Although the neuropsychological tests did not replicate Mattis's findings, and individually did not show much difference between affecteds and unaffecteds, the success of the discriminant analysis suggested that there was an underlying structure which differed for the two groups. One possible explanation for the difference between the results of the ANOVA tests and the discriminant analysis could be that a specific cognitive pattern existed in some, but not all, of the disabled readers; that is, that there was heterogeneity among the disabled readers. This could obscure a subgroup with significant deficits on the neuropsychological tests when the analysis of variance procedure was used, but the discriminant analysis may have detected more subtle differences and used them to correctly classify at least some of the disabled readers. Moreover, since we are assuming that the affected individuals in this population are etiologically similar in that they share a gene that is affecting their reading ability, it is crucial that we determine if they are phenotypically similar. If there are distinct subgroups within the affecteds, it could mean either that the tests are measuring abilities that are too distant from the primary gene effect, or that the population, in fact, is not genetically homogeneous.

To evaluate this possibility, cluster analysis was performed to see if reliable, phenotypically distinct subgroups were present. The methods and results of this analysis are reported in this paper.

MATERIALS AND METHODS

Data from the subjects described above were used in the cluster analyses. The entire population of 74 subjects was used in the first analysis, and a second analysis was done using only the 46 affected individuals and one undiagnosed person. Data describing this population are shown in Table 2. The Ward hierarchical method (Ward, 1963) was used for preliminary identification of the number of clusters present in the data and to obtain an initial solution to be used as input to the BMDP K-Means cluster analysis program (Dixon et al., 1981). The program EVAL (Huizinga, 1977) was used for internal evaluation of the clusters produced. For a given set of clusters, this program computes a number of evaluative statistics, including gamma and cluster homogeneity. Gamma is a measure of the degree to which an obtained set of clusters approximates an 'ideal' set. An 'ideal' set of clusters is defined as one in which any two members of the same cluster are more similar than the most similar pair of subjects who are members of different clusters. Clusters which satisfy this criterion are termed a compact and well-separated set of clusters. The potential values of gamma range from -1.0 to $+1.0$. A value of $+1.0$ indicates that all pairs of subjects satisfy this criteria, while a value of -1.0 is obtained when no such pairs meet the criteria. Cluster homogeneity compares

Table 2. Description of the population with one-way analysis of variance

	Affecteds (n = 46)				Unaffecteds (n = 27)				F significance
	min.	max.	mean	sd	min.	max.	mean	sd	
V IQ	81.0	131.0	109.9	13.5	101.0	138.0	118.8	9.9	$p < 0.01$
P IQ	90.0	131.0	111.4	11.3	87.0	140.0	113.6	11.7	n.s.
FS IQ	89.0	131.0	111.6	11.6	93.0	142.0	123.1	10.5	$p < 0.05$
Age	9.42	69.00	25.55	16.00	7.00	69.00	33.65	16.94	$p < 0.05$
Math[a]	-1.27	2.33	0.38	0.87	-0.93	2.07	0.60	0.76	n.s.
R Rec.	-2.33	1.67	-0.59	0.87	-0.73	2.07	0.54	0.69	$p < 0.001$
R Comp.	-2.33	1.47	-0.23	0.97	-0.80	1.67	0.63	0.66	$p < 0.001$
Spell.	-2.33	2.33	-0.89	0.96	-1.73	2.33	0.86	1.14	$p < 0.001$
Gen. Inf.	-1.47	1.87	0.47	0.78	-0.87	2.09	0.51	0.85	n.s.
WRAT Sp.	-2.76	0.84	-1.00	0.84	-1.73	1.58	0.22	0.81	$p < 0.001$
Gray[b]	1.20	16.20	6.42	4.37	1.70	15.80	11.87	3.36	$p < 0.001$
P Spd[c]	-14.81	7.77	-2.97	5.56	-12.80	12.16	0.13	6.23	$p < 0.05$
RQ[d]	0.44	1.07	0.74	0.14	0.74	1.33	0.97	0.16	$p < 0.001$

[a] Means expressed as z-scores.
[b] Means expressed as grade equivalents.
[c] Age-adjusted scores.
[d] Ratio of reading and spelling achievement to expected achievement.

the variance of each cluster with the overall variance present in the data set. A value of $+1.0$ is reached if there is no variation among members of a cluster, while negative values indicate that the variance is greater within the clusters than for the population as a whole. In addition, clusters were compared on the basis of age, sex, IQ, the achievement tests given previously, and the reading quotient. This quotient, which is a measure of the severity of the reading disability relative to overall ability, was adapted from Finucci (1978). For children, this was computed as:

$$\frac{\text{(Gray Oral Reading age equiv.} + \text{WRAT Spelling age equiv.)}/2}{\text{(Chronological age} + \text{age for grade} + \text{IQ age equivalent)}/3}$$

For adults, it was computed as:

$$\frac{\text{(Gray Oral Reading age equiv.} + \text{PIAT Spelling age equiv.)}/2}{\text{(Age for last grade} + \text{Mathematics age equiv.} + \text{Gen. Info. age equiv.)}/3}$$

Fourteen variables for which complete data were available were used in the cluster analyses. These were the Boston Naming test, Sentence Repetition test, Auditory Discrimination in Noise and Quiet, Sound Blending, Graphomotor coordination, Grooved Pegboard with dominant and nondominant hands, Oral Expression Verbal and Non-Verbal, Visual Retention, and three factors derived from the Weschler subtests: Perceptual Organization (PO: Block Design and Object Assembly), Verbal Comprehension (VC: Information, Similarities, Vocabulary, Comprehension), and Freedom from Distraction (FD: Arithmetic, Digit Span) (Cohen, 1952).

RESULTS

The Ward hierarchical method begins with each subject as a separate cluster. At each subsequent step, the two groups are combined which results in the minimum within cluster sum of squares. This procedure is continued until all subjects belong to one cluster. If the combining of n groups into $n-1$ groups results in a relatively large increase in the within cluster sum of squares, it is indicative of n clusters present in the data set. A plot of the sum of squares versus the number of groups is often useful for identifying such increases.

When the entire population was used, the Ward hierarchical method produced the groupings as shown in Figure 1. In Figure 1, a change is noted between two and one groups, so the K-Means analysis was done for two groups. This solution formed two clusters of 47 and 27 individuals respectively. These are summarized in Table 3 and Figure 2. The first cluster was composed of 26 affected and 21 unaffected individuals. There were 24 males and 23 females in the cluster. As can be seen in Table 3 and Figure 2, performance on the test battery was mixed, with somewhat lower scores in Auditory Discrimination, Sound Blending, and the Oral Expression tests. The second cluster

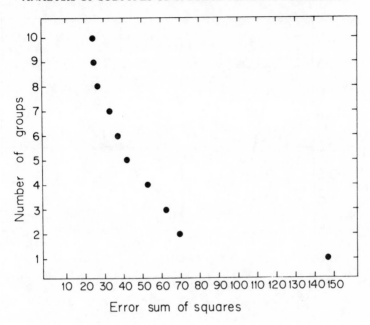

Figure 1. Results of Ward hierarchical analysis using the total population. The most evident change in the error sum of squares is seen with a two-cluster solution, which was then entered into the cluster analysis.

Table 3. Cluster mean scores for neuropsychological tests: affecteds and unaffecteds combined

Test	Cluster 1 ($n = 47$)	Cluster 2 ($n = 27$)	Significance
Boston Naming	0.31	−0.71	$p < 0.001$
Sentence Rep.	1.11	−0.47	$p < 0.001$
Auditory Discrim.			
Quiet	−0.33	−0.21	n.s.
Noise	−0.11	−0.75	$p < 0.01$
Sound Blending	−0.05	−0.59	$p < 0.001$
Graphomotor	0.38	−0.09	$p < 0.05$
Pegboard			
Dominant	0.36	−0.83	$p < 0.001$
Nondominant	0.52	−1.02	$p < 0.001$
Oral Expression			
Verbal	−0.02	−0.04	n.s.
Nonverbal	−0.03	0.25	n.s.
Visual Retention	1.23	0.21	$p < 0.001$
PO	0.72	0.29	$p < 0.001$
VC	1.23	0.21	$p < 0.001$
FD	0.45	−0.23	$p < 0.001$

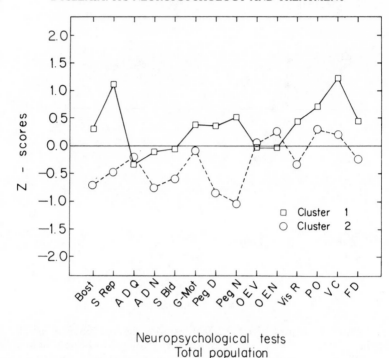

Neuropsychological tests
Total population

Figure 2. Comparison of the cluster mean scores on the neuropsychological battery.

Table 4. Cluster mean scores on achievement tests: total population

Test	Cluster 1 ($n = 47$)	Cluster 2 ($n = 27$)	Significance
PIAT Math[a]	0.72	0.01	$p < 0.001$
PIAT Reading Rec.	0.15	−0.72	$p < 0.001$
PIAT Reading Comp.	0.43	−0.49	$p < 0.001$
PIAT Spelling	0.11	−0.84	$p < 0.01$
PIAT Gen. Info.	0.73	0.06	$p < 0.001$
WRAT Spelling	−0.31	−0.94	$p < 0.01$
Gray Oral[b]	10.55	4.20	$p < 0.001$
Percept. Speed[c]	−1.55	−2.18	n.s.
RQ[d]	0.86 (−0.95)	0.81 (−1.27)	n.s.

[a] Means expressed as z-scores.
[b] Means expressed as grade equivalents.
[c] Age-adjusted scores.
[d] Ratio of reading and spelling achievement to expected achievement (converted to z-score with mean 1.0 and sd 0.15 for Figure 3).

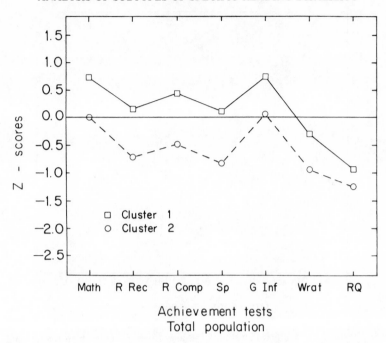

Achievement tests
Total population

Figure 3. Comparison of the cluster mean scores on the achievement and intelligence tests.

contained 20 affecteds and 6 unaffecteds and one unclassified male, and was made up of 18 males and 9 females. Overall, test performance was lower on all tests, with lowest scores on the same tests that were deficient in cluster 1, with the exception of the Pegboard (dominant) test. In addition, cluster 2 showed lower IQ scores on all three of the Weschler factors. There was no difference in age between clusters.

The clusters were also compared on the basis of their achievement test scores (Table 4; Figure 3). Cluster 2 mean scores were significantly lower on all tests except Perceptual Speed and the reading quotient. Interestingly, the reading quotient is the only measure that controls for IQ or overall ability.

Most importantly, tests for the internal evaluation of the clusters indicated that the clusters were not well separated or homogeneous. The value of gamma for three clusters was found to be -0.9682. Since a gamma of -1.0 indicates that members of different clusters are as alike as members of the same cluster, this statistic clearly indicates that there is little that distinguished the two clusters. The cluster homogeneity for cluster 1 was 0.221, and for cluster 2 was 0.022. This indicates considerable within-cluster variance. Thus both clusters were spread fairly wide and were fairly heterogeneous, with cluster 2 showing the most heterogeneity.

Cluster analysis was then performed using the same 14 variables, but only for the 46 affecteds and one undiagnosed individual. The results of the Ward

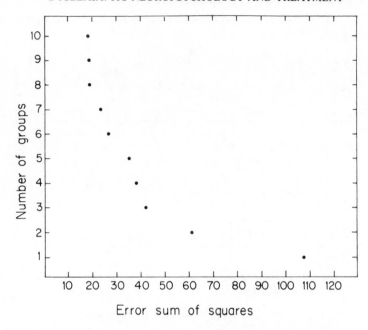

Figure 4. Results of the Ward hierarchical analysis using the disabled readers only. In this sample, a three-cluster solution was indicated.

Table 5. Cluster mean scores for neuropsychological test: affecteds only

Test	Cluster 1 ($n = 17$)	Cluster 2 ($n = 12$)	Cluster 3 ($n = 18$)	Significance
Boston Naming	−0.11	−1.26	0.06	$p < 0.01$
Sentence Rep.	1.15	−0.77	0.38	$p < 0.001$
Auditory Discrim.				
Quiet	−0.64	−0.71	0.15	$p < 0.05$
Noise	−0.51	−1.59	−0.16	$p < 0.001$
Sound Blending	−0.67	−0.73	0.19	$p < 0.001$
Graphomotor	−0.27	−0.02	0.88	$p < 0.001$
Pegboard				
Dominant	0.28	−1.06	0.14	$p < 0.01$
Nondominant	0.38	−1.56	0.18	$p < 0.001$
Oral Expression				
Verbal	0.14	−0.18	0.08	n.s.
Nonverbal	0.19	0.14	−0.10	n.s.
Visual Retention	0.67	−0.70	0.16	$p < 0.001$
PO	1.21	0.29	0.52	$p < 0.001$
VC	1.34	−0.17	0.56	$p < 0.001$
FD	0.55	−0.22	−0.30	$p < 0.001$

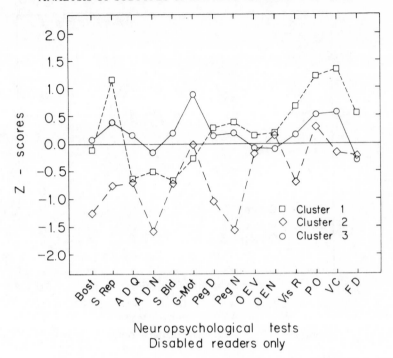

Figure 5. Comparison of the cluster mean scores on the neuropsychological battery: disabled readers only.

hierarchical test are shown in Figure 4. The best choice appeared to be for a three-cluster solution. The three clusters that were produced contained 17, 12, and 18 members respectively. These are summarized in Table 5 and Figure 5. These clusters were similar to those obtained in the analysis of the entire population, in that the second cluster showed general weakness in all tests, with the first and third clusters showing a variety of strengths and weaknesses, similar to that seen in cluster 1 of the previous analysis.

Internal evaluation of the clusters again showed considerable heterogeneity within clusters, with gamma equal to -0.9722 and cluster homogeneities of 0.227, 0.118, and 0.294 for clusters 1, 2, and 3 respectively. Cluster 2 showed the most heterogeneity. In addition, there was no consistency within family for cluster assignment, and no significant age or sex differences between clusters.

The means of the achievement tests and reading quotient for each of the clusters of affected individuals are shown in Table 6 and Figure 6. As is evident, there is no difference in the achievement profiles of the three clusters, with differences only in the severity of the reading scores. There were no significant differences in the RQs, indicating that the severity of the reading problems

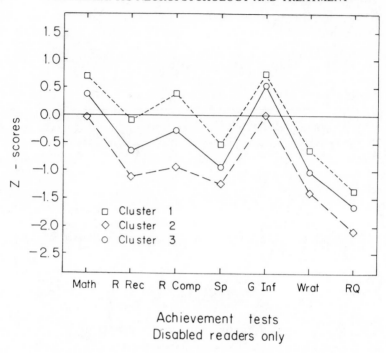

Figure 6. Comparison of the cluster mean scores on the achievement and intelligence tests: disabled readers only.

Table 6. Cluster mean scores on achievement tests: affecteds only

Test	Cluster 1 ($n = 17$)	Cluster 2 ($n = 12$)	Cluster 3 ($n = 18$)	Significance
PIAT Math[a]	0.70	−0.04	0.37	n.s.
PIAT Reading Rec.	−0.10	−1.12	−0.66	$p < 0.01$
PIAT Reading Comp.	0.39	−0.94	−0.29	$p < 0.001$
PIAT Spelling	−0.53	−1.24	−0.94	n.s.
PIAT Gen. Info.	0.74	0.01	0.53	$p < 0.01$
WRAT Spelling	−0.63	−1.39	−1.02	n.s.
Gray Oral[b]	8.84	3.15	5.76	$p < 0.001$
Percept. Speed[c]	−2.30	−2.48	−3.73	n.s.
RQ[d]	0.80 (−1.37)	0.69 (−2.09)	0.75 (−1.65)	n.s.

[a] Means expressed as z-scores.
[b] Means expressed as grade equivalents.
[c] Age-adjusted scores.
[d] Ratio of reading and spelling achievement to expected achievement (converted to z-score with mean 1.0 and sd 0.15 for Figure 3).

compared to overall ability was equivalent for the three clusters. There were no significant differences in achievement in either of the spelling tests for the three groups, or on the perceptual speed test.

DISCUSSION

The purpose of the cluster analysis was to detect any underlying heterogeneity among the disabled readers. The first analysis using the entire population classified almost all of the unaffected individuals in one cluster, but this cluster contained nearly as many disabled readers. Some relative weakness was seen in Auditory Discrimination in Quiet. The remainder of the affecteds and a few of the unaffecteds were classified into another cluster, which showed deficits in Auditory Discrimination in Noise and Sound Blending, as well as in most of the other tests, including the three WISC-R or WAIS factors. The most significant results, however, are that these subgroups were not at all homogeneous or distinct and did not show any difference in achievement profile or reading quotient.

Ideally, an autosomal dominant hypothesis would predict that the best solution for the total population would have been with two well-defined clusters; one of affecteds, and one of unaffecteds. However, this would assume that the neuropsychological variables are measuring underlying abilities that are directly related to reading ability. It should be recalled that the primary difference between the unaffecteds and affecteds in this population was that they differed on the presence or history of reading disability. The genetic hypothesis of an autosomal dominant gene was supported independently by the linkage analysis. Thus, the failure of the cluster analysis of the entire population to define clusters based on reading disability reflects on the relationship between the neuropsychological variables and the history of reading disability, and not on the genetic hypothesis. In this population, it appears that the neuropsychological variables that were measured were unrelated to past or present reading disability as indicated by the diagnosis and the reading quotient. Maturation was not a factor, since the clusters did not differ on age. These results could occur if the factor (or factors, ignoring the genetic hypothesis) involved in producing the reading disability is distal to the neuropsychological abilities. In this case, subtle differences may be seen between groups, but different types of tests may be required to find more basic differences. This is analogous to diagnosing pneumonia by measuring temperature; certainly a fever is associated with illness, but a much more definitive discrimination is made by microbiological methods.

Another factor which may have accentuated the similarities between affecteds and unaffecteds (and within affecteds) is the restricted range of variation imposed by the selection criteria, in that all subjects were of at least normal intelligence, from middle class backgrounds, had normal abilities in mathematics, and were from a relatively small gene pool (in that individuals were related). Thus other populations of disabled readers, even containing the same putative gene as in this population, may show more neuropsychological variation; however, this study would indicate that such variation would be influenced by other factors besides just the reading disability.

When only the disabled readers were analysed, three clusters emerged. Nearly all of the individuals in the second cluster were the same as in the second cluster of the first analysis, and the profile was basically the same. The first and third clusters corresponded fairly well to those in cluster 1 of the total analysis, with the first cluster showing more pronounced deficits in the Auditory Discrimination and Sound Blending tests, but also showing higher achievement in other areas, including IQ. The third cluster appeared to mirror the first, except with all scores moderated; the low scores were not as low, and the high scores were not as high. Thus the profiles did not seem distinctive, but rather appeared to be distinguished on the basis of severity. This was not related to age, sex, or family. The evaluation statistics again demonstrated that the clusters were not well-separated and compact, nor were they homogeneous. Finally, comparison of achievement test means for each cluster demonstrated that, again, the profiles were identical, only shifted on the basis of severity on the reading tests. The RQ indicated that all three groups were equally disabled on the basis of their discrepancy between reading achievement and expected abilities. Interestingly, all three groups were equally disabled on the two spelling measures. This would suggest that this is a persistent deficit in spite of overall intelligence, while reading is more modifiable. It may be, however, that more detailed tests of individual reading skills would indicate more persistent problems in all of the disabled readers.

As a whole, the cluster analyses did not reveal an underlying heterogeneity in the affecteds. Rather, it appeared that individuals with similar relative strengths and weaknesses were separated on the basis of overall ability. Certainly, IQ is correlated with performance on neuropsychological measures, and would be expected to influence one's ability to compensate for a reading disability. The affecteds appeared to resemble each other to a considerable extent, and about half of the affecteds showed even greater resemblance to the unaffecteds neuropsychologically. This is consistent with the hypothesis that the affecteds all do have the same genetic etiology for their reading disability which is not directly measured neuropsychological techniques. In those individuals with somewhat lower IQ, however, subtle but distinctive neuropsychological deficits are seen.

Interpretation of these subtle deficits is important in understanding the cognitive structure of the affected population. Cluster 1, and cluster 3 to some extent, appear to be the more 'specific' disabled readers. The pattern of deficits appears to mirror those seen with the analysis of variance results, primarily in Naming, Auditory Discrimination, and possibly Digit Span as seen in the lowered FD factor. The Sound Blending score did not show significant differences between affecteds and unaffecteds on the analysis of variance, but the cluster results suggest that about half of the disabled readers are deficient in this skill. This would support the hypothesis of an auditory processing deficit in the disabled readers, in perception or in short-term memory. The difficulties on the Boston Naming test suggest a problem with lexical retrieval, which may be in addition to the auditory processing problems, or as a result of poor auditory (that is, verbal) representations in the lexicon. The Verbal Comprehension factor was average, however, militating against a global language problem.

The members of cluster 2 showed a very similar pattern, except that they had other deficiencies in addition, primarily in motor areas. This may be a less specific group neuropsychologically, but it is important to note that visual abilities were still good, indicating that this is not a 'mixed' group. As is mentioned above, it is likely that the lowered neuropsychological profile corresponds to their somewhat lower (but still average) IQ.

The advantages of this analysis are that it indicates that there are not phenotypically distinct clusters in the data. Instead, it clearly shows the pattern of strengths and weaknesses common to most of the population. Thus, it can be treated as a single, homogeneous group. In that case, it is interesting to compare this population to the subtypes defined by other studies, to see if it is contained as a distinct type among other subtypes. However, it is difficult to compare the phenotype of this population with other studies, since the test battery and the population are not totally comparable. Still, some rough correspondence can be seen with other described subgroups. Lyon *et al.* (1982) described five subtypes on the basis of cluster analysis, and their second subtype, with deficiencies in sound blending, auditory discrimination and memory, naming, and receptive language comprehension, and with strengths in visual perceptual abilities, seems closest to our population. They equate their subtype with the Language Disorder of Mattis *et al.* (1975), which is in limited agreement with our findings. They also note that the members of this cluster were slightly older than in their other clusters, and certainly our population, with a mean age of 25.5, is much older. (It should be noted that the younger children were not different enough from their elders to constitute a separate cluster.) Lyon *et al.* also compared their subgroup 2 to the first subgroup of Petrauskas and Rourke (1979), which was described as showing impairments in sentence memory and verbal fluency, with some problems with memory for digits, word blending, and concept formation. While measures of verbal fluency and concept formation were not included in our battery, the remaining observations are consistent with ours. The authors noted that arithmetic ability was not decreased in that subtype, and also compared it with the Mattis *et al.* (1975) Language Disorder.

Lyon *et al.* (1982) further compared their subgroup 2 with the naming disorder subtype of Satz and Morris (1981). This population was not as similar to the one in the present study, being composed of children with more generalized academic difficulties. Their naming deficit group was low only in verbal fluency, and they described a separate subtype with a more global language disorder. Therefore it is difficult to see a direct correspondence with our population and one of their subtypes.

Of the three subtypes described by Doehring and Hoshko (1977) and Doehring *et al.* (1981), ours is most like their group O (impaired oral readers) with higher IQs and deficiencies in Digit Span. They suggest that there may be subtypes within this group. Perhaps this would reveal individuals with more auditory processing problems as well.

Watson *et al.* (1983) also used cluster analysis to define three subgroups of disabled readers. These were defined as (1) a visual processing disability, (2) a generalized language disorder similar to that of Mattis *et al.* (1975), and (3) a minimal deficit group with difficulties primarily in oral reading, auditory short-term memory, and visual–motor integration. Our population would seem to fit best with the minimal deficits group, which they also compare to Doehring and Hoshko's type O. However, they also compare it with an 'unexpected' subtype of Satz and Morris (1981). This group showed no deficits on any of the neuropsychological tests, and had low arithmetic as well as low reading scores. Thus our own population does not seem directly comparable, again probably because of the overall difference in subjects.

It is hoped that the preceding illustrates the difficulties in comparing studies with different populations and test batteries. Our results, along with those of others who have utilized statistical and other methods to validate their clusters (e.g. Watson *et al.*, 1983; Morris *et al.*, 1981; Satz and Morris, 1981) also emphasize the necessity for checking if the clusters actually describe important differences, since the programs will produce clusters out of even homogeneous data. Satz and Morris (1981) have already cautioned against inferring particular neurological abnormalities from the results of behaviorally defined clusters. We would further caution against assuming that the members of a given cluster have the same etiology or underlying deficits for their disability until this is somehow verified. If valid clusters are formed, cluster analysis can generate subpopulations for further research, but alone the procedure serves only to describe the characteristics of a given population on a given set of measures.

We have suggested the inclusion of genetic variables as a way to construct subgroups based on etiology. Several studies have attempted to assess genetic influences within their population in a cursory fashion. Mattis (1978) noted that there were individuals with positive family histories in all of their subtypes, and Satz and Morris (1981) used reading levels of parents to detect possible genetic contributions. Given the near certainty of genetic heterogeneity and adult compensation, such methods need to be replaced by more careful genetic analyses. At the very least, this would require the taking of a family history and testing of other family members, and some estimate of the possible mode of inheritance for each family. Confirmation that such family patterns are actually the result of genes will require formal genetic studies, either family studies with large sample sizes such as the Colorado Family Reading Study (cf. DeFries and Decker, 1982), or linkage studies.

ACKNOWLEDGEMENT

This work has been supported in part by NIH grants RO1 HD 13899 and 7F32 NF05761.

REFERENCES

Bakker, D. J., Teunissen, J., Bosch, J. (1976), Development of laterality-reading patterns. In: R. M. Knights and D. S. Bakker (Eds.), *The Neuropsychology of Learning Disorders: Theoretical Approaches*. Baltimore, University Park Press.

Boder, E. (1970), Developmental dyslexia: a new diagnostic approach based on the identification of three subtypes. *J. School Health* **40**, 289.

Boder, E. (1973), Developmental dyslexia: a diagnostic approach based on three atypical reading–spelling patterns. *Devel. Med. Child Neurol.* **15**, 663–687.

Brewer, W. F. (1963), Specific language disability: review of the literature and family study. AB Honors Thesis, Harvard College.

Camp, B., and McCabe, L. (unpublished), The Denver reading and spelling test, Research manual.

Cohen, J. (1952), Factors underlying the Weschler–Bellevue performance of three neuropsychological groups. *J. Abn. Soc. Psychol.* **47**, 359–365.

Decker, S. N., DeFries, J. C. (1981), Cognitive ability profiles in familial reading-disabled children. *Devel. Med. Child Neurol.* **23**, 217–227.

DeFries, J. C., and Decker, S. N. (1982), Genetic aspects of reading disability: a family study. In: R. N. Malatesha and P. G. Aaron (Eds.), *Reading Disorders: Varieties and Treatments*. New York, Academic Press.

Dixon, W. J., Brown, M. B., Engelman, L., Franc, J. W., Hill, M. A., Jennrich, R. I., and Toporek, J. D. *BMDP Stastical Software 1981*. Berkeley, University of California Press.

Doehring, D. G., and Hoshko, I. M. (1977), Classification of reading problems by the Q technique of factor analysis. *Cortex* **13**, 281–294.

Doehring, D. G., Trites, R. L., Patel, P. G., and Fiedorowicz, C. A. M. (1981), *Reading Disabilities: The Interaction of Reading, Language, and Neuropsychological Deficits*. New York, Academic Press.

Drew, A. L. (1956), A neurological appraisal of familial congenital word-blindness. *Brain* **79**, 440–460.

Dunn, L. M., and Markwardt, F. C. (1970), *Peabody Individual Achievement Test*. Circle Pines, Minn., American Guidance Service.

Finucci, J. M. (1978), Genetic considerations in dyslexia. In: H. R. Myklebust (Ed.), *Progress in Learning Disabilities*, Vol. IV. New York, Grune & Stratton.

Finucci, J. M., Guthrie, J. T., Childs, A. L., Abbey. H., and Childs, B. (1976), The genetics of specific reading disability. *Ann. Rev. Hum. Genet (Lond.)* **40**, 1–23.

Foch, T. T., DeFries, J. C., McClearn, G. E., and Singer, S. M. (1977), Familial patterns of impairment in reading disability. *J. Educ. Psychol.* **69**, 316–329.

Hallgren, B. (1950), Specific dyslexia (congenital word-blindness): a clinical and genetic study. *Acta Psychiatrica et Neurologica Scand.* Suppl., **65**.

Huizinga, D. H. (1977), *Cluster Analysis: Evaluation and dynamic typologies*. Unpublished doctoral dissertation, University of Colorado.

Ingram, T. T. S., Mason, A. W., and Blackburn, I. (1970), A retrospective study of 82 children with reading disability. *Devel. Med. Child Neurol.* **12**, 271–281.

Jastak, J. F., and Jastak, S. R. (1970), *Wide Range Achievement Test.* Circle Pines, Minn., American Guidance Service.

Johnson, D. J., and Myklebust, H. R. (1964), *Learning disabilities: educational principles and practices.* New York, Grune & Stratton.

Lewitter, F. I., DeFries, J. C., and Elston, R. C. (1980), Genetic models of reading disability. *Behav. Genet.* **10**, 9–30.

Lyon, R., Stewart, N., and Freedman, D. (1982), Neuropsychological characteristics of empirically derived subgroups of learning disabled readers. *J. Clin. Neuropsychol.* **4**, 343–365.

Mattis, S. (1978), Dyslexia syndromes: a working hypothesis that works. In: A. L. Benton and D. Pearl (Eds.), *Dyslexia. An Appraisal of Current Knowledge.* New York, Oxford University Press.

Mattis, S., French, J. M., and Rapin, I (1975), Dyslexia in children and young adults: three independent neuropsychological syndromes. *Devel. Med. Child Neurol.* **17**, 150–163.

Morris, R., Blashfield, R., and Satz, P. (1981), Neuropsychology and cluster analysis: Potentials and problems. *Clin Neuropsychol*, **3**, 79–99.

Morton, N. E. (1956). The detection and estimation of linkage between the genes for elliptocytosis and the Rh blood groups. *Am. J. Hum. Genet.*, **8**, 80–96.

Nie, N. H., Hull, C. H., Jenkins, J. G., Steinbrenner, K., and Bent, D. H. (1975), *Statistical package for the social sciences.* New York, McGraw-Hill.

Omenn, G. S., and Weber, B. A. (1978), Dyslexia: search for phenotypic and genetic heterogeneity. *Am. J. Med. Gen.* **1**, 333–342.

Ott, J. (1974), Estimation of the recombination fraction in human pedigrees: efficient computation of the likelihood for human studies. *Am. J. Hum. Genet.* **26**, 588–597.

Pennington, B. F., Smith, S. D., McCabe, L. L., Kimberling, W. J., and Lubs, H. A. (1983), Developmental continuities and discontinuities in a form of familial dyslexia. In: R. Emde and R. Harmon (Eds.), *Continuities and Discontinuities in Development.* New York, Plenum Press.

Petrauskas, R. J., and Rourke, B. P. (1979), Identification of subgroups of retarded readers: a neuropsychological multi-variate approach. *J. Clin. Neuropsychol.* **1**, 17–37.

Robinson, A. R., Lubs, H. A., and Bergsma, D. (1979), Sex chromosome aneuploidy: prospective studies on children. *The National Foundation: March of Dimes Birth Defects: Original Article Series*, Vol. XV (1). New York, Alan R. Liss.

Robinson, H. M. (1963), *Gray Oral Reading Test.* Indianapolis, Bobbs-Merrill.

Satz, P., and Morris, R. (1981), Learning disability subtypes: a review. In: F. J. Pirozzolo and M. C. Wittrock (Eds.), *Neuropsychology and Cognitive Processes in Reading.* New York, Academic Press.

Smith, S. D., Kimberling, W. J., Pennington, B. F., and Lubs, H. A. (1983a), Specific reading disability: identification of an inherited form through linkage analysis. *Science* **219**, 1345–1347.

Smith, S. D., Pennington, B. F., Kimberling, W. J., and Lubs, H. A. (1983b), A genetic analysis of specific reading disability. In: C. L. Ludlow and J. A. Cooper. *Genetic Aspects of Speech and Language Disorders.* New York, Academic Press.

Ward, J. H. (1963), Hierarchical grouping to optimize an objective function. *J. Am. Stat. Assoc.* **58**, 236–244.

Watson, B. U., Goldgar, D. E., and Ryshon, K. L. (1983), Subtypes of reading disability. *J. Clin. Neuropsychol.* **5**, 377–399.

Zahalkova, M., Vrzal, V., and Klobovkova, E. (1972), Genetical investigations in dyslexia. *J. Med. Genet.* **9**, 48–52.

CHAPTER 14

Language Structure, Dyslexia, and Remediation: The Czech Perspective

Z. MATĚJČEK and J. STURMA
Postgraduate Medical Institute, Praha, Czechoslovakia and
Child Psychiatric Clinic, Dolni Pocernice, Czechoslovakia

READING IN CZECH

Reading and spelling in Czech may be considered relatively easy when compared, for example, with English, as it is phonetically very consistent.

Even the first *Glagolitic* alphabet, devised by Saints Cyril and Methodius, the Greek apostles of the Slavs in the middle of the ninth century AD, was phonetically very well adapted to the Slavonic because its spelling was phonetic.

The original Glagolitic was then replaced by Cyrillic which was in turn replaced by Roman type and script in the early Middle Ages. At the beginning of the fifteenth century, Jan Hus, the church reformer and rector of Prague University, ingeniously revised Czech spelling. He introduced diacritical marks to supplement the basic Latin alphabetic characters so that each sound had a corresponding letter making Czech spelling phonetically consistent. Of the European languages, Finnish is comparable in this respect, and Spanish very similar.

This phonetic consistency lends itself nicely to an analytic–synthetic method of teaching reading and writing. As soon as the Czech child learns the letters of the alphabet the acquisition of the basic ability of joining words in text is not far behind. Comprehension of written text is limited only by the developing vocabulary, which by school age is usually several thousand words and not too different from the spoken vocabulary. Towards the end of the second grade or the beginning of the third grade Czech children reach the 'socially acceptable level' of reading, i.e. the speed of approximately 60 to 70 words per minute. Children begin to enjoy books and are able to learn by reading. Reading speed, under these circumstances, is the best individual indicator of reading development. Other indicators such as accuracy and comprehension correlate highly with speed. For example, teachers may claim that they assess their pupils' reading not by speed, but by the quality of reading. The tests, however, showed a highly positive correlation between the speed of a child's reading and his teacher's assessment: $r = 0.882$ in the 2nd grade, $r = 0.826$ in the 4th grade. The number of mistakes made, on the other hand, changes little after second grade.

HISTORY

Interest in specific learning disability in the Czech lands dates from the beginning of this century. The first article to be published was by a professor of neurology at Charles University in Prague, Heveroch (1904). The incentive was a case of an eleven-year-old girl referred to him by her school teacher. After examining the case of 'Alexia' he felt that other similar cases are comparatively frequent in school practice—but feared that they would not attract the same attention from pedagogists as they would from neurologists. He was correct, for the first special school classes for disabled readers were not established until 1962 in Brno. Prague followed in 1965—and since then there has been a steady development. There are special classes in almost every large town in Czechoslovakia and special remedial centers are functioning in every regional district—so that special help is now accessible to almost all children suffering from reading and spelling disorders.

SPECIAL CARE

Special care for disabled readers is carried out on five different levels:

(1) For the mildest cases of reading disability the remedial work is part of the normal curriculum and is carried out directly in ordinary elementary schools by classroom teachers. The child is taught somewhat differently and receives additional remedial exercises. The main condition for success is the teacher's familiarity with remedial methods and ability to put them into practice—and to adapt them to the individual needs of each child.

(2) In case of more pronounced difficulties which cannot be overcome during the normal classes, special remedial treatment takes place out of school. The remedial treatment is carried out by specially trained persons, either clinical psychologists or special pedagogists in child psychiatric centers or in psychopedagogic centers which are found in every district. The therapist sets the course and both the child and its parents receive detailed instructions for homework. The therapist then checks progress regularly and provides encouragement to the child and parents when they progress. The parents are heavily involved—they become the actual therapists for their own dyslexic child. The experiment with a large-scale involvement of parents in the remedial treatment of their dyslexic children in Great Britain, newly reported by Young and Tyre

(1983), is very similar to the approach in Czechoslovakia. Even the results referred to by Young and Tyre are very similar to what the follow-up studies show in Czechoslovakia. It may be also mentioned that Saunders (personal communication, 1984) in the USA has experimented with the same procedures, especially with children and their fathers. He reports very similar outcomes.

(3) The third level, which is becoming more and more popular in Czechoslovakia, is the resource room technique. The therapist, who has a special room and special equipment in school, does the remedial treatment with dyslexic children either individually or in groups of two, three, or four children during the school hours but out of class, daily or several times a week. There is less involvement of parents and more involvement of the professional therapist than in the previous case, the success being largely dependent on the latter's professional qualities.

(4) The fourth level of treatment includes special classes for dyslexic children, whose operation is largely oriented towards the correction of reading difficulties of their pupils. These classes (within normal schools) provide an atmosphere of 'undeserved' school failures. There are no more than 12 of these children in such a class. Here, the success may be due to the favourable 'psycho-therapeutic' attitude of the teachers and to the teachers' creative practices and imagination. Classes for dyslexic children, of course, have not any outward designation as such, being only sections of each grade.

(5) Children suffering from the most severe forms of dyslexia, or children who cannot go to special classes because they live too far off in the country, are subjected to concentrated therapeutic care in special residential centers within child psychiatric clinics. These clinics are, of course, a state service, whose care is provided without cost to the parents. Dyslexic children usually stay there for a period of several months up to a year or more.

When suitable remedial methods for an individual child are found, the child can move into higher and higher levels of remedial care: into special classes, into remedial treatment done by parents and directed by the therapist, and finally into normal classes without any further special help.

MILIEU

The environment that forms the background to our study of dyslexia can be summed up as follows:

(1) Phonetically very consistent spelling.
(2) Uniform school system.
(3) Uniform teaching methods, uniform and obligatory syllabus, uniform textbooks (the ideal of school inspectors is, say, for all fourth-grade children in all elementary schools to be on the same page of the same textbook on the same day).

(4) Workers making the diagnosis usually conduct the remedial treatment as well; which, in the words of one of our leading people in the field, the late O. Kučera (1959) 'constitutes a continuous diagnostic-therapeutic experiment'.

This situation, of course, has both advantages and disadvantages. The question to ask is what can be gained from this structured educational system in terms of our general knowledge about specific learning disorders. By comparing the clinical picture of disorders under different 'life' conditions can we come to know what, in fact, is generally valid so that the pedagogy of Czechoslovakia can be evaluated.

The following are just a few selected examples of the work being done in Czechoslovakia. They are more indicative of hesitation than certainty—more of ignorance than knowledge; but we feel they are not unusual.

CHILDREN FROM CHILDREN'S HOMES

In the 1950s, our work with dyslexics began. We knew next to nothing about psychological deprivation. The first boy that we treated remedially for dyslexia had been brought up in a succession of children's collective institutions since his birth: he had never lived in a family. In the years to come we were to treat more of such children—more, it seemed, than could be reasonably expected from their representation in the child population. We were puzzled. The treatment was difficult and only partially successful. We were fighting a universally unfavourable complication—lack of motivation.

Today we know that it was quite natural and inevitable. New findings from neonatal psychology have shown that the child is born with the ability to distinguish sound frequencies of the human voice from nonvocal frequencies. The child in an infants' home is chronically 'undernourished' in terms of human speech stimuli. And neuropsychology teaches us that in such cases it is likely that the brain's left hemisphere is, in fact, functionally and chronically under-stimulated. The inactivity of speech functions leads to a certain functional atrophy—we may recall the extreme case of the girl child Genie (Curtis, 1977). Children brought up in children's homes consistently lag behind other children in their speech development—and the highest deficit is about the third year of age. By the time of school entrance, the deficit, measurable by tests, is usually made up for to a certain degree.

The study of psychological deprivation has brought us to the realization that the problem is not just in the deficit of one function, but that the child also usually channels his interest, motivation, and then his skills and gratification (which again is a motivational factor) from the sphere of the deprived function to that of another function which has not suffered from deprivation, for our particular case to the visual–perceptual sphere—which, as a rule, means predominantly right-hemisphere.

Our findings about these children fit in completely with the typology that Bakker (1979) derived from his neuropsychological studies. These children were stumbling readers, making no glaring mistakes and inversions; but their reading was painfully slow, uncertain, and halting. Today we know that they were unable to provide speech content for what they perceived quite well visually. In the remedial treatment it is necessary both to train and develop speech, keyed to orthography, and find the motivational/emotional key to spoken communication.

Rourke and Strang's (1981) hypothesis states that the development of a relative brain hypofunction on the one hand and the development of a hyperfunction on the other hand are closely related with the child's interaction with his social environment, i.e. especially with his family environment and with the exchange of emotional stimuli.

What is the point of talking about institutional children? Well, our aim is to show through experience with these children that the future of a better understanding of learning disabilities lies in the imaginative interaction of various approaches, and dyslexia, undoubtedly, is a model example of a need for cooperative relationships of neonatal psychology, interactional psychology, neuropsychology, and the theory of deprivation.

SPECIFIC DYSLEXIC PATTERNS

During the 1950s we examined the reading skills of 300 randomly selected children, 350 'poorest' readers in their classes, and 200 children in special schools for the mentally retarded in Prague. The findings were compared with those of Bennett (1942), whose research was very similar to ours. The relative frequencies in some types of reading mistakes by Czech and American, i.e. English-speaking, children were practically identical.

For example, topographically there were the same percentages of mistakes in endings, in first syllables of words, and in the middle of words. On the other hand, there were some marked differences. For example, reversals formed 12 per cent in the repertory of mistakes by American children. In Czech children, reversals were found in 4 per cent of second-graders, and in fourth grade they represented a mere 1.5 per cent of all mistakes. Mistakes in mid-word vowels were made by 15 per cent of the American children, while Czech children showed no more than 6.5 per cent, and only the youngest at that. These and other error comparisons between Czech and American children are shown in Table 1.

The conclusion at that time was that the so-called specific mistakes are most probably merely an accentuation and fixation of particular tendencies in the given language and of the methods of teaching it, and occur both in the normal and the dyslexic school population.

It was not until recently that a Czech psychologist, Jošt (1983), began to compare the incidence of inversions and reversals in children of different ages,

Table 1. Types of reading errors. Czech and English-speaking children

Errors	Czech children (%) 2nd Grade	5th Grade	English children (%)
A	36.1	29.0	31
B	12.4	13.6	16
AB/A	18.4	24.1	6
AB/B	11.3	13.6	4
AB	4.9	4.3	8
Median vowel	6.7	4.3	15
Reversals	4.6	1.5	12
Final 's'	—	—	5
Substitutions	2.8	8.7	3
Softening of consonants	2.8	0.9	—

A = unlike ending, B = unlike beginning, AB/A = more like letters at the beginning of the word than at the end, AB/B = more like letters at the end of the word than at the beginning, AB = errors in the middle part of the words, 'Median vowel' = errors in median vowels only, 'Final s' = omissions or additions of final 's' were sole errors

dyslexics, and normal readers, both in visual reading and tactile reading, i.e. without control by sight. He concludes that reading is affected by some sort of factor X that is influenced by either the inclination of resistance of the perceptual apparatus to inversions. This X factor is found in both normal and dyslexic readers, both in visual and tactile reading, and is only partially a function of age. In non-dyslexics this X factor is a relatively isolated phenomenon and can be easily compensated for, while in dyslexics it is connected with other peculiarities and as a result it is difficult to correct. In itself, however, it is not specific for dyslexics. Even in Czech preschool children and in school beginners one frequently notes a tendency to reverse, which is often spontaneously and readily corrected. Some of the dyslexics however, do not 'outgrow' the tendency. Further definition of the X factor is needed to determine its pedagogical implications and whether this new hypothetical construct will serve further useful purposes.

AUDITORY PERCEPTION AND SYMBOLIC ASSOCIATION

The process of relating visual impressions to sounds and of understanding the symbolic significance of visual perceptual forms is essentially the same in English and in Czech, since in both spelling patterns are largely phonetic. It is only the degree to which they are phonetic that is different. As the phonetic nature of the spelling becomes crucially important, the significance of auditory perception is increased, and the disorders and difficulties in auditory perception must of necessity manifest themselves in spelling deficiencies.

Thus in Czech we are forced to give special critical attention to relations between auditory perception and articulatory characteristics of speech and to relationships between reading and writing in both the diagnosis and the remedial treatment of dyslexia. We have arrived at the conclusion that we have to deal with a certain articulatory and perceptual clumsiness which is characteristic of one type of dyslexia—a type relatively common in the Czech dyslexic population.

Only after having made this observation did we conduct a historical probe into the methods of elementary teaching of reading from the end of the eighteenth century to the present. We were surprised to discover how some methodologists, on purely empirical grounds, emphasize the training of auditory analysis and synthesis, while others concentrate on training visual perception. We were surprised at the periodical prominence of one approach at the expense of the other. It is obvious that one method works better for one kind of difficulty, the second for another. The almost regular desertion of one or the other was a reaction to the inevitable failure of either approach in some of the child readers and spellers.

The second probe concerned the methods for preschool preparation of children. In Czechoslovakia, more than 80 per cent of children at preschool age attend nursery schools (at the age of 5 to 6 almost 100 per cent of children will have undergone 'preschool education'). Preschool methods are largely dominated by exercises in visual perception, whereas exercises of auditory perception directed towards later reading and spelling are very much in the background. Our observations on the need for both will aid in reforming preschool experience.

SYLLABLES

The remedial treatment of dyslexics has shown the syllable to be the suitable starting-point. From dichotic listening research it is known that the syllable is the most useful phonetic unit of speech. One of our colleagues (R. Nahlovsky, unpublished) has been intensely studying the problem of syllables and text analysis. To summarize his findings: seven children's books total 50,000 words of which more than 6,300 are recurring; the first 100 words include 73 new ones, but after reading 10,000 words we find that the proportion is 10 new words for each 100 words; the 500 most frequently used words cover 57 per cent of text.

Syllables present a somewhat different picture. At first they repeat frequently. The 150 most frequent syllables occupy 75 per cent of any Czech text and 336 syllables can cover 98 per cent of the text, while the remaining of 2 per cent of the syllables rarely occur.

After going through three million syllables, Nahlovsky found 9716 individual syllables. This number is probably nearing the final count for Czech.

All children in Czech schools are taught, from the very beginning, to use the basic decoding and encoding (phoneme–grapheme correspondence) techniques. Given the phonetically consistent spelling, the perfect mastery of this technique is a question of several months in the first grade in most children. Even dyslexic children are usually well up to mastering the technique, even though they take longer to do so. Their stumbling-block in reading, however, is combining letters in syllables and words. Here syllable training helps.

Accordingly, in remedial treatment we teach our dyslexics fluent syllable reading. Our 'window' techniques are specially directed towards it. Now we can at last explain why this method is so successful: in syllable reading we still remain within the functional scope of one hemisphere, i.e. the left hemisphere. The 150 most frequent syllables that cover 75 per cent of text are quite enough to allow the child relatively quick progress, even if the remaining 25 per cent of syllables must be still 'deciphered'. Remedial exercises, as a result, receive a positive motivational impulse.

One other interesting point: the Japanese script Kana consists of exactly 150 individual syllabic signs, the syllables being formed either by a mere vocalic sound or by a simple combination of consonant–vowel. Professor Tsunoda (1981) states that the Japanese employ the left hemisphere to a greater extent than peoples speaking and writing different languages; interestingly, it seems that among Japanese there are fewer dyslexics than in other languages except perhaps among Scandinavians.

LETTER CONFUSIONS

The point of departure for Matějček and Vokounová (1982) is the problem of Norwegian dyslexics and normal readers addressed by von Tetzchner et al. (1978) at the University of Oslo. In their experiment 65 children from special third and fourth grades for dyslexics — and 85 children of corresponding age and school grade without reading difficulties were shown slides tachistoscopically for 500 ms, each one with a random pattern of four letters selected from the total set of nine letters (b, d, f, g, k, m, n, p, t). Errors made by the children in the reproduction of the letter sequences were assessed. The same asymmetries in the frequencies of substituted and substituting letters are found in the Norwegian and Czech dyslexics and the normal readers alike.

As might be expected, the dyslexics differ from the normal readers in the number of correctly reproduced patterns. This is, however, due not so much to the letter confusions as to the number of 'other mistakes'. Even if errors in letter recognition are more frequent in dyslexics than in normal readers, the differences are mostly unimportant and unconvincing. Nor do the changes in the pattern of exposed letters particularly distinguish between them.

However, what does actually differentiate between Czech and normal readers is the number of letter omissions. Dyslexics more frequently (on the whole with great statistical significance) fail to reproduce the whole pattern of letters and simply skip one or more letters. (It is only rarely that they miss all of the four letters. Most frequently they perceive just one or two while two or three go unnoticed.)

Table 2. Letter confusions in Czech fourth-grade children

'Other mistakes' in normal readers and dyslexics

		Number of mistakes per one child				
		Normal readers	Dyslexics	chi^2	d.f.	p
1.	Number of incorrect letters in set					
1	letter incorrect	32.2	40.4	6.67	3	n.s.
2	letters incorrect	27.1	27.8	4.24	3	n.s.
3	letters incorrect	8.9	13.1	13.75	3	0.01
4	letters incorrect	2.5	3.0			n.s.
2.	Mistakes in sequences of letters					
1	letter incorrectly located	12.2	15.2	25.01	3	0.001
2	letters	13.6	11.6	3.40	3	n.s.
3	letters	1.2	1.1			n.s.
4	letters	2.5	0.2			n.s.
3.	Letters omitted					
1	letter omitted	12.2	15.2	9.63	3	0.02
2	letters omitted	13.6	54.3	23.82	3	0.001
3	letters omitted	18.9	38.9	27.11	3	0.001
4	letters omitted	8.6	13.5	16.41	3	0.001

These data suggest a certain generalized perceptual 'clumsiness', slowness, and unreadiness typical of dyslexics. Data for fourth graders regarding other types of mistakes are summarized in Table 2.

Another remarkable differentiating characteristic of our dyslexics is the confusion in the test of projected letters with letters which were not, in fact, presented in the original set of nine letters. (In pretest practice all children were assured that the choice of letters in slides is limited and that besides the nine letters there will be no others.)

In the group of normal readers there appeared, on average, 3.0 of such mistakes per child (33 children of this group, i.e. 39 per cent, avoided them completely). The group of dyslexics, on the other hand, made 12.2 mistakes per child, that is, four times the normal readers. (Only 11 dyslexics, i.e. 17 per cent, avoided the mistakes.) In all probability these findings indicate that dyslexics lack the usual feedback control of percepts and that the 11 dyslexics who made no errors were of a separate typology from the others.

The tendency to letter omissions and intrusions of letters not actually presented is the most striking of all. The possible explanation may be that perceptual processes in dyslexics are slower and that the internal censorship of feedback control does not operate reliably enough. The child is seemingly incapable of coordinating multiple thought processes (Goldstein, 1974).

There seem to be some links with the latest findings from a completely different field. Pavlidis (1981, 1985) in his revealing studies of eye movements ascribes the dyslexic's erratic eye movements to one or more of the following factors: (1) oculomotor control problems, (2) sequential inability, (3) attentional problems, (4) prediction/synchronization problems.

The perceptual slowness and clumsiness found in the dyslexics of our study are in agreement with the eye movement findings of Pavlidis (1981, 1985). It also seems that all these findings are quite in keeping with Luria's basic scheme of brain functioning. According to Luria (1973) every complex mental activity is a functional system that requires the concerted action of three principal units. One regulates the tone and alerts the brain; a second collects, processes, and stores information; and a third unit programs, regulates, and verifies mental activity. All three of them are interrelated (see also Frostig and Maslow, 1979). In this case, we seem to be concerned with a certain functional inefficiency of this three-phase system. The moment one of the component units is pressured, the other two malfunction under a type of law of limited effort.

The logical conclusion is that to explain dyslexic difficulties we must look for the causes in the imperfect cooperation of the cerebral functional complexes, i.e. in complex dysfunctions rather than in specific dysfunctions of individual brain structures that outwardly look like individual specific symptoms. In actual fact what we have found so far are relatively wide-ranging, general, and complex dysfunctions of multiple and interacting origins whose external manifestations are the typical polysymptomatology of dyslexia.

BOYS AND GIRLS

The proportion of boys to girls in our dyslexic classes and in outpatient care is 6 or 7:1. Recently we examined normal readers in fourth grades and fourth-grade dyslexics in special classes by means of SPAS (Student's Perception Ability Scale) Boersma and Chapman (1979). In SPAS the child self-grades his academic successfulness on six scales: General Ability, Arithmetic, School Satisfaction, Reading/Spelling, Penmanship, and Confidence.

The dyslexics in special classes ($N = 135$) had, of course, significantly poorer school results than the control children from normal classes ($N = 105$), and on the whole objectively, they rated satisfaction with themselves as schoolers significantly lower. In the group of normal readers, the girls score significantly higher than boys in all indicators, but—and this is important—the girls in the group of learning disabled children score as low as the boys and are not significantly different. The dyslexic boys show greater self-confidence and apparently respond more positively to the conditions of special classes. In fact, they do not particularly depart from the self-assessment of the boys in normal classes. By contrast, the dyslexic girls in special classes quite significantly differ from the girls in normal classes in all scales. Obviously, their reaction to the situation is different.

The factors in play are probably many. If affected, girls exhibit greater dysfunction than boys; with only a mild form of learning disability girls are more likely to cope in normal classes than boys. In special classes girl dyslexics form a minority, in fact an exception. Boys and girls each present their specific mentalities; generalities are inappropriate and special need is of ultimate importance.

CONCLUSION

Dyslexia as a specific disorder of language communication process seems to be universal — we encounter it wherever children learn to read and write. At the root of it we find brain mechanisms, suggesting that dyslexia is a dysfunction inherent in the human species. Nonetheless, it manifests itself only when mankind has arrived at a certain level of culture and civilization. The disorder is manifest at a certain stage of individual mental maturity and only in confrontation with the educational demands of society. Dyslexia has undoubtedly a number of forms, types, and modalities, depending on individual languages, systems of spelling, and grapheme–phoneme correspondences, but also on different educational methods and policies, sociocultural conditions, etc. Our contribution aims to draw attention to these interdependences. Dealing with dyslexia, we should always bear in mind it is a practical problem involving real children. Dyslexia is not just another scientific conundrum — there is a standing need for actual help to be given to these suffering children, each one *individually*.

REFERENCES

Bakker, D. (1979), Dyslexia in developmental neuropsychology: hemisphere specific model. International Conference on 'Psychology and Medicine', Swansea, Great Britain, July 1979.

Bennett, A. (1942), An analysis of errors in word recognition made by retarded readers. *J. Educ. Psychol.*, **33**, 25.

Boersma, P. J., and Chapman, J. M. (1979), *Student's Perception Ability Scale* — Manual. Edmonton, University of Alberta.

Curtis, B. (1977), *Genie*. New York, Academic Press.

Frostig, M., and Maslow, P. (1979), Neuropsychological contributions to education. *J. Learn. Disab.* **12**, 538.

Heveroch, A. (1904) About specific reading and spelling difficulties in a child with excellent memory (In Czech). Praha, Česká škola.

Jošt, J. (1984), Vision and touch in the development of reading skill and reversal tendency (In Czech). *Čs. psychol.*, **28**.

Kučera, O. (1959), Specific reading disabilities in Czech children (In Czech). *Čs. psychiat.* **55**, 14.

Kučera, O., Matějček, Z., and Langmeier, J. (1963), Dyslexia in children in Czechoslovakia. *Amer. J. Orthopsychiat.* **33**, 448.

Luria, A. R. (1973), *The Working Brain*. New York, Basic Books.

Matějček, Z. (1965), The care of children with reading disability in Czechoslovakia. *Bull. Orton Soc.* **15**, 24.

Matějček, Z. (1971), Dyslexia: diagnostic and treatment findings. *Bull. Orton Soc.* **21**, 53.

Matějček, Z. (1976), Dyslexia in Czechoslovakian children. In: L. Tarnopol and M. Tarnopol (Eds.), *Reading Disabilities: An International Perspective*. Baltimore, University Park Press, pp. 131–154.

Matějček, Z., and Vokounová, A. (1982), Letter confusions in Norwegian and Czech children. *Remed. Educ.* **14**, 47.

Pavlidis, G. Th. (1981), Sequencing, eye movements and the early objective diagnosis of dyslexia. In: G. Th. Pavlidis, and T. R. Miles (Eds.), *Dyslexia Research and its Applications to Education*. Chichester, John Wiley, pp. 94–154.

Pavlidis, G. Th. (1985), The diagnostic significance of eye movements in dyslexia. *J. Learn. Disab.* **18**, 42–50.

Rourke, P. B., and Strang, J. D. (1981), Subtypes of reading and arithmetic disabilities: a neuropsychological analysis. In: M. Rutter (Ed.), *Behavioral Syndromes of Brain Dysfunction in Children*. New York, Guilford.

Saunders, R. (1984), Personal communication.

Tetzchner, S. von, Martinsen, H., and Ottem, E. (1978), Asymmetries in confusions of letters among dyslexic, deaf and normally hearing children. Oslo, University of Oslo.

Young, P., and Tyre, C. (1983), *Dyslexia or Illiteracy? Realizing the Right to Read*. Milton Keynes, The Open University Press.

CHAPTER 15

Personality and Situational Factors in Learning Disabilities

TANIS BRYAN
University of Illinois at Chicago, USA

INTRODUCTION

Medical Disease Model of Dyslexia

Theories and research in dyslexia have been dominated by the medical disease model. In this model it is believed that biological functions intrinsic to the individual transcend social and cultural influences. Dyslexia is perceived as a symptom of some biological disturbance. Explanations for dyslexia revolve around damage to particular parts of the brain, uneven maturation or maturational lags in brain development, and/or genetic influences. While these hypotheses are seductive, they have not yielded definitive information about the causes, the physiological or psychological processes in dyslexia; much less have they generated useful prescriptions to cure dyslexia.

Interactional Model

More promising both to our understanding of the causes and treatment of dyslexia is theory and research generated by an interactional model. In this model, human development is perceived to be the result of an interaction between the individual's genetic disposition and the individual's experiences (Endler and Magnuson, 1978). While this model recognizes the significant contributions of biology, human learning, and behavior are considered to be the result of a continuous, reciprocal relationship between person and situation variables. What is important is that research which has examined the relative influence of person and situation variables has shown that there is greater predictive power from analyses which incorporate both in the design. Research in medicine, psychology, and education all show significant person–situation interactions (Bandura, 1977;

Cronbach and Snow, 1977; Baron *et al.*, 1974), and this model will be the major focus of this chapter.

Dyslexia and Learning Disabilities

This chapter reviews studies which examine person and situational variables which have been shown to be important to our understanding of learning disabled children. The focus is on the learning disabled rather than the dyslexic simply because the related research has been limited to the learning disabled. Since learning disabilities represent heterogeneous groups of children, most of whom have reading problems, it is assumed that dyslexics would form a sizable subgroup within such samples. Hence it is believed these studies are relevant to dyslexia and provide at least a peek into how reading disabled youngsters differ from normally achieving readers on personality and situational factors.

While the term 'dyslexia' has been used for more than 100 years the term 'learning disabilities' is the newest in childhood psychopathology, in use since the late 1960s. The term has generated considerable controversy, in part because the number of children so labeled mushroomed in a very short period of time. Since 1975 the number of identified learning disabled children increased 20 per cent each year to reach 1.5 million in 1983. Controversy also stems from school districts' use of this category as a generic umbrella to provide special services to children who show considerable heterogeneity in type and severity of learning difficulties. However these children differ from one another, they share in common the experience of prolonged school failure. To the extent that the common experience of failure is predictably related to affective, cognitive, and behavioral responses, we may be able to describe learning disabled (and dyslexic) children in spite of learning differences. With this in mind the question asked is: do certain personality correlates of reading failure serve as a common denominator across varying samples of learning disabled children?

PERSONALITY FACTORS IN SCHOOL FAILURE

Self-concept

Teachers long have recognized the relationship between the experience of school failure and negative self-concept, and most strive to improve self-esteem, motivation, and reading achievement through the use of verbal praise and exhortations. By and large it is believed that improvements in reading lead to improvements in self-regard.

Unfortunately, the assumption of a unidirectional cause and effect relationship between reading success and positive self-esteem has not been supported by research. Studies find that there are students who are unresponsive to the experience of success (Thomas, 1980) and these same students fail to take personal credit and satisfaction from their achievements. In addition there are students who appear to benefit from failure, to interpret failure as a discriminative stimulus to engage in problem solving (Dweck and Reppucci, 1973). Moreover, there are students who are unresponsive to teacher exhortations to try harder in the face of failure, seemingly as a result of students beliefs that it is ability, not effort, which counts (Covington and Beery, 1976). Furthermore, studies designed to improve self-concept and achievement motivation, such as failure-free instruction, equal access to academic rewards, and/or nongraded classrooms have not resulted in the emotional improvements for which they were designed (Thomas, 1980).

These seemingly paradoxical findings led to the hypothesis that children's perceptions of events, their interpretations, intentions, and expectations may be as important as the event itself (Thomas, 1979; Covington and Beery, 1976). Thus, interest has grown in assessing learning disabled children's self-perceptions and cognitions as they relate to academic competence. This in turn has led to concern for how these perceptions might influence children's responsiveness to variations in teaching strategies. In the following sections of this chapter studies are reviewed which have focused on learning disabled students' self-perceptions and their responses to variations in instruction.

A number of studies compared learning disabled and non-disabled youngsters on measures of self-concept. The data show that younger learning disabled children in grades three through six rate themselves more negatively than classmates (Black, 1974; Chapman and Boersma, 1980). However, studies of older students in grades five through twelve do not show that the learning disabled differ from the non-disabled in their self-concepts (Pearl and Bryan, 1982; Tollefson et al., 1982). A comparison of the instruments used in the studies suggest that these age differences may be spurious. The instruments used with younger children are weighted with items related to academic performance (e.g. 'I'm not doing as well in school as I'd like to' — Coopersmith, 1967). Instruments administered to older students are weighted with items which focus on general feelings of self-worth (e.g. 'I feel that I have a number of good qualities' — Rosenberg, 1965). Thus, a reasonable interpretation of inconsistent findings across ages may be that the learning disabled have negative self-judgments which are specific to academic achievement but also believe they have personal attributes which make them worthy individuals. The provision of special education services may indeed help the learning disabled limit their negative self-evaluations to the academic domain. However, while the learning disabled may judge themselves as having redeeming features, findings in the self-concept studies suggest that their negative self-concepts extend broadly across performance-related activities. The learning disabled rate themselves as doing more poorly than classmates in school subjects and on tasks on which they have had little (Chapman and Boersma, 1980) or no experience (Butkowsky and Willows, 1980). It may be that they associate any performance-related task with negative self-expectations. A second related finding is that the learning disabled express less optimism about the likelihood of future improvements in performance than the non-disabled (Chapman and Boersma, 1980; Butkowsky and Willows, 1980; Dunn, Pearl, and Bryan, 1981) and recall doing worse than they actually did (Pearl, Bryan, and Herzog, 1983). Their consistently negative, pessimistic perceptions have led to the hypothesis that the learning disabled are at risk for the learned helplessness found in adults (Seligman, 1975) and children (Dweck, 1975).

Attributions: Locus of Control and Learned Helplessness

Many of these studies have been based on Weiner's (1974) two-dimensional taxonomy of attributions, explanations for success and failure. One dimension refers to internality vs. externality. A belief in internal control means that outcomes are interpreted as the result of factors over which the individual has control such as one's effort and ability. A belief in external control means that outcomes are interpreted as the result of luck, others, task difficulty, and other factors over which the individual has no control. The second dimension in the taxonomy refers to stability. Ability and task difficulty are viewed as stable factors while effort and luck may be relatively unstable over time and situations. There is a considerable literature which shows that there is a positive relationship between adopting an internal locus of attributions and academic achievement. Individuals who believe in internal control show greater persistence on tasks, select unfinished rather than finished tasks, delay gratification, and are more likely to actively seek, retain, recall, and reproduce information (Stipek and Weisz, 1981; Dweck, 1975; Bialer, 1961).

In contrast, individuals who hold learned helpless attributions believe that events are the result of uncontrollable factors. This belief is associated with lack of persistence and withdrawal from challenging tasks, even when successful completion of the task is possible. Passivity, lack of persistence, negative self-attitudes about intellectual performance, and lower self-esteem has been associated with learned helplessness in adults (Seligman, 1975) and children (Dweck and Reppucci, 1973). The parallels between descriptions of learned helpless attitudes and behaviors and descriptions of the learning disabled are striking. Descriptions of the learning disabled as holding negative academic self-concepts, expressing less optimism about future accomplishments, and discounting actual success has led to the hypothesis that these children do not believe they have control over their environment, that they would display learned helpless attitudes and behaviors. If the learning disabled do not believe success is under their control, there would be no reason for them to have high hopes for future success, nor to attribute failure to controllable events. The experience of prolonged school failure may lead the learning disabled to increasingly believe they are not in control of their destinies.

Research assessing learning disabled youngsters' locus of attribution supports the notion that the learning disabled hold attitudes similar to those found in learned helplessness. Across a wide age span, using different measures, there are consistent differences between learning disabled and achieving students. Using a generalized locus of control (Nowicki and Strickland, 1973), learning disabled 9- and 10-year-olds (Fincham and Barling, 1978) and junior high students (Hallahan *et al.*, 1978) were more external than achieving students. Using a scale which assesses internality for success and failure, the Intellectual Achievement Responsibility Questionnaire, IARQ, (Crandall, Katkovsky, and Crandall, 1965), third through sixth and third through eighth graders were found more external than normal achievers in attributions for success but not failure (Chapman and Boersma, 1980; Pearl, Bryan, and Donahue, 1980) while learning disabled junior high students were more external than non-disabled classmates (Hallahan *et al.*, 1978).

Since distinctions between the factors of ability, effort, task difficulty, and luck have been linked to learned helplessness (Dweck and Reppucci, 1973) studies have also examined attributions more specifically. Dweck and Reppucci (1973) showed that attributions about effort were particularly significant as learned helpless students discounted the importance of effort following the experience of failure. Hence, learning disabled students attributions for the importance of effort relative to ability, task difficulty, and luck have been of interest. Pearl (1982) asked first through eighth grade learning disabled and normal achieving students to rate the importance of the four factors for success and failure in reading, in social situations, and in doing puzzles. Although groups did not differ in their ratings of the importance of effort for success, the learning disabled were less likely than the normal achievers to consider not trying hard enough an important reason for their failures. Further, while normal achievers rated task difficulty as equally important in success and failure, the learning disabled rated task difficulty more important for success than failure. They believe that success is more likely to occur because tasks are easy than that failure is likely to occur because tasks are difficult. Finally, while normal achievers considered task difficulty more important to performance in reading than in social situations or in doing puzzles, the learning disabled believed task difficulty of equal importance across domains. In sum, the evidence shows the learning disabled do hold attitudes similar to those described in the learned helplessness literature. They have negative self-perceptions about their likely success on performance-related activities and do not interpret success as an indication they have control of their destinies.

These studies show that normal achievers are likely to attribute success to internal factors, like ability and effort, and failure to factors like effort or task difficulty. In contrast, the learning disabled are less likely than normally achieving classmates to take credit for their success, to perceive success as related to their own ability, and they are more likely to attribute failure to a lack of ability. Failure is attributed to stable factors and success to factors other than their ability.

Test Anxiety and Fear of Evaluation

A personality factor which has been studied very little is that of test anxiety. The only study to date on learning disabled is by Bryan, Sonnefeld, and Grabowski (1983). The results indicate that the learning disabled express more test anxiety than normally achieving classmates. Since test anxiety has been associated with fear of failure, one hypothesis about the learning disabled is that they are motivated to avoid failure. It might be noted that the motive to avoid failure has been found to have a greater impact on student performance than the motive to succeed (Bryan *et al.*, 1983). An experiment by Gottlieb (1982) addressed test anxiety in students described as educationally handicapped. Students were asked to read aloud orally and told either that their reading would be evaluated by a teacher or that they were just practicing. The educationally handicapped youngsters made more oral reading errors in the evaluative than in the non-evaluative condition. These test anxiety and/or fear of failure data may be relevant to explain the depressed performance of the learning disabled.

One motive of the learning disabled may be to avoid failure. Any situation which involves evaluation of performance may be interpreted as a potential source of failure and increase error. This suggests that the achievement and performance of the learning disbled may be differentially affected by situational variables. While studies have shown that ability and achievement tend to be stable across time and situations (Endler and Magnuson, 1978), the performance of the learning disabled is more likely to be influenced by external factors than the performance of normally achieving children. We turn now to those studies which have compared learning disabled and non-disabled children's learning and/or behavior in different situations.

SITUATIONAL FACTORS

Audience

One simple situational factor which may influence performance may be the presence of an audience. While no data are available regarding the learning disabled and audiences, social comparison research has found that the learning disabled in mainstreamed classes have lower self-concepts than learning disabled who spend at least some time in segregated classes with other handicapped students (Strang, Smith, and Rogers, 1978). Being surrounded by higher achieving students may make the children judge themselves more harshly and have a depressing effect on performance. Gottlieb (1982) found educationally handicapped students made no more errors when reading aloud to nonreading kindergarteners than when they read alone; however, there is some question as to whether younger children represent a salient audience. Nonetheless, knowing the learning disabled's greater anxiety about evaluation suggests more research is needed.

Responses to Success and Failure Experiences

A number of studies have examined learning disabled children's attributions and behavior in response to the experience of success vs. failure. An early study (Keogh, Cahill, and MacMillan, 1972) used the interrupted task paradigm to study academically handicapped (learning disabled + behavior disorders) boys explanations of failure. Boys were interrupted while doing a perceptual motor task having been told they would be stopped if they were working too slowly and not doing well (failure condition) or if they were doing well (success condition). Interviewed afterwards the 9-year-olds attributed failure to complete the task to experimenter explanations while 12-year-olds blamed themselves irrespective of experimenter explanations. Pearl, Bryan, and Herzog (1983) assessed learning disabled and non-disabled students' responses to high or low success, based on the ratio of winning to losing game points on a laboratory bowling game. Results show no differences in attributions when students had high success. In the low success condition, the normal achievers responded by generating task strategies while the learning disabled responded with vague, undifferentiated responses. Furthermore, the learning disabled reported having obtained fewer high scores than they actually had, and predicted they would do more poorly should they play the game again than did the non-disabled students.

Butkowsky and Willows (1980) had fifth grade poor, average, and good readers do a reading anagram and tracing task under success (solvable) and failure (unsolvable) conditions. Results show that the poor readers, in contrast to both average and good readers, predict they will do fewer problems, spent about 40 per cent less time on the unsolvable problems, and were particularly pessimistic about future performance after the failure experience. Similar results were obtained by Tollefson et al., (1982) in a study of junior high seventh through ninth grade learning disabled students. Before doing a spelling lesson, learning disabled students were asked to predict the number of easy, moderately difficult, and difficult words they would spell correctly. After taking a spelling test, they were interviewed about why they had done well or poorly and asked to predict how many words they would spell if given another similar list. Learning disabled students attributed success on the easy list to ease of task, success or failure on the moderately difficult words to effort, and failure on difficult words to either lack of ability or task difficulty. Learning disabled students were highly variable in their predictions for future spelling performance, either over- or underestimating relative to their actual performance. In sum, learning disabled students appear to be particularly reluctant to take credit for their successes, opting for ease of task as an explanation. Moreover, learning disabled students are likely to blame themselves, naming lack of ability, for their failures.

These results were essentially replicated by Aponik and Dembo (1983) in a study of adolescents' attributions for success and failure, in response to easy, moderate, or difficult tests. Learning disabled and non-disabled adolescents were given the IARQ, and three tasks consisting of verbal analogies graded *a priori* as easy, moderate, or difficult. After doing each task the students were given success or failure feedback and then asked to attribute causality to ability, effort, task difficulty, or luck. On the IARQ, the normal achievers were more internal than the learning disabled for success and failure items. Measure of students' attributions for the three tasks found the non-disabled adolescents attribute success to their own ability more than did the learning disabled students who perceived ability more a factor in failure. The learning disabled students also consider luck to be more important than non-disabled students across the different levels of difficulty. As task difficulty increased in the success conditions the non-disabled increased both effort and ability attributions; under failure, they increased attributions to task difficulty and decreased their emphasis on ability and effort. The learning disabled, as task difficulty increased in the success condition, placed greater importance on luck, while under failure, ability attributions were stable for each level of task difficulty.

Responses to High vs. Low Classroom Structure

Locus of attribution theory suggests that children who differ in their beliefs should respond differently to different instructions. Students who hold internal beliefs should respond better in low structure situations, those in which they have control. Students who hold external beliefs should learn better in high structured situations, those in which others have control (Baron *et al.*, 1974; Rotter, 1966). Learning disabled students who are external should, therefore, perform better in high vs. low teacher structures.

Pascarella and Pflaum (1981) assigned reading groups to one of two reading intervention programs which varied in the degree of structure provided by the teacher. The reading program was designed to teach students to detect their errors while reading orally and to correct these errors. Reading groups comprising learning disabled and other poor readers were randomly assigned to one of two modes of teacher responding. In the teacher-determination-of-error (TDE) the teachers explicitly and directly told students in their small reading groups whether or not their answers were correct. In the other mode, the student-determination-of-error (SDE), teachers encouraged students to figure out for themselves if their answers fitted. Students were administered the IARQ and pre-post tests of reading achievement. On the IARQ the learning disabled scored less internal than other poor readers. Further, students who scored high in internality showed significantly higher post-test reading scores in the SDE than the TDE condition. In contrast, students who scored low in internality, that is, who held external beliefs, showed significantly higher post-test reading scores in the TDE than the SDE condition. Thus, the learning disabled students scored significantly higher in externality and made greater reading progress in the highly structured TDE than the SDE mode.

While this study showed that a fit between student attribution and teacher response mode can have a significant impact on student reading progress, no attempts were made in this study to change student attribution. A few studies have shown it is possible to increase student persistence on various tasks after attribution retraining (Dweck, 1975; Chapin and Dyck, 1976; Fowler and Peterson, 1981). Efforts in this regard using learning disabled students, however, have not been particularly successful in showing changes in student attributions. Pascarella *et al.*, (1983) extended the Pascarella and Pflaum (1981) study to examine the generalizability of attribution retraining of learning disabled students using the reading error detection and self-correction program. A third teacher mode was added to the design. In this transition condition, the first lessons were like the TDE, the last lessons were like the SDE, but the middle lessons shifted to include increases in the number of teacher exhortations for the students to try harder. Since students were in their regular reading groups they not only received their teachers' exhortations immediately after naturally occurring failures, but they also observed them when their group-mates made errors. The results show the same attribution by treatment interaction pattern as reported in the Pascarella and Pflaum (1981) study, but there were no significant effects for the transition condition. Efforts to alter student attributions, and to shift them from the high to low structure condition were not successful. A similar lack of success was reported by Schunk (1981).

In the Schunk study, children showing low arithmetic achievement received either modelling of division operations or didactic instruction in which they studied and practiced on their own. During the practice phase of the treatment, the trainer attributed their success or failure to high vs. low effort. Post-test measures consisted of math accuracy, persistence, and self-efficacy. Children in both treatment groups judged themselves more efficacious, persisted longer, and solved more problems than a no-treatment control group. Treatments, however, did not differentially affect self-efficacy, or persistence, although the modelling condition resulted in greater gains in math accuracy. The effort attributions had no effect on perceived efficacy or on arithmetic performance. Perceived efficacy was a significant predictor of arithmetic performance across conditions.

The results of these studies suggest that the effects of attribution retraining may be influenced by the performance context in which they occur (Chapin and Dyck, 1976; Schunk, 1981). On the one hand, if children learn they can succeed despite a history of prolonged failure, they may show high persistence irrespective of teacher feedback. However, if they fail after spending considerable effort, especially if that effort is known to others, attribution retraining which emphasizes effort may be threatening to feelings of self-worth, since this would imply the student lacks ability (Schunk, 1981).

Modeled after the Pascarella and Pflaum study on performance, the impact of external control was extended to physical fitness tasks. Bryan and Smiley (1983) had learning disabled and non-disabled boys do sit-ups and the shuttle run in a neutral condition or one in which they were given an external rationale for performance. In this case students were told that drinking apple juice prior to performing would give them extra energy to do well. In the neutral condition they were told the juice would prevent thirst. Results found that neither the external nor neutral explanations influenced the learning disabled; but the performance of the non-disabled was depressed in the external rationale condition. In a follow-up study, Pearl, Bryan and Smiley (in preparation) had boys do the sit-ups and the shuttle run in one of three rationale conditions. In the internal rationale they were told that based on an earlier performance they were the type of person who if they really tried hard would do very well. The external rationale and neutral conditions were the same as in the earlier study. Results showed that the learning disabled performed as well as the normal achiever in both the external and internal rationale conditions. In the neutral condition the learning disabled performed significantly worse than the achieving boys.

The results of these varied studies show that we can influence the learning and performance of the learning disabled by matching teacher response mode with student attribution style. There is considerably less evidence that we can influence their thinking about the causes of their performance. In the short run it may be expeditious simply to match instructional style to student beliefs. Yet, because self-generated learning, in the face of temporary failure, may be a significant educational goal, considerably more research exploring the interaction of attribution and response to instruction and feedback are needed. Furthermore, while the results concerning the interaction of attribution and responses are quite consistent across these studies, alternative explanations for findings should be considered. Given the strategy deficits of the learning disabled (Wong, 1980; Torgesen, 1975) and the verbal information processing limitations of the learning disabled (Vellutino, 1980), these findings might reflect learning/memory differences rather than motivational/attributional differences between learning disabled and other students. For instance, the Bendell *et al.* (1980) and the Pascarella *et al.* (1983) data could result from limitations in information processing skills among external learning disabled students relative to internal learning disabled students. Teachers providing spelling strategies and/or correct responses may reduce the load on student working memory, and thus increase their likely correct responses. Failure to obtain attribution shifts following attribution training may, therefore, be the result of true learning differences among learning disabled students.

Group Reward Structures

The impact of the organization of the classroom on achievement has received considerable attention recently. Those classroom structures commonly used include cooperative, competitive, and individualized goal structures. *Cooperative* goal structures are those in which incentives are based on group products. *Competitive* goal structures distribute incentives based on the individual's performance relative to others. *Individual* goal structures base incentives on the performance of the individual using some set standard. There is a large database showing that cooperative goal structures have a positive impact on many types of task performance and interpersonal attitudes. Cooperative goal structures appear to have a positive effect on tasks which involve problem solving, cognitive rehearsal, and group productivity (Slavin, 1977). Children in cooperative structures report greater peer support and encouragement, and more positive attitudes toward their teachers, task, and other group members, and feel that others like them better than children in competitive or individualistic groups (Johnson and Johnson, 1979).

Classroom instruction organized around cooperative reward structures is distinctly different from that used in special education. In resource programs, and in segregated classrooms for the handicapped, the reward structures emphasize individualized goals and incentives. The Individual Education Plan (IEP) mandated by PL 94–142 requires that the handicapped child's education be based on an assessment of that individual child's educational needs. Special education programs do not consider the child in the context of the classroom where children are grouped for various instructional purposes. Given the positive results found in studies which have compared cooperative vs. individual goal structures, Johnson and Johnson (1979) have argued that cooperative goal structures would enhance both the learning and social acceptance of handicapped youngsters. Yet the research conducted has failed to discriminate between cooperative instructions vs. incentives, and, it has not examined the achievement of individual children in groups. To find that group products are better than individual products does not tell us the contribution and/or learning of the individual child. To compare the performance of individuals in group structures based on cooperative vs. individual goals, Cosden, Bryan, and Pearl (1983) and Bryan, Cosden, and Pearl (1983) conducted a number of studies. They first assessed the impact of cooperative instructions and incentives and individualized instructions and incentives on learning disabled and non-disabled youngsters. The performance of students in four types of dyads was compared: (a) a learning disabled and non-disabled partner received instructions and incentives to cooperate; (b) two normal achieving students received instructions and incentives to cooperate; (c) a learning disabled and normal achieving student received instructions and incentives based on individual performance; and (d) two normally achieving students received the individual instructions and incentives. Students performance on a reading task and their interactional behaviors during a study period were analyzed.

The results show that learning disabled boys' performance was largely unaffected by goal structures. But the normal achieving boy with a learning disabled partner showed a performance decrement in the cooperative condition. Normally achieving partners in the cooperative structure showed the best performance. Performance differences seem related to study behaviors. The learning disabled boys and their normally achieving partners engaged in less interactive study behavior than the non-disabled dyads. Assessment of attributions found that boys in the cooperative condition rated themselves somewhat higher in ability than boys in the individual condition. Students who wanted to work with their partner again attributed higher levels of ability, effort, and luck to their partners.

Learning disabled girls also tended to do worse on the reading performance measure than normally achieving girls. However, the normally achieving girls did not show a performance decrement as a function of having a learning disabled partner. Indeed analyses of study behaviors showed considerable positive interactions between the learning disabled girls and their achieving partners. On the attribution measure, the learning disabled girls rated their partners ability as higher than their own. Girls in the cooperative condition believed their partners put more effort into their performance than girls in the individual condition. Girls in the cooperative condition reported more partner satisfaction than girls in the individual condition.

Because the learning disabled — normally achieving male dyads failed to engage in appropriate study behaviors in the cooperative condition, a second study examined whether showing the boys a model of cooperative behaviors would increase adaptive study interactions. The study was repeated with a third condition added in which a short videotape of two boys engaging in interactive study behaviors was shown prior to the dyads being given the cooperative instructions and incentives. The results showed that while the learning disabled still did more poorly than the normal achievers on the performance measure, the normal achieving boys in the model plus cooperative incentives condition did not show a performance decrement. Both modeling plus cooperative instructions/incentives resulted in an increase in positive interactive study behaviors. Hence the results of these two studies show that the learning disabled do more poorly than normally achieving students irrespective of goal structures and that they may not have the performance skills to benefit from cooperative group structures without some additional coaching on how to interact with peers in the group. Yet, showing a short film which depicts correct, adaptive behaviors was highly effective in eliciting appropriate study behaviors, and in improving the interactions between learning disabled and normally achieving males. Females are largely unaffected by goal structures and seem to engage in considerable interactive study behaviors under both sets of instructions and incentives.

SUMMARY

Several personality and situational factors have been discussed, although none have been thoroughly researched. The results show that each is deserving of systematic study to sort out the factors influencing the learning disabled student. Nonetheless, across these studies the data show that the learning disabled differ on personality variables found important to academic achievement. Self-concept, self-esteem, locus of attributions differentiate the learning disabled from achieving students, and in each case, the learning disabled hold the more maladaptive attitudes. Insofar as such attitudes affect student behavior, it is critical that such beliefs be taken into account when working with the learning disabled. Persistence, choice of tasks, and willingness to engage in cognitively challenging activities are behaviors associated with these attitudes. Thus, it is not surprising that the learning disabled are described as learned helpless. They show the attitudes and behaviors associated with learned helplessness. It may well be that many of the performance decrements of the learning disabled are falsely identified as learning problems when in fact these represent motivational problems. A passive learning style and failure to respond to tasks with problem-solving strategies have been interpreted in the learning disability literature as problems in metacognition, memory, learning, and/or language. It may be that the primary motive for the learning disabled is to avoid failure which they do by allowing teachers to play dominant roles in the teacher–learner relationship. Not expecting to be in control of learning, the learning disabled may wait to be rescued. Given the belief that one is not in control of one's destiny, that increased effort will not help one face adversity, there is no reason to seek alternate strategies when faced with difficulty.

Overall, the results of these studies suggest the following. First, it appears that these are students who have a primary motive to avoid failure. Much of their behavior and attitudes in response to performance situations would suggest this. Second, these are students who do not take personal credit for success. How to convince them that their ability and effort is accounting for their achievement, and not that of kind teachers giving them easy work, has not been resolved by the literature. To date, the only resolution that has been effective has been to match student attribution and teacher mode. While the learning disabled do make greater reading progress in a highly structured than low structured teacher response style, this resolution does not move the learning disabled toward motive to achieve.

Another major issue is related to learning disabled students' responses to failure. Special education dogma dictates that teachers should provide learning disabled students with success experiences. Yet, it is responses to coping with

228   DYSLEXIA: ITS NEUROPSYCHOLOGY AND TREATMENT

failure that may be critical in determining students' willingness to persevere when learning is difficult. Instruction programmed to teach the learning disabled such coping strategies has not yet been designed or evaluated.

Thus, the research on the interaction between personality and situational factors in influencing the performance of the learning disabled demonstrates that definitions of the learning disabled which focus only on cognitive variables will not be effective in describing the learning disabled. To the extent that affective and motivational variables are ignored, the assessment and treatment of the learning disabled may be sorely limited in effectiveness. While it may well be that constitutional factors contribute significantly to learning disability, the exclusion of personality and situational factors from consideration may well sabotage our efforts to understand and intervene. It is therefore deemed imperative that interactional approaches to research between discipline be taken.

REFERENCES

Aponik, D. A., and Dembo, M. H. (1983), LD and normal adolescents' causal attributions of success and failure at different levels of task difficulty. *Learning Disability Quarterly* 6, 31-9.

Bandura, A. Self-efficacy: toward a unifying theory of behavioral change. *Psychological Review* 84, 191-215.

Baron, R. M., Cowan, G., Ganz, R. L., and McDonald, M. (1974), Interaction of locus of control and type of performance feedback: considerations of external validity. *Journal of Personality and Social Psychology* 30, 285-292.

Bendell, D., Tollefson, N., and Fine, M. (1980), Interaction of locus-of-control orientation and the performance of learning disabled adolescents. *Journal of Learning Disabilities* 13, 83-86.

Bialer, I. (1961), Conceptualization of success and failure in mentally retarded and normal children. *Journal of Personality and Social Psychology* 29, 303-320.

Black, W. F. (1974), Self-concept as related to achievement and age in learning-disabled children. *Child Development* 35, 1137-1140.

Bryan, T., and Smiley, A. (1983), Learning disabled boys' performance and self assessments of physical fitness tests. *Perceptual and Motor Skills* 56, 443-450.

Bryan, T., Cosden, M., and Pearl, R. (1983), The effects of cooperative goal structures and cooperative models on LD and NLD students. *Learning Disability Quarterly*, 5, 415-421.

Bryan, J. H., Sonnefeld, L. J., and Grabowski, B. (1983), The relationship between fear of failure and learning disabilities, *Learning Disability Quarterly*, 6, 217-222.

Butkowsky, I. S., and Willows, D. M. (1980), Cognitive-motivational characteristics of children varying in reading ability: evidence for learned helplessness in poor readers. *Journal of Educational Psychology* 72, 408-422.

Chapin, M., and Dyck, G. (1976), Persistence in children's reading behavior as a function of N length and attribution retraining. *Journal of Abnormal Psychology* 85, 511-515.

Chapman, J. W., and Boersma, F. J. (1980), *Affective Correlates of Learning Disabilities*. Lisse, Swets & Zeitlinger.

Coopersmith, S. (1967), *The Antecedents of Self-esteem*. San Francisco, W. H. Freeman.

Cosden, M., Pearl, R., and Bryan, T. (1985), The effects of cooperative vs. individual goal structures on learning disabled students, *Exceptional Children*, 52, 103-114.

Covington, M. V., and Beery, R. G. (1976), *Self-worth and School Learning*. New York, Holt, Rinehart & Winston.

Crandall, V. C., Katkovsky, W., and Crandall, V. J. (1965), Children's beliefs in their own control of reinforcement in intellectual–academic situations. *Child Development* **36**, 91–109.

Cronbach, L. J., and Snow, R. E. (1977), *Aptitudes and Instructional Methods: A Handbook for Research on Interactions*. New York, Irvington/Naiburg.

Dunn, G., Pearl, R., and Bryan, T. (1981), Learning disabled children's self evaluations. Chicago Institute for the Study of Learning Disabilities, University of Illinois, Chicago.

Dweck, C. S. (1975), The role of expectations and attributions in the alleviation of learned helplessness. *Journal of Personality and Social Psychology* **31**, 674–685

Dweck, C. S., and Reppucci, N. D. (1973), Learned helplessness and reinforcement responsibility in children. *Journal of Personality and Social Psychology* **25**, 109–116.

Endler, N. S., and Magnuson, D. (1978), Toward an interactional psychology of personality. *Psychological Bulletin* **83**, 956–974.

Fincham, F., and Barling, J. (1978), Locus of control and generosity in learning disabled, normal achieving, and gifted children. *Child Development* **49**, 530–533.

Fowler, J. W., and Peterson, P. L. (1981), Increasing reading persistence and altering attributional style of learned helpless children. *Journal of Educational Psychology* **73**, 251–260.

Gottlieb, B. W. (1982), Social facilitation influences on the oral reading performance of academically handicapped children. *American Journal of Mental Deficiency* **87**, 153–158.

Hallahan, D. P., Gajar, A., Cohen, S., and Tarver, S. (1978), Selective attention and locus of control in learning disabled and normal children. *Journal of Learning Disabilities* **11**, 47–52.

Hiasama, T. (1976), Achievement motivation and locus of control of children with learning disabilities and behavior disorders. *Journal of Learning Disabilities* **9**, 58–62.

Johnson, R. T., and Johnson, D. W. (1979), The social integration of handicapped students into the mainstream. In: M. Reynolds, R. Hlidek, D. W. Johnson, R. Johnson, N. Sprinthal and F. Wood (Eds.), *Social Acceptance and Peer Relationships of the Exceptional Child in the Regular Classroom*. Reston, Virginia, Council for Exceptional Children.

Keogh, B. K., Cahill, C. W., and MacMillan, D. L. (1972), Perception of interruption by educationally handicapped children. *American Journal of Mental Deficiency* 107–118.

Nowicki, S., and Strickland, B. R. A locus of control scale for children. *Journal of Consulting and Clinical Psychology* **40**, 148–154.

Pascarella, E. T., and Pflaum, S. W. The interaction of children's attribution and level of control over error correction in reading instruction. *Journal of Educational Psychology* **73**, 533–540.

Pascarella, E. T., Pflaum, S. W., Bryan, T. H., and Pearl, R. (1983), Interaction of internal attribution for effort and teacher response mode in reading instruction: a replication note. *American Educational Research Journal* **20**, 269–276.

Pearl, R. (1982), LD children's attributions for success and failure: a replication with a labeled LD sample. *Learning Disability Quarterly* **5**, 173–176.

Pearl, R., and Bryan, T. (1982), Learning disabled children's self-esteem and desire for approval. Paper presented at the international conference, Association for Children and Adults with Learning Disabilities, Chicago, Ill., 1982.

Pearl, R., Bryan, T., and Donahue, M. (1980), Learning disabled children's attributions for success and failure. *Learning Disability Quarterly* **3**, 3–9.

Pearl, R., Bryan, T., and Herzog, A. Learning disabled and nondisabled children's strategy analysis under high and low success conditions. *Learning Disability Quarterly* **6**, 67–74.

Pearl, R., Bryan, T., and Smiley, A. (1982), Effects of experimenter-induced attributions on physical fitness tasks. Child, University of Illinois at Chicago.

Rosenberg, M. (1965), *Society and the Adolescent Self-image*. Princeton, NJ, Princeton University Press.

Rotter, J. B. (1966), Generalized expectancies for internal vs. external control of reinforcement. *Psychological Monographs* **80**, whole issue.

Schunk, D. H. (1981), Modeling and attributional effects on children's achievement: self-efficacy analysis. *Journal of Educational Psychology* **73**, 93–105.

Seligman, M. E. (1975), *Helplessness*. San Francisco, Freeman.

Stipek, D. J., and Weisz, J. R. (1981), Perceived personal control and academic achievement. *Review of Educational Research* **51**, 101–138.

Strang, L., Smith, M. D., and Rogers, C. M. (1978), Social comparison, multiple reference groups and the self-concepts of academically handicapped children before and after mainstreaming. *Journal of Educational Psychology* **70**, 487–497.

Thomas, A. (1979), Learned helplessness and expectancy factors: implications for research in learning disabilities. *Review of Educational Research* **49**, 208–221.

Thomas, J. W. (1980), Agency and achievement: self-management and self-regard. *Review of Educational Research* **50**, 213–240.

Tollefson, N., Tracy, D. B., Johnsen, E. P., Buenning, M., Farmer, A., and Barke, C. R. (1982), Attribution patterns of learning disabled adolescents. *Learning Disability Quarterly* **5**, 14–20.

Torgeson J. (1975), Problems and prospects in the study of learning disabilities. In: M. Heatherington (ed.), *Review of Child Development Research*, Chicago: University of Chicago Press, Vol. 5.

Vellutino, F. R. (1980), *Dyslexia: Theory and Research*. Cambridge, Mass., MIT Press.

Weiner, B. (1974), *Achievement Motivation and Attribution Theory*. N. J. General Learning Press.

Wong, B. Y. L. (1980), Activating the inactive learner: use of questions/prompts to enhance comprehension and retention of implied information in learning disabled children. *Learning Disability Quarterly* **3**, 29–37.

CHAPTER 16

Learning Disability among Seriously Delinquent Youths: A Perspective

HARRIET E. HOLLANDER
CMHC-UMDNJ, Rutgers Medical School, Busch Campus, Hoes Lane, Piscataway, NJ 08854, USA

The chapter compares the prevalence of Specific Developmental Disorders (SDD) and Attentional Deficit Disorders (ADD) with other diagnosable clinical conditions found in two hundred juvenile offenders consecutively admitted to state correction institutions. It reports on their family status and economic background, as well as their previous history of evaluation and remediation (Hollander and Turner, 1985). The association of Specific Developmental Disabilities and other diagnosable clinical conditions with violent crime is analyzed. The results are considered in the framework of the current debate over whether learning disabilities and delinquency are causally linked.

Clinical research carried out in juvenile court settings has drawn attention to the high prevalence of learning and attentional disorders in delinquent youths. Prevalence statistics have been used as evidence that a causal link exists between learning disorders and delinquency even if the mechanism that links them is unknown (Weiss, 1971; Cantwell, 1978; Campbell, 1974). Support for early interventions to thwart a delinquent outcome has been advocated (Berman, 1972; Poremba, 1975).

Critics have warned against prematurely concluding that learning disabilities and delinquency are causally linked on the basis of prevalence statistics. They have pointed to methodological flaws in the procedures used to estimate prevalence. They argue that many studies fail to adhere to a rigorous definition of learning disabilities, set forth in Federal regulations (Public Law 94–142, 1977). These regulations designate the learning handicapped child as one whose failure to learn cannot be attributed to low IQ, social disadvantage, emotional disorder, or poor motivation. These criteria have been incorporated into the new Diagnostic and Statistical Manual of the American Psychiatric Association.

DSM-III classifies Specific Developmental Disorders and Attention Deficit Disorders (with and without hyperactive syndrome) as separate conditions.

A second criticism has focused on the failure of research investigators, who advocate the concept of a causal link, to take into account the salience of environmental factors, such as poverty and family disorganization (Glueck and Glueck, 1970; Andry, 1971; Offord, 1978). Compared to the impact of these factors, Murray (1977) argues that learning disabilities occupy only a small piece of territory in the causal map.

The present research was primarily designed to create a profile of the incarcerated delinquent. A profile approach avoids the dilemma of deciding which of many significant variables is pre-eminent in precipitating a delinquent outcome. It does not, and indeed cannot, given the state of the art, specify whether familial, economic, or individual developmental factors are primary in creating social deviance or increasing the risk of incarceration.

However, a broader perspective on the statistical relationship of learning disabilities and delinquency can be obtained by investigating the following questions:

(1) What type of clinical disorders generally characterize a population of serious juvenile offenders?
(2) What is the family status and economic background of these offenders?
(3) What is the prevalence of Specific Developmental Disorders relative to other clinical disorders?
(4) How prevalent is reading retardation among institutionalized offenders, as differentiated from the prevalence of Specific Developmental Disabilities defined as reading below the third grade level, despite an IQ of 85 or above?
(5) To what extent are Specific Developmental Disabilities associated with serious emotional disorders, such as Schizotypal, Borderline, and Paranoid Personality Disorders?
(6) Is having a Specific Developmental Disorder and/or Attention Deficit Disorder associated with committing violent crimes?
(7) Have delinquent adolescents diagnosed as having Specific Developmental Disorders or Attention Deficit Disorders ever had diagnostic and/or remedial treatment through special classes or tutoring?

SURVEY OF THE LITERATURE

Definitional issues continue to be central to efforts to determine the prevalence of learning disabilities and of Attention Deficit Disorders among delinquent youths. Estimates of prevalence vary according to the definitional criteria used to sample and classify subjects.

Reading failure and other disabilities according to Federal guidelines, denote a discrepancy between IQ score level and expected performance for chronological age. Attention Deficit Disorders, which are more prominent in children than in adolescents and which often overlap with learning disabilities (Silver, 1981), are diagnosed from observation of a pattern of impulsivity, hyperactivity, inattentiveness, and resistance to discipline.

Delinquency is not defined clinically, but legally. A delinquent is a minor who has committed a felony. Delinquents differ from status offenders who are not felons, but truants, runaway, and 'incorrigible' children who cannot be managed at home. Delinquents vary according to the degree they penetrate the judicial system. For example, in 1979, the police in the state of New Jersey made 120,000 arrests (New Jersey Uniform Crime Reporting, 1979). Seriously delinquent youths probably comprise only 6 per cent of this court-involved population, but it is estimated that they account for up to 50 per cent of arrests for serious juvenile crime (Wolfgang et al., 1972).

Some studies, in which learning disabilities are related to delinquent outcome, use fairly broad criteria to define learning disability and attention disorders as well as delinquency. For example, merely backward readers may be counted as learning disabled. Felons and status offenders may both be defined as court-involved delinquents. It is, therefore, not surprising that in recent reports in the literature authors, who considered the prevalence evidence, arrived at different conclusions regarding the link between learning disabilities and delinquency. For example, Poremba (1975) estimated that 50 per cent of the court-involved adolescents he studied had symptoms of minimal brain damage. In other studies reviewed by Poremba (1975), prevalence estimates range from 32 per cent (Duling, 1970) to 58 per cent (Berman, 1972) to 90.4 per cent (Compton, 1974) among subjects defined as delinquent.

Murray et al., (1979), reviewing these studies and others for the Office of Juvenile Justice and Delinquency Prevention (OJJDP) took a closer look at the statistical evidence. He concluded that most of the quantitative studies had been too poorly designed for prevalence estimates to be considered as reliable, or as supporting the hypothesis that learning disabilities and delinquency are causally linked. Studies were particularly faulted for their lack of adherence to a rigorous definition of learning disability. For example, Compton (1974), who found that 90 per cent of delinquents were learning disabled, counted any evidence of psychological or social disadvantage as a learning handicap.

Critchley (1968) and Hurvitz et al. (1972), followed more rigorous experimental procedures and obtained more conservative estimates. Critchley found that 60 per cent of 477 institutionalized delinquents were retarded in reading. However, the number of youths with IQs over 91 who had specific dyslexia was only 19.8 per cent. Critchley suggested that a link between delinquency and violence exists. He cites anecdotal evidence portraying E. Harvey Oswald, who assassinated Kennedy, as a dyslexic.

Hurvitz and Bibace (1972) found that both learning disabled and delinquent boys performed more poorly than normals on a test of motor development.

Delinquents also performed more poorly than a normal control group on tasks of sensorimotor and symbolic sequencing. However, these authors noted that the distribution of social class was skewed in their subjects. They suggested that lower class children with learning disabilities were more likely to be labeled delinquent than middle class children with learning disabilities.

Following the publication of Murray's (1975) review, Campbell and Varvariz (1979) at the Educational Testing Service were funded by OJJDP to direct a project to investigate the prevalence rates of learning disabilities among 1103 court-adjucated delinquents and non-delinquent school children aged 12–15 years. Groups were equated for socioeconomic status. An IQ cut-off score of 80 was adhered to in this sample. Their carefully designed study precisely specified the definitional boundaries for classifying learning disability.

Decision rules for a positive diagnosis included behavioral evidence of hyperactivity, poor performance on perceptual motor tasks, uneven achievement scores, and discrepancies in ability tests. The results indicated that 38.2 per cent of adjudicated delinquents had learning disabilities compared to 19.1 per cent learning disabilities among officially non-delinquent peers. Significant interaction between delinquency and intelligence level was found among the learning disabled youths. Juveniles in the borderline range of intelligence with SDD's appeared to have a greater risk of adjudication. When data were analyzed to exclude subjects with a lower level of intellectual ability, the incidence of learning disability was 27.7 per cent among delinquent boys.

It appears that in the literature, definitional boundaries have not been clearly established with regard to the often overlapping clinical symptoms of learning disorders, attention deficit and hyperactivity. Kinsbourne (1982) suggests that when attention, as concentration, cannot be maintained, hyperactivity results. Deficient concentration is manifested as inability to selectively attend to the relevant stimulus and underlying learning disability. The basic disorder can, therefore, be considered a disorder of attention. Pavlidis (1981), proposes that abnormal eye movements may be used for the objective diagnosis of such deficient attention.

Pirozollo and Hansch (1982) have reviewed the large body of evidence indicating that neurological and neurophysiological abnormalities exist in children with developmental dyslexia. However, they also point out that developmental dyslexia is not a homogeneous entity.

Are conditions such as attention deficit disorder, hyperactivity, and learning disability independent or overlapping? Silver (1981) explored the relationship between hyperactivity and/or attention deficit and learning disability. Of 110 S's diagnosed as learning disabled, 26 per cent were hyperactive, 41 per cent were distractible, and 24 per cent were both hyperactive and distractible. Of 100 S's diagnosed as hyperactive, 92 per cent were found to have learning disabilities. In a third group, (N = 100) where emotional disorder was the primary diagnosis, 3.5 per cent of children were found to have learning disabilities, 12 per cent were hyperactive, 3 per cent were distractible, and 8 per cent were both hyperactive and distractible.

It appears that although not all hyperactive children will be found to be distractible, most will have learning disabilities. Not all learning disabled children will have symptoms of hyperactivity and distractibility. When learning disabled children become delinquent, the antisocial behavior may be attributed to the underlying distractibility and poor impulse control associated with the attention deficit and/or hyperactive condition (Silver, 1981).

The specific relationship between hyperactivity and delinquency has been investigated by a number of authors. Weiss (1971) followed 64 non-psychotic children with mean IQs above 84. They were first diagnosed at an average age of 8 years and were reassessed at an average age of 13 years. Hyperactivity was no longer the chief complaint, although the majority continued to be distractible. Those who were found to be antisocial had families who were rated as significantly more pathological than those who were not antisocial. Huessy (1974) found that, in a sample of 84 hyperkinetic children, the risk of being institutionalized was 20 per cent greater than in the general population.

Cantwell (1978) considers that the hyperkinetic disorder runs in families and expressed in various patterns of deviance. He cites one of his earlier investigations (Cantwell, 1972) in which he found that hyperactivity in child subjects was associated with parental sociopathy in 16 per cent of mothers and with maternal alcoholism in 8 per cent of cases.

Lewis (1979) reports that violent delinquents are distinguished from less violent juvenile offenders by both major and minor neurological signs. Violent delinquents may also present paranoid symptomatology, visual, auditory, olfactory, or gustatory hallucinatory experiences and bizarre behavior, especially among those who have witnessed violence. She suggests that violent behavior may result when a child is impaired and has witnessed violence.

One research study, carried out to evaluate the impact of learning disabilities on subjects who were not delinquents, points to family status as a key variable affecting adult social adjustment. Spreen (1982) studied predominantly middle class adults who had been disabled readers. His subjects had average or better than average IQs and were free of psychiatric disorders. Those subjects who came from a lower socioeconomic group seemed to have had advantageous family backgrounds, since they had secured entrance to select private schools which provided educational remediation. Most subjects had been extensively treated for their disability. Spreen (1982) found that these subjects compared favorably in level of academic and vocational adjustment with their non-reading disabled adult peers.

Socioeconomic status itself seems to be related to reading achievement. Tarnapol (1971) reports that youths from lower socioeconomic circumstances read at the fifth grade level on the average. Feinberg (1980), summarizing the more recent results of Clark's study on non-delinquent inner-city school children in Newark, reports that ninth graders, aged fifteen, from socially disadvantaged families, read at the sixth grade level.

In summary, the literature provides evidence that reading disability or reading backwards is prevalent among delinquents, along with neurological soft signs reflected in impaired motor, sensorimotor, or sequencing function. However, correlating a clinical condition with delinquent outcome, does not establish causation. Factors such as low IQ, history of family stress, low socioeconomic status, presence of psychiatric disorder, combined with criminality in other family members, or lack of remedial experience, must be taken into account. Unless these factors are shown to have no relationship to social deviance, the assumption that learning disability plays a primary role in a delinquent outcome, remains open to question.

The design of the present study lent itself to the taking of a broad, rather than a narrow, perspective on learning disabilities and delinquency. Specific Developmental Disorders were not singled out for investigation, but were assessed in the context of other profile characteristics. The presentation of the diagnostic classifications for all subjects permitted the comparison of the relative frequency of SDD/ADD to other developmental handicaps.

Socioeconomic status and history of remedial experience were analyzed to fill out the profile of the delinquent.

Reading backwardness, which can be attributed to poor motivation, or inadequate schooling was differentiated from disability in learning, which can be attributed to genetic, or neurophysiological factors. The basis for this differentiation is described more fully in the methodology section.

METHOD

Two hundred juveniles, consecutively admitted to state correctional facilities during a ten-week period, who ranged in age from 12 to 18.9 years, with a mean age of 15.5, were the subjects of this research. Ethnically, 57 per cent of the youths were Black, 35 per cent were Caucasian, and 5.7 per cent were Hispanic.

A profile was compiled on each juvenile consisting of a number of variables. These included results of IQ tests, the determination of diagnostic classification according to DSM-III, including classification for Specific Developmental Disabilities or Attention Deficit Disorder, the assessment of family background, and economic status, and the investigation of each child's previous evaluation and treatment history. Information was supplemented by a standardized individual interview with each juvenile, coded for computer analysis.

Diagnostic classification for all developmental disorders was based on case records which contained previous psychiatric, psychological, and neurological evaluations, on intake psychological testing, which included the WISC, or WAIS, or Army Beta, the MMPI (read aloud to poor readers), the Bender-

Gestalt, the Draw-A-Person, the Sentence Completion and a Rorschach (when appropriate), a Structured Interview coded for computer analysis, and a brief mental status examination.

Pre-screening diagnoses were carried out in the following manner for Specific Developmental Disabilities and Attention Deficit Disorders. Juveniles were considered *suspect* for learning disability if they met at least one of the following criteria: significant retardation in reading (e.g. below third grade level), despite a Verbal, Performance, or Full Scale IQ score of 85 or above on the WISC or WAIS or on the Army Beta, significant discrepancies of 15 points or more between Verbal IQ and Performance IQ, poor performance on the Bender-Gestalt, or self-reported reading problems. If a clear diagnosis, supported by previous evaluations, could not be made, adolescents were individually tested by a disability specialist with such tests as the Learning Aptitude, the Durell Spelling Test, the Peabody Individual Achievement Test, or Botel Word Recognition and Word Opposites.

In addition, results were analyzed for a subsample of 57 juveniles, who had completed tests for school placement within the institution. General level of reading and arithmetic ability was determined for each subject in the subsample, using the WRAT as a locator test, and/or Primary, Intermediate, or Advanced Forms of the Stanford Achievement Tests.

A reading age was derived for each subject. The reading age (R.A.) was his reading achievement grade, plus five years, four months, which represented age of school entrance. By this method, a fourteen-year-old, who read at the eighth grade level, would be considered an 'average' reader. A fourteen-year-old who read at the fifth grade level, could be considered 'backward', although not dyslexic. If the discrepancy between R. A. and C. A. (chronological age) was less than three years, the juvenile was considered to have reading backwardness. If he read below the third grade or more than three years below grade level, he was considered dyslexic.

DSM-III is a multi-axial system designed to include all significant clinical conditions. The criteria require that the primary classification reflect the reason for referral or institutionalization. Principal diagnoses, usually coded on Axis I, include Conduct Disorders, Adjustment Disorders, Attention Deficit Disorders, Retardation, and Schizophreniform Disorders. They are defined as follows:

Attention Deficit Disorder (ADD) is manifested in such signs as inappropriate attention, impulsivity and hyperactivity, and may include stubbornness, negativism, low frustration tolerance, mood lability, lack of response to discipline, temper outbursts, and neurological soft signs.

Conduct Disorders (CD) refer to repetitive and persistent patterns of difficulty at home or in the community in which the basic right of others or community norms are violated.

Adjustment Disorders (AD) of Emotion and Condition refer to dysfunctional reactions, including antisocial behavior, traceable to a recent external stress. Among Axis I classifications, where both conditions exist, Conduct Disorder is given precedence over Adjustment Disorder as the primary diagnosis.

Axis II classifications refer to conditions such as Personality Disorders (PD) or Specific Developmental Disorders (SDD) which frequently occur in conjunction with other conditions. They are coded on a secondary axis to ensure that they are not overlooked.

Personality Disorders include: the Borderline Personality, manifested by symptoms of identity confusion, chronic feeling of boredom or emptiness, evidence of self-destructive behavior such as gambling, theft, substance abuse, or self-mutilation, mood changes, manipulativeness, inappropriate displays of anger; the Schizotypal Personality manifested by recurrent visual or auditory illusions (but not prominent hallucinations), magical thinking, ideas of reference, odd (but not incoherent) speech, social isolation, and hypersensitivity to criticism; and the Paranoid Personality manifested by symptoms of hypervigilance, guardedness or secretiveness, avoidance of blame, pathological jealousy, restricted affectivity, and expectation of trickery or harm.

Specific Developmental Disorders refer to deficient performance in reading, writing, spelling, arithmetic, understanding, and the expression of language, given consideration of an individual's tested intelligence level and educational opportunity.

In this study, SDD was classified under the following conditions. A *low* threshold was set for defining average intelligence, e.g. any score in the average range on a verbal or nonverbal standard measure obtained during intake testing or reported in the case record. A *high* threshold (below third grade) was set for diagnosing learning disability in reading, in order to exclude backwardness attributable to poor schooling or lack of motivation. Thus, a severely backward reader with spuriously a low IQ score (one with much scatter) who appeared to have average intellectual ability, was not overlooked.

DSM-III also contains V codes described as conditions not attributable to mental disorders which are a focus of treatment or concern. The V code used in this study was 'Borderline Intelligence', defined as IQ below 85 and above 69 based on either intake testing or reported scores in the case record.

RELIABILITY

Reliability of screening diagnoses was carried out by referring to appropriate outside specialists four groups of juveniles, each containing ten randomly selected adolescents, who had (1) Personality or Adjustment Disorders;

(2) Specific Developmental Disorders; (3) Attention Deficit Disorders or (4) Borderline IQs. Each group, as appropriate to their disorder, was re-evaluated by either a child psychiatrist, by a learning disability specialist, at a cerebral dysfunction clinic, or by a psychologist. The specialists could not be blind to the likelihood of an Axis I diagnosis of Conduct Disorder since juveniles are required to wear uniforms, and to be accompanied by security escorts under all circumstances.

Granted these constraints, the child psychiatrist confirmed seven out of ten classifications, changing three classifications of Adjustment Disorder to Conduct Disorder with Borderline Personality Features. The learning disability specialist upheld all classifications of Specific Developmental Disability. Test re-test reliability for the IQ tests was 0.79. The Cerebral Dysfunction Clinic supported ADD screening diagnoses in seven out of ten cases. They recognized a significant history of seizures in the eighth subject and minor neurological soft signs in the remaining two cases.

RESULTS

As Table 1 indicates, seriously delinquent, incarcerated youths are a heterogeneous group. Most of 185 wards (84.8 per cent) were primarily classified as having Conduct Disorders since DSM-III gives priority to the diagnosis that

Table 1. Classification of juvenile offenders ($N = 185$)

Undersocialized Conduct Disorder				
	%		%	
Aggressive Type	18.4	Non-Agressive Type	10.8	
with Personality Disorder (PD) (Borderline, Schizotypal Paranoid)	23.8		2.2	
Specific Development Disorder and/or Attention Deficit Disorder and PD	5.9		0.0	
SDD/ADD	5.9		2.2	
Socialized Conduct Disorders				
	%		%	%
Aggressive Type	2.2	Non-Agressive Type	7.0	
with Personality Disorder	0.0		1.6	
Specific Development Disorder and/or Attention Deficit Disorder and PD	0.0		0.5	
SDD/ADD	0.5		3.8	
Adjustment Disorder				9.2
Schizophreniform Disorder				2.2
Other				3.8

specified the reason for institutionalization. But nearly half (46.4 per cent) had an associated developmental disorder. An additional 15.2 per cent had primary developmental handicaps such as an Adjustment Disorder of Emotion and Conduct (9.2 per cent) or Schizophreniform Disorder (2.2 per cent).

The most prevalent handicap (47 per cent) associated with the diagnosis of Conduct Disorder was Borderline IQ, listed as a V code in DSM-III. A diagnosis of Borderline IQ reflected an IQ score below 85, and was assigned only if *none* of the intake intelligence test scores, or previous scores in the case record were above that level.

Black Ss scored significantly below White Ss on the Army Beta, but Full-scale and Performance scores on the WISC were comparable for Black and White Ss. The IQ distribution for all Ss was positively skewed. In fact, only 5.3 per cent of juveniles had IQs above 110.

Psychiatric disorders were widespread; 27.6 per cent of juveniles with Conduct Disorders also had Borderline, Schizotypal, or Paranoid Personality Disorders. These adolescents were not overtly psychotic, but had symptoms of self-destructive behavior, mood swings, and chronic feelings of restlessness or boredom. They were physically assaultive, suspicious, had histories of brief psychotic episodes, recurrent visual or auditory hallucinatory experiences, strange thoughts, and magical thinking and other bizarre behaviors.

Learning disabilities were found among significant numbers of juvenile offenders, but are certainly not the most prevalent developmental handicap in this group. Only 18.8 per cent of these juveniles had a Specific Developmental and/or Attention Deficit Disorder. Of these adolescents, 6.4 per cent also had an associated Personality Disorder.

What accounts for the discrepancy between the present prevalence data on Specific Developmental Disabilities (SDD)/Attentional Deficits (ADD), and higher estimates reported by some other investigators? One explanation is that low prevalence estimates of SDD in this study are a function of definition and procedure. The present investigators differentiated between Ss who had clear-cut learning impairments, despite average intelligence, and Ss who had general reading backwardness. Although SDDs were found in only 18.8 per cent of Ss, reading backwardness was pervasive in the sample. The average reading level was fourth grade, as was the average math level. Only 6.4 per cent of 62 adolescents tested at expected grade level.

The data were analyzed to determine whether low IQ in Ss contributed to the general phenomenon of reading backwardness. However, as Table 2 shows, low IQ cannot be the major factor in reading backwardness, since reading backwardness occurs in Ss with low average IQs whose reading performance should have been more adequate.

It was hypothesized that the finding of reading backwardness (rather than dyslexia, with its genetic, neurophysiological basis) might be attributed to the poor quality of schools attended by inner city youths. While not all subjects were 'inner city' minority youths, most did come from adverse family

Table 2. Reading ability by IQ level ($N = 57$)

Level	IQ 85 and above	IQ 84 and below	Total	Percentage
Backward (R.A. 3 years below expected level)	25	0	25	43.9
Specific Development Disorder (R.A. below 3rd grade)	8	0	8	14.0
Normal (R.A. within 3 years of grade level)	12	12	24	42.1
Total	45	12	57	100.0

Reading age (R.A.) is reading achievement level plus five years, four months.

circumstances. In this sample, 74.5 per cent came from families broken by divorce and separation, compared to a national average of 24.5 per cent of Caucasian children and 43.9 per cent of Black children. There were 51 per cent of boys from families who had once been on welfare; 37.5 per cent were from families presently supported by welfare.

Thirty-five per cent of juveniles reported criminality in other family members, 24.5 per cent reported alcoholism in the family, and 22 per cent reported a history of child abuse (distinguished from spanking for misdeeds). These stressful family situations were undoubtedly related to high truancy rates and low rates of school enrollment. Only 34.6 per cent of juveniles were enrolled in school and were attending classes when apprehended. Absence from school certainly would suppress achievement levels in reading and mathematics even if learning disabilities were not present.

Compared to delinquents with Borderline IQs or to other juveniles, subjects who had SDDs or ADDs were among the least likely to commit violent crimes (even when Ss with Personality Disorders were included). Juveniles who committed crimes against persons (murder, assault, robber, rape, arson), were likely to have a diagnosis of Undersocialized Aggressive Conduct Disorder or a Personality Disorder rather than a learning disability.

Low IQ was implicit in the diagnosis of Undersocialized Conduct Disorder, Aggressive Type, and was significantly associated with violence. As shown in Table 3, Ss with Borderline IQs were more likely to be sentenced to a reformatory for violent rather than property offenses ($\chi^2 = 19.77$, d.f. $= 6$, $p < 0.003$).

Poremba (1975), Berman (1972), and Silver (1981) have suggested that intervention directed to the remediation of learning disabilities might thwart a delinquent outcome. Juveniles in this sample could have had the benefit of legislation in effect in New Jersey, since 1966, to identify and provide education for learning handicapped students (N. J. Stat. Ann. 18: A: 7B-1 et seq. (West 1985) originally enacted L. 1966, Ch. 29, S5). Educational,

Table 3. Developmental problem and type of crime committed ($N = 174$)

Developmental Problem	Crimes Against Property and Non-Victim Crime		Crimes Against Persons		Total
	N	%	N	%	N
Undersocialized Conduct Disorder, Aggressive Type	16	47.0	18	52.9	34
Specific Developmental Disorder and/or Attention Deficit Disorder and Personality Disorder	24	68.5	11	31.4	35
All adjustment disorders	12	70.5	5	29.4	17
Personality Disorders (without SDD and/or ADD)	27	52.9	24	47.1	51
All other Conduct Disorders	28	75.7	9	24.3	37
Total	107	61.5	67	38.5	174

Likelihood ratio $\chi^2 = 9.833$, d.f. = 4, $p < 0.04$.

remedial, psychological, and community services should have been available for adolescents who were severely handicapped, both developmentally and socially.

Did they receive such help? We searched case records and carried out probes as part of the structured interview to find out. Unlike Spreen's intellectually able subjects, who had the advantage of special treatment programs and who were comparable to non-learning disabled peers as adults, the delinquents in this study had not been exposed to intensive or remedial interventions.

Only 49.3 per cent of juveniles had had diagnostic evaluation by Child Study Teams, a learning specialist, or mental health professional prior to their admission to a correctional setting. There were no differences based on diagnostic categories. Only 39 per cent of these adolescents had even had special services in the form of tutoring or special classes. The youths most likely to have had special education experiences were not those who were clearly learning disabled or even those most cognitively handicapped (with IQs below 80). Less than 40 per cent of the learning disabled or cognitive impaired received such help. However, 80 per cent of youths with IQs of 80 to 90 were likely to have had special placement.

DISCUSSION

It is readily apparent from the present results that delinquency is not a unitary clinical entity. Although delinquents are classified in DSM-III as having Undersocialized or Socialized Conduct Disorders with Aggressive or Non-Aggressive features, their most distinctive clinical characteristics are their multiple psychiatric, neurological, and intellectual handicaps.

Almost half of these incarcerated adolescents (47 per cent) have below average IQs. Among their other developmental handicaps are Borderline, Schizotypal, Paranoid Personality Disorders (27 per cent) Schizophreniform Disorder (2.1 per cent) and Specific Developmental Disorders or Attentional Disorders (18.8 per cent), and both SDD and Personality Disorder in 6.4 per cent of the sample.

Since other developmental disorders in these delinquents are more prevalent than learning disorders and are associated with more serious patterns of crime, the present results do not justify the conclusion that learning disabilities are uniquely associated with a delinquent outcome.

It may be argued that the present findings are attributable to the narrow standard employed for defining delinquency and learning disorders. It may indeed be the case that definitional boundaries account for differences in our findings and those of Poremba (1975). However, a 19.8% prevalence rate of dyslexia, similar to our rate of 18.87 was obtained by Critchley (1968) in juvenile offenders with average intelligence.

The present study may have underestimated the prevalence of residual attentional disorders. When they were children, such disorders may have been present in juveniles now diagnosed as Undersocialized and Aggressive. Many children with Borderline IQs often have minor neurological soft signs. By early and mid-adolescence, however, clear signs of ADD are no longer present (Weiss, 1971; Silver 1981). These Attentional Disorders are difficult to diagnose retrospectively with any confidence. Among adolescents, the presence of a few neurological soft signs may not meet DSM-III criteria for positive diagnosis. Symptoms of impulsivity, negativism, and resistance to discipline can overlap with symptoms of Personality Disorder and Conduct Disorder. These symptoms, positively identified by other investigators as 'soft signs' of ADD/SDD, we may have classified in other diagnostic categories.

Although the present results indicate that most delinquents have a developmental handicap, the results should not be interpreted to mean that a developmental disorder in and of itself is associated with a delinquent outcome. Delinquency appears to be associated with having a developmental handicap in the context of severe family disorganization—divorce, separation, alcoholism, child abuse, reliance on public welfare, criminality among other family members. The sequence is one where genetic, familial, neurophysiological factors as well as substandard education and psychiatric limitation can lead to reading failure as well as to delinquent outcome.

Two facts stand out in sharp contrast to each other. On the one hand, data show that at least half the delinquents in the study had never been professionally evaluated, and that only 39 per cent had ever received treatment. Those with specific developmental disorders of reading and average IQs were *least* likely to have received special interventions. On the other hand, Spreen (1982) has shown that children who have been placed in remedial settings (presumably by supportive parents) have achieved levels of adult adjustment similar to their non-learning disabled peers. The presence or absence of a parental support system and effective treatment is a critical variable impacting on adult adjustment when learning disabilities are present. The risks of a delinquent outcome are probably increased for children who are untouched by meaningful remedial intervention on the part of the school, community, or mental health systems.

Few correction settings provide well-run educational and remediation programs that are combined with re-education efforts. So we do not know whether genuinely appropriate remediation programs for the nearly one out of five delinquents with learning handicaps can reduce recidivism. Nor do we know if early interventions can prevent delinquent outcomes.

It does appear that the correction system is the repository for inadequately served mentally, intellectually, and educationally handicapped children of the poor.

REFERENCES

Andry, R. G. (1971), *Delinquency and Parental Pathology*. London, Staples Press.

Berman, A. (1972), Neurological dysfunction in juvenile delinquents: implication for early intervention. *Child Care Quarterly* 1 (4), 264–271.

Campbell, P. B., and Varvariz, D. S. (1979), *Psychoeducational Diagnostic Services for Learning Disabled Youth*. Princeton, NJ, Educational Testing Service.

Cantwell, P. (1978), Hyperactivity and antisocial behavior. *Journal of the American Academy of Child Psychiatry* 17 (2), 252–262.

Cantwell, P. (1980), The diagnostic process and diagnostic classification in child psychiatry—DSM-III. *American Academy of Child Psychiatry* 19, 345–355.

Clark, K. (1980), *Effective Urban Secondary Education: Review of the Literature*. Unpublished draft manuscript. New York.

Current Population Reports Special Studies p. 23 No. 80 (1979), *Social and Economic Status of the Black Population 1970–1978*. US Dept. of Commerce: Bureau of the Census, Washington, D. C., 003–024 01659–1.

Critchley, E. M. R., (1968), Reading retardation, dyslexia and delinquency. *American Journal of Psychiatry* 115, 1537–1547.

Compton, R. (1974), Diagnostic evaluation of committed delinquents. An address to the Symposium Youth in Trouble. Academic Therapy Publications. Cited in Poremba (1975).

Diagnostic and Statistical Manual of Mental Disorders. 3rd edn. Washington, DC, American Psychiatric Association.

Duling, F., Eddy, E., and Risko, V. (1970), Learning disabilities of juvenile delinquents. Morgantown, West Virginia Department of Educational Services. Robert E. Kennedy Youth Center. Cited in Poremba (1975).

Feinberg, (July 9, 1980), Scores of Inner City Youth. *Washington Post*, Washington, D.C.

Glueck, S., and Glueck, E. (1970), *Toward a Typology of Juvenile Offenders*. New York, Grune & Stratton.

Hollander, H., and Turner, F. Characteristics of incarcerated delinquents. *Journal of the American Academy of Child Psychiatry* 24, 221–226.

Huessy, H., Metoyer, M., and Townsend, M. (1974), 8–10 year follow up of 84 children treated for behavioural disorders in rural Vermont, *Acta Paedopsychiat.* 10: 230–235.

Hurvitz, I., and Bibace, R. M. (1972), Neuropsychological function of normal boys, delinquent boys, and boys with learning problems. *Perceptual and Motor Skills* 35, 387–394.
Kinsbourne, M. (1982), The role of selective attention in reading disability. In: Malatucha, R. V., and Aaron, P. G. (Eds.), *Reading Disorders, Varieties and Treatment*. New York, Academic Press. pp. 199–214.
Lewis, D. O., and Balla, D. A. *Delinquency and Psychopathology*. New York, Grune & Stratton.
Lewis, D. O., Shanok, S., Pincus, J., and Glaser, G. H. (1979), Violent juvenile delinquents. *Journal of American Academy of Child Psychiatry* 18, 307–319.
Loehlin, J. C., Lindzey, G., and Spuhler, J. N. (1975), *Race Differences in Intelligence*. San Francisco, W. H. Freeman and Co.
Murray, C. A. (1966), The link between learning disabilities and juvenile delinquency. Task Force Report 76JN-99-0009. Washington, DC, National Institute for Juvenile Justice and Delinquency Prevention.
New Jersey State Facilities Education Act of 1979 L 1979 C 207 (N. J. Stat. Ann. 18: A: 7B-1 *et seq.* (West 1985) originally enacted L. 1966, Ch. 29, S5).
New Jersey Uniform Crime Reporting (1979), January. West Trenton.
Offord, D. R., Poushinsky, M. F., and Sullivan, K. (1978), School performance, IQ and delinquency *Brit. J. Criminol.* 18, 110–126.
Pavlidis, G. Th. (1981), Sequencing, eye movements and the early diagnosis of dyslexia. In: Pavlidis, G. Th., and Miles, T. R. (Eds.), *Dyslexia Research and its Application to Education*. Chichester, John Wiley.
Pincus, J. J., and Tucker, G. T. (1978), Violence in children and adults: a neurological view. *Journal of the American Academy of Child Psychiatry* 17, 2, 277–288.
Pirozollo, F. J., and Hansch, E. C. (1982), Neurobiology of developmental reading disorder. In: Malatesha, R. N., and Aaron, P. G. (Eds.), *Reading Disorders: Varieties and Treatments*. New York, Academic Press.
Poremba, C. D. (1975), In: Helmar R. Myklebust (Ed.), *Learning Disabilities, Youth and Delinquency: Programs for Intervention in Progress in Learning Disabilities*, Vol. III. New York, Grune & Stratton, pp. 123–149.
Public Law 94–142, *Public Law of the General Education Provision Acts as Amended 20 USC 1232d*. Federal Register Vol. 42, No. 163, Tues., August 23, 1977.
Robins, L. N. (1966), *Deviant Children Grown Up*. Baltimore, Williams and Wilkins.
Silver, L. B. (1981), The relationship between learning disabilities, hyperactivity, distractibility and behavioral problems. *Journal of the American Academy of Child Psychiatry* 20, 385–397.
Spreen, O. (1982), Adult outcome of reading disorders. In: Malatesha, R. V., and Aaron, P. G. (Eds.), *Reading Disorders: Varieties and Treatment*. New York, Academic Press, pp. 199–214.
Tarnopol, L. (Ed.), Proceedings of the panel on medication: medicating children with learning disabilities, Part I. In: London, Little Brown & Co., pp. 119–208.
Weiss, G., Minde, K., Werry, J., Douglas, D., and Nemeth, E. (1971), Studies on the hyperactive child. *Arch. Gen. Psychiat.* 24, 409–414.
Wolfgang, M. E., Figlio, R. M., and Sellin, T. (1972), *Delinquency in a Birth Cohort*. Chicago, University of Chicago Press.

Treatment

Dyslexia: Its Neuropsychology and Treatment
Edited by G. Th. Pavlidis and D. F. Fisher
© 1986 John Wiley & Sons Ltd.

CHAPTER 17

Remediation for Dyslexic Adults

Doris J. Johnson
Northwestern University, Evanston, Illinois, USA.

The purpose of this chapter is to review several factors regarding reading instruction for adults with dyslexia. The discussion includes psychological and vocational issues as well as those related to remediation since an understanding of the goals, backgrounds, and overall psychoeducational characteristics of the individual is needed in order to plan a program. Because of the heterogeneity of the population, reading instruction should be person-orientated rather than method-bound.

At the outset, it is important to consider the nature of the population to be served. Northwestern University has had a diagnostic and remedial clinic within the department of Communicative Disorders for over thirty years. As a part of the professional preparation and research program, both children and adults come to the campus for assessment and instruction. While hundreds of dyslexics have been evaluated, only a limited number of adults come for remediation. This is due, in part, to the fact that the Learning Disabilities program is devoted to research and teacher training as well as service. Furthermore, not all adults request remediation; some merely want a better understanding of their problems.

In general, the adults in the program are well motivated. Many are self-referred and may be somewhat different from school-aged dyslexics who are required to participate in Special Education. Others were referred by their employers, when there was a question about promotion or job maintenance, or by college instructors or vocational rehabilitation workers. In a few instances a spouse or family member encouraged the adult to seek help.

Before scheduling an evaluation, the adults were asked to write a letter (uncorrected) describing the nature of their difficulties and stating why they wanted help. While a few were reluctant to write because of their poor reading and spelling skills, they all complied with the request. Occasionally it was necessary for a family member to address the envelope or send a translation if the writing was illegible. These letters were useful in understanding the nature of the problems and helpful in making a diagnosis. Through their writing, the adults clearly conveyed the idea that dyslexia is not simply an academic handicap. It is a life problem that interferes with many aspects of social and vocational mobility as well as education.

Their letters, together with the extensive case history done at the time of the evaluation, revealed that all of the dyslexics had a history of chronic reading and learning problems. Most were identified during kindergarten or early elementary school. And most said that, at one time, they felt either retarded or 'bad' because they could not learn as well as others. While many said they had problems related to self-esteem, they frequently had developed ingenious coping strategies to use at school, work, or in social situations. Some had found ways to avoid reading menus, signs, and other material at work. A few had never told their children they were unable to read and were becoming embarrassed when a child came to them and asked for help with school work. In other instances, the dyslexics had told a few friends, co-workers, or teachers about their difficulties and felt comfortable asking for help.

An analysis of the case histories and chief complaints indicated that the adults wanted to be tested for various reasons. Approximately one-third of a group of ninety had never been evaluated; therefore, they wanted to find out why they had difficulty learning. Basically, they wanted a differential diagnosis and information regarding intelligence and achievement. Another third had been diagnosed as learning disabled or dyslexic but they wanted a clearer definition of the problem. They wanted to know more about their levels of performance in order to make more informed decisions regarding future employment and education. The final third wanted remediation so they could pursue further education or make a job change. Several were very inefficient readers and were exhausted because of the time it took to complete reading or writing assignments in school or at work.

Many in the group had received remedial reading or special education during their early school years, and most said remediation had been helpful but it had not been available during secondary school, having been discontinued when they were twelve or thirteen years old. It was of interest to note that many had maintained their level of performance but had not made any gains after remediation was terminated. Thus, many of the dyslexics were reading between a fifth and seventh grade level (10 to 13 year age range). Those who had received limited help in school could not read more than a few words.

Despite the problems, the majority were employed. However, as expected, their work required limited reading and writing. This meant that some with high average mental ability were employed as stockmen, as messengers for companies, or in skilled labor jobs. Those who were performing at higher levels did read and write at work but they frequently had to spend extra time completing their work.

Because of the frustrations associated with their reading problems, approximately one-third of the group had been referred for counselling or psychotherapy. In part, there was hope that the counselling would be useful in 'removing a reading block'. The adults reported that the counselling helped them deal with feelings of inadequacy but it did little to facilitate their reading performance.

While many dyslexics were eager to try remediation, others were ambivalent. They wanted to improve but they also were fearful of another failure. One young woman said, 'I had fourteen years of phonics and I still can't read; I just worry about getting my hopes up again'. Others expressed fears about revealing weaknesses to teachers again since they had painful memories of school. Still, many want to try. One man who was not reading above a seven-year level wrote in faulty script, 'I want to learn to read and write so I can go on with my learning'. Those who were reading at higher levels wanted remediation because they were exhausted from spending so much time on their assignments. One man who was reading at a nine-year level said it often took him two hours to write a short memo at work because he had to look up most of the words in the dictionary. Another in a junior college said he had no social life because he had to spend every minute studying.

These comments are meant to suggest that one does not simply give the adults a test battery and plan a program of remediation. One must be sensitive to their hopes and fears as well as their goals. We are neither overly optimistic nor pessimistic and generally begin remediation on a three-month trial basis to determine whether the adults want to continue and to obtain some data regarding progress and prognosis. It is our feeling that no one should engender false hopes for a 'quick cure' among a group of sensitive people who have already experienced repeated failures. Nevertheless, adult dyslexics can make significant gains in reading and writing.

GENERAL CHARACTERISTICS OF THE POPULATION

All of the adults in the program are seen for an intensive two-day psychoeducational study which includes a lengthy case history, an evaluation of auditory and visual acuity, both verbal and nonverbal intelligence, many aspects of oral language, reading, spelling, written language, mathematics, and various nonverbal cognitive functions such as spatial orientation. The test battery is similar to that we use with adolescents; however, specific tests are selected according to the individual's age and abilities (Johnson, Blalock, and Nesbitt, 1978).

An analysis of ninety case records indicate that the age range of the group tested extended from twenty to forty-two years with the majority being in their late twenties and early thirties. Approximately one-third were in school (junior college, university, or trade school) while the others were employed. A few were unemployed while waiting to change jobs or enter school. Many had fine work records and had held the same position for several years. All recognized the significance of work and wanted to be as independent as possible.

The socioeconomic levels of the group varied from lower middle to upper middle class. All had come from families in which schooling, at least through high school, was expected. All except two spoke standard English.

The interests and background experience of the group varied as one might expect with any population. Some preferred sports and outdoor activities; others enjoyed art and music; and said they spent their free time with families. Several, however, commented on their limited social life and were concerned about their isolation. A few had joined groups for the learning disabled as a means of understanding their problems and an opportunity for making friends.

In general, we find it is important to consider background interests and experience as well as academic achievement when selecting materials for remediation since the reading of familiar content tends to be easier than that which is unfamiliar.

All of the dyslexics in this population met the criteria for the diagnosis of learning disabilities. Auditory acuity was within normal limits and visual acuity was either normal or corrected with glasses. All had at least average mental ability on either verbal or performance measures. No person with a full scale IQ below 89 was included. The mean IQ for the group described here was 102. The range extended from 89 to 127. These findings are similar to clinical studies we have done on dyslexic children (Johnson and Myklebust, 1965).

READING AND RELATED LEARNING PROBLEMS

The reading achievement levels for the group varied considerably. Those with the most severe disorders could not read more than a few words while others were performing at a twelfth grade level. The mean reading grade level for a group of eighty was 8.2. On the surface, this might suggest that the reading problems were not severe since many were not totally illiterate. However, when adults with above-average intellectual functions are unable to read their secondary school textbooks they clearly have difficulty mastering their programs independently. Furthermore, even though many were reading at a twelve- or thirteen-year grade level, none could be classified as efficient readers. While they managed to 'get by' in many situations, they had not automatized the basic subskills necessary for reading. When given series of experimental word lists that are typically mastered by the age of nine, even the adults who were reading at a twelfth grade level made mistakes. Thus, they may be similar to the subjects described by Guthrie (1973) and Samuels (1976). Guthrie reported that one source of disability among poor readers was a lack of mastery of subskills, with subsequent interfacilitation of subskills into higher-order units.

Although the focus of this paper is on reading problems of adults, it is important to emphasize that reading problems rarely occur in isolation. Both clinical observations and research on subtypes of dyslexia indicate that oral language problem tend to co-occur with reading disabilities (Myklebust and

Johnson, 1962; Mattis, French, and Rapin, 1975; Denckla, 1977; Lyon, 1983). For example, dyslexics frequently have disorders of phonemic discrimination, comprehension, memory span, retrieval, syntax, and linguistic awareness in addition to their reading difficulties (Johnson, 1980). In our adult population, well over half of the group had some problems with oral language. This is in keeping with the proportions described in an earlier study with children (Johnson and Myklebust, 1965).

If one views reading as a visual symbol system which is superimposed on oral language, then it is evident that a disturbance in the latter may interfere with one or more aspects of reading. For example, the student who fails to comprehend spoken language will typically have reading comprehension problems. Similarly, the student with defective oral syntax may be unable to make good predictions when reading in context (Goodman and Goodman, 1977). On the other hand, some children with auditory verbal disorders are aided by reading. They may be able to abstract certain linguistic rules visually that they cannot acquire auditorially (Johnson, 1982).

In certain instances, dyslexics have difficulty with all aspects of symbolic behavior, including nonverbal representation (Eisenson, 1984). Thus, in some cases, we need to investigate skills such as picture interpretation, and nonverbal communication. Generally, one can expect to find written language problems among dyslexics since writing follows reading developmentally. In a few instances, some aspects of spelling may be easier than oral reading because there is no need for re-auditorization. Nevertheless, all of the dyslexics we have studied had difficulty with written formulation of ideas.

The assessment of reading includes a minimum of four achievement tests— not simply to determine grade level, but to note the conditions under which the person gives the best and poorest performance. One of the purposes is to ascertain whether there are differences according to forms of input, mode of response, and unit of discourse (e.g. word, sentence, or context). The tests include (1) oral reading of single words, (2) oral reading of context, (3) silent reading of single words, i.e. vocabulary, and (4) silent reading comprehension. Many findings indicate that students with verbal expressive disorders read better silently than orally. In other instances, students can only read and comprehend orally, and those with attention disorders actually improve during oral reading because they are required to attend to all of the words.

Throughout the reading assessment and diagnostic teaching we also try to learn as much as possible about the strategies used by the reader. For this we incorporate concepts from Gray (1947) who suggested that one needs to use several strategies in order to be an efficient reader. These include (1) word form or configuration, i.e. rapid sight recognition, (2) phonetic analysis, (3) structural analysis, i.e. identification of words by noting derivatives, word endings, and prefixes, and (4) context. It is evident that various cognitive and linguistic skills are needed for each of these strategies. For example, quick recognition of sight words requires visual perception, memory, and verbal meaning. Phonetic analysis, on the other hand, requires more linguistic skills including analysis and synthesis. Structural analysis requires more knowledge of morphosyntax and an understanding of the meaning-bearing units within words. Contextual cues may be derived either from background knowledge and experience or from linguistic skills. Hence, it is interesting to select reading passages with familiar and unfamiliar content as well as passages that vary in syntactic complexity. Some dyslexics do not realize that they can use all of these strategies, whereas others cannot use multiple strategies. Still others have weaknesses in particular aspects of reading, such as phonetic analysis.

In general, the dyslexic adults in our population tried to use all of Gray's strategies but they were not totally efficient in the use of any. It was not uncommon for an adult to misread a simple one-syllable word or to reverse an occasional letter. This does not mean that remedial programs for visual perception or primary decoding skills were needed, but it appears that many reading behaviors are not automatized (LaBerge and Samuels, 1974). A detailed inspection of error patterns provided further insights into the instructional needs of the group.

Word Identification

In order to gain information about the reading of single words, we use both standardized achievement tests and a series of experimental tasks which include lists of high frequency nouns, CVC words organized according to vowel patterns, words with relatively regular phoneme–grapheme correspondence which have consonant clusters in the initial and final position, lists which have the potential for reversals and transpositions of letters, words organized into semantic groups such as fruits and vegetables, and high frequency functor words such as 'the, where', etc. Our preliminary findings indicate that the dyslexics with the most severe problems (i.e. those reading below a 7- or 8-year level) tend to read high frequency nouns with the greatest success. They appear to be using holistic strategies together with meaning and memory to identify these words. Their poorest performance tended to be on the short vowel words that contained consonant clusters in the initial and final position. It is hypothesized that there were various reasons for these errors. Some in the group had very poor phonemic segmentation and synthesis skills. Others seemed to be using faulty scanning techniques and others appeared to have difficulty with temporal ordering (Bakker and Schroots, 1981). It is of interest to note, however, that some of the dyslexics could spell words with regular phoneme–grapheme patterns more accurately than they could read them. This is in keeping with the findings of Bryant and Bradley (1980).

On the word lists containing the potential for reversals and transpositions of letters, none of the dyslexics manifested any consistent error but those with the most severe problems had occasional reversals and sequencing errors (from/form; big/pig). The errors they did make tended to be on the medial portion of the word rather than on the consonants. These findings tend to support the findings of Vellutino (1977) who stated that poor readers have few visual perceptual disorders and that their primary problems are related to verbal coding.

Phonetic Analysis

The ability to decode multisyllabic words in isolation is a major problem for most dyslexics. An inspection of approximately one thousand errors made by the adult dyslexics indicated that they tended to identify words on the basis of the first sound and, in most instances, the final sound. Errors were made on the medial portions and vowels in the word. Similar findings were reported by Shankweiler and Liberman in their studies with children (1972). As one might expect, these decoding problems also tend to interfere with reading comprehension (Perfetti, 1977).

The adults with poor phonetic analysis on reading tasks performed below expectancy on tasks of phoneme segmentation. For example, they had difficulty saying words slowly — syllable by syllable or by phoneme. The impact of this segmentation problem was noted even more on spelling. They tended to write words in a nonphonetic manner, frequently omitting syllables or sounds in writing (Boder, 1973). A detailed analysis of their writing indicated that the higher the spelling grade level, the better the performance on the phoneme segmentation tasks.

Structural Analysis

The adults were given both word lists and contextual material in order to investigate their use of structural analysis. Word lists with high frequency words such as the following were prepared: 'jump, jumps, jumping, jumped, jumper', 'cover, uncover, recover'.

The findings revealed that the dyslexics were generally able to read words with simple inflected forms but they had difficulty when there were marked pronunciation shifts as in 'apply–application'. This problem was not always limited to reading; some dyslexics could not pronounce multisyllabic words easily but knew the meanings. Most had difficulty on tasks which required them to derive an inflected form with nonsense words (e.g. troppy–troppier). Similar problems of metalinguistic awareness were reported by Vogel (1975) and by Hook and Johnson (1978). When the adults in remediation were asked to explain the significance or meaning of word endings and prefixes those with the most severe problems were confused about the meaning. A 25 year-old said he thought 'pre' meant after; he also said that 'bi' meant three times.

Our observations during remedial sessions indicated that dyslexics made rapid progress when they realized they could identify words by searching for meaning units. Some had been emphasizing the 'sound structure' or only phonetic analysis. This was also evident in their spelling as they focused on sounds rather than meaning units (desizhun/decision; jumpt/ jumped).

Failure to attend to word endings was noted in spontaneous written language also. An analysis of syntactic error patterns on the Picture Story Language Test (Myklebust, 1965) indicated that the most frequent mistake was omission of word endings. It is hypothesized that at least some of the errors are due to the fact that the adults tend to read by looking at a few key words and making hypotheses from context. If they do not attend to word endings while reading they will not hold the proper image for purposes of writing. In other cases, the written language errors reflect faulty oral syntax. They wrote as they spoke.

Context

As stated above, the adults tend to use their background knowledge when reading. This can be demonstrated by asking them to read both familiar and unfamiliar material. For example, a college student read unfamiliar material at approximately a third grade level but performed much better when asked to read an article from a psychology journal. She was interested in the topic and made good predictions because of her background knowledge. Needless to say, this type of observation is important for remediation. Adults who are required to read word lists or unfamiliar material may become discouraged and not even realize how well they can read if they make good hypotheses. At least some of their reading material should be related to their work and interests since this will afford them with an opportunity to read for confirmation (Chall, 1979). As they improve in other word attack strategies they can do more reading for learning.

When preparing materials for reading in context it is important to select passages of varying lengths. Too often standardized tests consist of only one paragraph. Such passages limit the reader's opportunity to use previous context when making predictions. As good readers become engaged in the content they make fewer errors. Thus, we see more errors within the first paragraph than in other portions of the discourse. For all of these reasons, we find it helpful to follow the procedures for preparing materials and analyzing errors according to the Goodman design (Goodman and Burke, 1972). They suggest that the reader be given stories or trade books which have not been read previously. The materials should have the potential for eliciting at least twenty-five errors.

Monitoring

Throughout all of the reading tasks we are interested in knowing how well dyslexics monitor for meaning and for syntax. Thus, when we listen to them read single words we want to know if they self-correct and/or realize they may have said something that is not a real word. Similarly, when reading context, we note their self-corrections and ability to monitor for both semantics and syntax. An inspection of over one thousand errors on tests of single word reading indicated that the dyslexics could monitor for meaning up to the fourth or fifth grade level. After that they frequently uttered nonsense words. This may be a reflection of both poor decoding skills and a limited spoken vocabulary.

In our work with both children and adults we have found that some dyslexics cannot monitor for meaning while reading aloud; they are overloaded with too much stimulation (Johnson and Myklebust, 1967). Therefore, we tape-record their reading; then we ask them to listen to the tape with no printed material in front of them and note if they can hear any mistakes. Later they are asked to listen and mark the errors and finally to re-read the passage in order to become more adept at monitoring. This type of training frequently results in marked progress in oral reading. It also aids attention to details.

In summary, the adult dyslexics generally try to use the various strategies described above but they are not proficient with any of them. They tend to look at the first and last letters of words and then guess from context. Most continue to have difficulty with higher level phonetic and structural analysis skills.

REMEDIATION OBJECTIVE

The goal of remediation is to help the dyslexic become a more efficient reader and to use as many strategies as possible. The ultimate objective is to close the gap between potential and achievement in order to foster as much educational, social, and vocational mobility as possible. We recognize, however, that we may not be able to achieve these objectives and, in working with the severe cases, we begin reading for protection, survival, and basic communication in the environment. As dyslexics make progress, more reading for information and pleasure is introduced. Those in higher education are helped to deal not only with the content of the courses but the reading and writing skills needed for independent learning.

The results of these objectives is not via any single method. Rather the programs are designed according to individual needs and the types of strategies the person can or cannot use. While it is possible to categorize methods according to their primary emphasis (e.g. alphabetic, look–say, etc.) (Naidoo, 1981), these terms are limiting because they do not define all of the critical features of the instructural system (Johnson, 1978). Methods that focus on one or more sensory systems (e.g. visual, multisensory) are equally limiting. It is my impression that the term 'method' should include such factors as the nature of the orthography, the vocabulary, the sentence structure, and the nature of the content. One should note whether the method is primarily analytic or synthetic and whether rules are learned implicitly or explicitly. We also are concerned with the types of sensory input, the modes of response, and the role of writing in reading. Considering the complexity of the reading process, and the individual variations in ability and performance, it is evident that no single set of materials can be used with such heterogeneous groups.

At the outset of remediation, we try to help the dyslexics realize that they can use multiple strategies for reading and we discuss those which they seem to be using most and least effectively. Through such discussions the adults become more proficient just because they have become more conscious of ways in which they can use what they know. We emphasize the importance of structural analysis since some have not been aware of the ways in which they can identify words by looking for meaning units. Some have overemphasized phonics. We also try to show how to use multiple strategies simultaneously. For example, with a word like 'recorder', the dyslexic might use either phonetic or structural analysis.

In most lessons, we try to achieve a balance between work on subskills or specific strategies and context. Just as the athlete or musician needs work on exercises as well as games or music, so also the reader needs a combination of activities in each lesson.

Remediation for rapid word identification usually begins with high frequency nouns and verbs. Miles (1981) indicated that most dyslexics need a good basic sight vocabulary. We emphasize high content, high imagery words because they tend to be more easily retained than the high frequency function words (the, there). Moreover, we feel the severe dyslexic needs a vocabulary of words he can use each day like names of food, clothing, street signs, etc. We also find that students with severe oral expressive problems can use recognition responses with these words by matching pictures to words even though they cannot recall them for rapid oral reading.

The high frequency functor, non-content words like 'the, then, with' are taught in context with other words the student has already learned. Occasionally it is necessary to provide minimal training on rapid visual perception of new words to improve scanning and consistency. Thus a word like 'there' might be written in several different ways (ther; theer; therre) and the adult is asked to find the one like the model and explain why the others are not correct. Verbalizing these differences seems to aid both perception and memory. Emphasis is given to position, order, and number of letters.

Remediation for phonetic analysis, in severe cases, tends to begin with words that have relatively consistent phoneme–grapheme correspondence and which vary in length from two to six letters. We find this type of training can be used to enhance phoneme segmentation, temporal organization, visual scanning, and crossmodal integration as well as reading *per se*. Thus, rather than using only CVC words or word families (e.g. hop, mop, top), we find it more beneficial to present the words 'an, and, sand, stand, strand' and ask the reader to find similarities and differences. We also emphasize auditory–visual integration by asking questions such as 'Does this say "sand"? Why not?'. We include work on spelling by manipulating letter tiles and/or writing. These latter activities are particularly helpful for enhancing linguistic awareness and phoneme segmentation.

The procedures for decoding multisyllabic words are similar to those we use with children (Johnson and Myklebust, 1967). Words are presented as wholes and in syllables with spacing between each syllable (e.g. napkin nap kin). Words are said as wholes then by syllable. At times syllables are presented on separate cards so the dyslexics can combine them to create new words. We use word lists devised by specialists in the field of reading and reading disabilities but we use very few explicit rules (Gillingham and Stillman, 1940; Orton, 1937; Steer, Peck, and Kahn (1971)). Instead, we attempt to improve rule abstraction by asking the dyslexic to inspect words and note patterns. We rarely ask dyslexics to draw lines between syllables because the line simply becomes another feature in the word. Our goal is to help them visually and auditorially analyze words by presenting words with spaces between syllables and by orally segmenting them. Then the units are recombined into whole words.

As the dyslexics learn new words structural analysis is emphasized by adding various verb endings, prefixes, and suffixes. Practice is provided in lists, phrases, and context. Since many dyslexics have difficulty with oral language we use sets of words for reading and syntax. Sentences with words such as 'apply, applies, applying, application' are prepared. Whenever possible, efforts are made to combine work on oral language, reading, spelling, and written language.

While I have said little about reading comprehension in this paper, meaning is central to all symbolic behavior. There is little merit in learning to decode words we do not understand. In the initial stages of reading we use familiar vocabulary to make certain that the dyslexics are bringing background knowledge to the task; later however, they are taught how to read for new meanings. They note, for example, synonyms, parenthetical expressions, and structural devices in the text. Because of numerous language problems among dyslexics one must always be concerned about the best means of assessing comprehension. Those with oral formulation difficulties may comprehend material but they cannot recall words or organize ideas when asked to summarize the content. Therefore, they may need more opportunities for recognition responses. In addition, many with mild to moderate decoding difficulties lose meaning during the process of reading. Thus we encourage them to read and reread the material before asking comprehension questions.

Progress varies with the adults as it does with children. Our earlier clinical investigations indicated that some children made as little as six months' progress in a year whereas others made four years' progress in the same time period (Johnson, Blalock, and Nesbitt, 1978). The amount of success varies with motivation, effectiveness of instruction, intensity of instruction, and the severity of the problem. Unfortunately, we have not been able to provide *intensive* remediation for many adults because of their schedules and the nature of our program. Nevertheless, some have made significant gains in 90-minute periods each week. One man, for example, made four years' gain in three years and has been able to start his own business. Others at the upper level made sufficient progress to manage college or trade school programs independently. Even one grade progress can make a difference in levels of independence and in the type of work that adults can do. It is particularly exciting to observe the high levels of achievement attained by some adult dyslexics. We, like Rawson (1968), have seen several go on to professional schools, but the residuals of the problems persist.

In our work with both children and adults we frequently use the Vineland Social Maturity Scale (Doll, 1953) as a guide for measuring both problems and progress. This scale was designed to investigate the ability of an individual to care for himself and others. By doing a careful Vineland, it is clear that a reading disability can interfere with independence. For example, the mean social quotient for a group of sixty dyslexics in an earlier study was 86 (Johnson and Myklebust, 1965). Thus, dyslexia is clearly not a school problem. One cannot pass certain items pertaining to the use of the telephone unless one can alphabetize and use the phone book. Certain locomotion items require reading timetables and maps. By using the Vineland as a guide for certain aspects of remediation we can foster independence. Reading and writing should also be used for communication, work, and leisure time.

REFERENCES

Bakker, D., and Schroots, H. (1981), A study of dyslexic weaknesses and the consequences for teaching. In: G. Th. Pavlidis and T. R. Miles (Eds.), *Dyslexia Research and its Applications to Education*. Chichester, John Wiley.

Boder, E. (1973), Developmental dyslexia: a diagnostic approach based on three atypical reading–spelling patterns. *Developmental Medicine and Child Neurology* 15, 663–687.

Bryant, P., and Bradley, L. (1980), Why children sometimes write words which they do not read. In: U. Frith (Ed.), *Cognitive Processes in Spelling*. New York, Academic Press.

Chall, J. (1979), The great debate: ten years later with a modest proposal for reading stages. In: L. Resnick and P. Weaver (Eds.), *Theory and Practice of Early Reading*, Vol. 1. Hillsdale, NJ, Erlbaum.

Denckla, M. (1977), Minimal brain dysfunction and dyslexia: beyond diagnosis by exclusion. In: M. E. Blaw, I. Rapin, and M. Kinsbourne (Eds.), *Topics in Child Neurology*. Jamaica, NY, Spectrum Publications.

Doll, E. (1953), *Measurement of Social Competence*. Circle Pines, MN, American Guidance Service.

Eisenson, J. (1984), *Aphasia and Related Disorders in Children*, 2nd edn. New York, Harper & Row.

Gillingham, A., and Stillman, B. (1940), *Remedial Training for Children with Specific Disability in Reading, Spelling and Penmanship*. New York, Sackett and Wilhelms.

Goodman, K., and Goodman, Y. (1977), Learning about psycholinguistic processes by analyzing oral reading. *Harvard Educational Review*, 47, 317–333.

Goodman, Y., and Burke, . (1972), *Reading Miscue Inventory*. New York, Macmillan.

Gray, W. (1947), *On Their Own in Reading*. Chicago, Scott Foresman.

Guthrie, J. (1973), Models of reading and reading disability. *Journal of Educational Psychology* 65, 9–18.

Hook, P., and Johnson, D. (1978), Metalinguistic awareness and reading strategies. *Bulletin of the Orton Society* 27, 62–78.

Johnson, D. (1978), Remedial approaches to dyslexia. In: A. Benton and D. Pearl, *Dyslexia: An Appraisal of Current Knowledge*. New York, Oxford University Press.

Johnson, D. (1980), Persistent disorders in young dyslexic adults. *Bulletin of the Orton Society* 30, 268–276.

Johnson, D. (1982), Programming for dyslexia: the need for interaction and analyses. *Annals of Dyslexia* 32, 61–70.

Johnson, D., Blalock, J., and Nesbitt, J. (1978), Adolescents with learning disabilities: perspectives from an educational clinic. *Learning Disability Quarterly* 1, 24–36.

Johnson, D., and Hook, P. (1978), Reading disabilities: problems of rule acquisition and linguistic awareness. In: H. Myklebust (Ed.), *Progress in Learning Disabilities*, Vol. 4. New York, Grune & Stratton.

Johnson, D., and Myklebust, H. (1965), Dyslexia in childhood. In: J. Hellmuth (Ed.), *Learning Disorders*, Vol. 1. Seattle, Special Child Publications.

Johnson, D., and Myklebust, H. (1967), *Learning Disabilities: Educational Principles and Practices*. New York, Grune & Stratton.

LaBerge, D., and Samuels, S. (1974), Toward a theory of automatic information processing in reading. *Cognitive Psychology* 6, 293–323.

Liberman, I. (1973), Segmentation of the spoken word and reading acquisition. *Bulletin of the Orton Society* 23, 65–77.

Lyon, G. R. (1983), Learning-disabled readers: identification of subgroups. In: H. Myklebust (Ed.), *Progress in Learning Disabilities*, Vol. 5. New York, Grune & Stratton.

Mattis, S., French, J., and Rapin, T. (1975), Dyslexia in children and adults: three independent neuropsychological syndromes. *Developmental Medicine and Child Neurology* 17, 150–163.

Miles, E. (1981), A study of dyslexic weaknesses and the consequences for teaching. In: G. Th. Pavlidis and T. Miles (Eds.), *Dyslexia Research and its Applications to Education*. Chichester, John Wiley.

Myklebust, H. (1954), *Auditory Disorders in Children*. New York, Grune & Stratton.

Myklebust, H. (1965), *Development and Disorders of Written Language*, Vol. 1, *Picture Story Language Test*. New York, Grune & Stratton.

Myklebust, H., and Johnson, D. (1962), Dyslexia in children. *Exceptional Children* 29(1), 14–25.

Naidoo, S. (1981), Teaching methods and their rationale. In: G. Th. Pavlidis and T. Miles (Eds.), *Dyslexia Research and its Application to Education*. Chichester, John Wiley.

Orton, S. (1937), *Reading, Writing and Speech Problems in Children*. New York, W. W. Norton.

Perfetti, C. (1977), Language comprehension and fast decoding: some psycholinguistic prerequisities for skilled reading comprehension. In: J. Guthrie (Ed.), *Cognition, Curriculum, and Comprehension*. Newark, DE, International Reading Association.

Rawson, M. (1968), *Developmental Language Disability: Adult Accomplishments of Dyslexic Boys*. Baltimore: The Johns Hopkins Press.

Samuels, J. (1976), Hierarchical subskills in the reading acquisition process. In: J. Guthrie (Ed.), *Aspects of Reading Acquisition*. Baltimore, The Johns Hopkins University Press.

Shankweiler, D., and Liberman, I. (1972), Misreading: a search for causes. In: J. Kavanagh and I. Mattingly (Eds.), *Language by Ear and by Eye: The Relationships between Speech and Reading*. Cambridge, MA, MIT Press.

Steer, A., Peck, C., and Kahn, L. (1971), *Solving Language Difficulties: Remedial Routines*. Cambridge, MA, Educators Publishing Service, Inc.

Vellutino, F. (1977), Alternative conceptualizations of dyslexia: evidence in support of a verbal deficit hypothesis. *Harvard Educational Review* **47**, 334–354.

Vogel, S. (1975), *An Investigation of Syntactic Abilities in Normal and Dyslexic Children*. Baltimore, University Park Press.

CHAPTER 18

Single Case Methodology and the Remediation of Dyslexia

BARBARA WILSON and ALAN BADDELEY
Rivermead Rehabilitation Centre, Oxford,
UK and MRC Applied Psychology Unit, Cambridge, UK

This chapter concentrates on the remediation of *acquired* dyslexia but it is hoped that the strategies described for evaluating treatment will also be valuable for those working with developmental dyslexics. Clearly, the effectiveness of teaching strategies needs to be investigated in both areas. Whenever treatment or remediation is attempted for any problem or condition it is important to know whether the intervention itself causes change or whether changes are due to some other factor not directly related to treatment. In the case of acquired dyslexia, changes could be due to spontaneous recovery or natural change over time.

Sometimes research findings from large group studies may be helpful in indicating which remediation techniques work. Group studies, however, are of limited value in evaluating the effects of treatment. In group studies it is usually the case that (a) two or more groups of people are subjected to different treatments or (b) one group is subjected to two or more treatments. The results are typically described in terms of the average or mean response of each group under each condition. Despite the fact that individual differences are common, group studies rarely indicate those persons who have improved, those who have deteriorated, or those who remain the same as a result of the treatment. Such individual responses are obscured by taking the mean scores. In addition, group studies frequently confuse clinical significance with statistical significance. It is possible to obtain a statistically significant result which makes little, if any, difference to the lives of the people in the study. Conversely, it is possible for the results to be declared nonsignificant and yet some of the people in the study may find that the treatment procedure influences their everyday functioning in a demonstrably constructive manner.

Consider the following hypothetical examples: (a) a drug may be found to significantly improve eye movement characteristics in poor readers. Their reading skills, however, remain unchanged. This would be a case of statistical without clinical significance; (b) relaxation training could be given to a group of children to see whether their rate of reading increases. The results may not be significant although a few children in the group may improve their reading rate to normal levels. In such a case clinical significance would occur for some of the group members.

Single case experimental designs avoid many of the problems inherent in group studies. The treatment can be tailored to the individual's particular needs and his or her responses to treatment or intervention strategies can be continuously evaluated whilst controlling for the effects of spontaneous or improvements over time. Many of the examples of single case designs to be found in the literature come from drug studies and from the field of behaviour modification or behaviour therapy. Recently, however, case studies have been employed in neuropsychology and remediation of cognitive deficits (e.g. Gianutsos and Gianutsos, 1979; Wilson, 1982). The earliest of the single case designs were no more than descriptions of individual patients (e.g. Freud and Breur, 1974). These can, of course, be illuminating both from the point of view of describing the natural history of certain rare and intriguing syndromes (e.g. Broca, 1861) and in producing theoretical understanding of particular disabilities (Shallice, 1979; Baddeley and Wilson, 1983).

One case of acquired alexia which responded to remediation, illustrates the usefulness of the natural history type of approach. The subject D.C. (Wilson, White, and McGill, 1983) was a young man who was shot in the head in 1977 at the age of 23 years. The bullet entered the left occiput and lodged in the left temporal area. Following a difficult post-operative period including four operations and persistent meningitis for several months he was found to be severely intellectually impaired. When assessed, prior to treatment for alexia, he was found to have a full-scale IQ of 56 on the Wechsler Adult Intelligence Scale (Wechsler, 1955). He was unable to read any words, letters, or digits. He was unable to sort real words from nonsense words or write to dictation. He could sort digits from letters, tell if letters were upside down or not, copy letters and printed words and match pairs of printed words provided they were both written in the same case (i.e. upper or lower). He could spell, orally, a few three-letter words but made frequent errors. His speech was fluent and grammatical but some word-finding problems and perseverations were evident. His performance on both the Peabody Picture Vocabulary Test (Dunn, 1965) and the Token test (DeRenzi and Vignolo, 1962) was normal. He could not name colours or point to the correct colour named by the examiner. He was, however, able to match colours. Although no formal record of his premorbid reading ability could be traced he had passed examinations to enter the Royal Air Force and therefore must have been at least an average reader.

In October 1980, 3 years after the gunshot wound, an attempt was made to teach D.C. to read again. The first approach was a 'look-and-say' or whole word method. Six words (ladies, gentlemen, exit, and his three names D...., P...., C....) were selected. These were introduced one at a time. For the first twelve treatment sessions (each lasting 30 minutes) an attempt was made to teach D.C. to read the words aloud. In the second thirteen treatment sessions (also lasting 30 minutes) an attempt was made to teach D.C. to recognize, i.e. point to the correct words. D.C. failed to identify any of the six words above chance level.

At that time all of those working with D.C. believed he would never read again. He refused to accept this, however, and persisted in asking for reading tuition. In October 1982, i.e. five years after his injury, a phonetic approach was tried. The procedure was as follows:

(1) *Sounds* of the letters of the alphabet were taught one at a time from A–Z in order. Upper case letters were taught before lower case.
(2) Letters were presented in random order and D.C. was required to say the sounds.
(3) D.C. was taught to select the vowels from an array of letters.
(4) Two- and three-letter regular words were introduced.
(5) Irregular words were introduced.

In December 1982, formal teaching ceased and D.C. worked alone at his reading. In May 1983 his reading age was 9 years and 1 month (he had failed to score prior to treatment). He still read almost every word phonetically, remembering very few words as whole units. Almost all errors were with irregular words and he appeared to have changed from an alexic to a surface dyslexic. However, he used context to help him and frequently deciphered an irregular word in a page of text. If, after several attempts, he failed to make sense of a word, he asked someone to help him. His spelling was also phonetic. As many young children read like surface dyslexics before going on to learn irregular words as whole units, it is possible that D.C. might follow this pattern and become a more 'normal' reader in time.

Case descriptions like that of D.C. are informative, particularly when the improvements are as dramatic as they were in this case. For more subtle measures, however, when changes are perhaps less striking, then an experimental design is required. The simplest of the experimental designs is the reversal or ABAB design. An example of this design is described by Zlutnick, Mayville, and Moffat (1975). A 17-year-old mentally handicapped girl was having several attacks of motor epilepsy each day despite anticonvulsant medication. The seizures were preceded by a characteristic chain of events. Following a baseline period, treatment was introduced which consisted of interrupting the chain very early in the sequence. The number of seizures fell from an average of 16 a day to less than one a day. When baseline conditions were reinstated the number of daily seizures increased. With the reintroduction of treatment they fell to a near-zero level once more.

Although the reversal design is simple, its application to treatment programmes is limited for three main reasons. Firstly, it is usually impossible to revert to baseline conditions. Suppose a reading impaired person has been taught to read some new words, then she cannot 'unlearn' these. Secondly, there may be occasions when it is unethical to revert to baseline conditions. This is less likely, perhaps, in dyslexia but it is a very real problem in some situations. For example, if a child is successfully treated for severe self-injurious behaviour then it would be unacceptable to reintroduce the self-injury. Thirdly, it is frequently impracticable to revert to baseline conditions. If, for example, a poor reader is taught to spend some time each day on his reading homework, then parents or teachers will not appreciate reverting back to a situation in which he refuses to do his reading.

Perhaps one occasion where a reversal design might be appropriate in reading remediation is when one wishes to know the effectiveness or otherwise of feedback. Let us imagine that a stroke patient with unilateral neglect frequently omitted the beginnings of words, e.g. read 'chocolate' as 'late' and 'handbag' as 'bag' (this is sometimes described as attentional dyslexia). Information or feedback on the number of errors made in a column of 50 words could reduce the error rate. The baseline period (or A phase) here would consist of measuring the error rate say on five separate occasions. The treatment (or B phase) would involve feedback on the number of errors. If the error rate should drop, the chances are that the feedback or treatment procedure would be responsible. There would be a small chance, however, that the improvement could have occurred because of other reasons. Hence, to reduce the possibility of this, information on error rate could be withheld for a period (reversal to baseline conditions). Suppose the error rate increased once again and only fell following the reintroduction of the feedback procedure. In this case it would be very unlikely that natural recovery or some independent factor had been responsible for the change.

Variations on the ABAB design are frequently made in behavioural approaches, so one might, for example, have included a C phase or C + D phases in the programme. The C phase could have been positive reinforcement in the shape of tokens or money and the D phase could have been both feedback and money. These designs are more fully described in Hersen and Barlow (1976) and Yule and Hemsley (1977).

Because of the limitations of reversal designs it is usually more appropriate to use a multiple baseline design as an evaluative procedure in cognitive remediation. There are three main kinds of multiple baseline designs: (1) multiple baseline across behaviours, (2) multiple baseline across settings, and (3) multiple baseline across subjects. (While it is true to say that (3) is not a proper *single* case design, it is included here because the kinds of research difficulties encountered with small groups of subjects are similar to those found with a single subject.)

(1) Multiple baseline across behaviours design. In this design several different behaviours or problems are selected for treatment. Baselines are taken on all the behaviours but only one is treated at a time. Again, this method enables

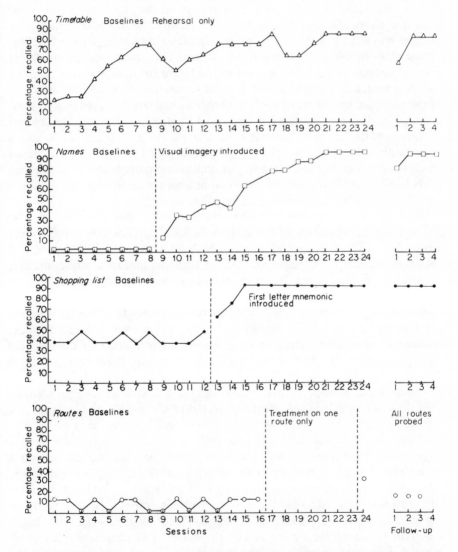

Figure 1. A multiple baseline across behaviours design. A baseline is established for the performance of an amnesic patient across four tasks. Treatment is then introduced, and its effect on performance plotted.

the researcher to separate out the effects of treatment from the effects of general improvement. An illustration of this design is provided by Wilson (1982). The patient was a 51-year-old man who had suffered a bilateral stroke affecting both posterior cerebral arteries. This had left him with a classic amnesic syndrome. Four problems were selected for treatment: remembering (i) his daily timetable, (ii) the names of staff he came into regular contact with, (iii) a shopping list, and (iv) short routes. Baselines were taken on all the problems but only one treated at a time. During the first week of treatment he was able to remember more of his daily timetable simply by extra practice in recalling it. The baselines on the other problems remained stable. During the second week of treatment a visual imagery procedure was used to teach him the names of staff. During the third week a first letter mnemonic strategy was introduced to improve recall of the shopping list. Three of the four problems had now been reduced to some extent. Finally, several strategies were used in attempts to teach him a short route around the rehabilitation centre. None of the strategies improved his ability to remember the route. It can be seen from Figure 1 that the results cannot be explained by spontaneous recovery or improvement over time, as all problem areas would have improved together — or at least the improvement would not have been coincidental with the intervention strategy.

Later in this chapter we describe how this design was used to teach a dyslexic girl to learn letters of the alphabet. This multiple baseline across behaviours design is flexible and adaptable for many problems, both behavioural and cognitive. It could, for example, be used in an attempt to teach a surface dyslexic to read ten irregular words. Baselines could be taken which show that she never pronounces any of the words correctly. One new word could be tackled each session while baselines are taken on the remaining words. After ten sessions seven words may be consistently read correctly. As improvement would appear to have occurred *after* intervention, it could be concluded that the teaching strategy would be responsible for improvement rather than some unrelated factor.

The multiple baseline across settings design is used when one problem or behaviour is treated but the effects of treatment are investigated in successive settings. It is a useful design when situation specific effects may occur. For example, Carr and Wilson (1983) used it with a spinal patient who did not lift himself frequently enough from his wheelchair with the result that pressure sores developed. A lift was defined as the man's buttocks leaving the seat of the wheelchair for 4 seconds. One lift every 10 minutes was considered desirable (the man was required to push himself up with his arms). It can be seen from Figure 2 that following baselines in four different settings — the workshops, lunch times, tea/coffee breaks, and on the ward — a machine was fitted to his wheelchair in one setting only (the workshops). The machine recorded the number of lifts made. Once it had been attached to the chair, the number of lifts dramatically increased but only in this particular setting. In the next stage

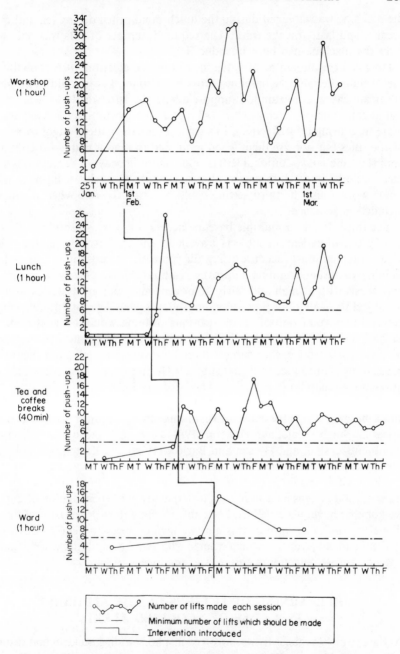

Figure 2. A multiple baseline across settings design. A treatment programme to increase the frequency with which the patient lifts from his wheelchair was introduced successively across different environmental settings.

the machine was attached during the lunch break, then during tea and coffee breaks, and lastly on the ward. The required number of lifts was only made *after* the machine had been introduced.

How can this design be of value in reading remediation? It is probably less useful than the multiple baseline across behaviours, but it could be employed in certain cases. For example, suppose a letter-by-letter reader is being taught sound combinations such as $s + h =$ sh and $a + y =$ ay. Initially one might teach these rules using printed letters. In such a setting the patient might *learn* many of the rules but not *use* them when requested to read a real word containing both the 'rule' and additional letters, e.g. 'shop' or 'pay'. The second 'setting' then could be to teach the person to use the rule when she or he encountered single words, and the third setting could be using the rule when words were included in sentences.

The third design, a multiple baseline across subjects, is useful when only a small group of patients or subjects is available and one wishes to test the efficacy of an intervention procedure using all subjects. Suppose it is believed that training in visual scanning improves reading ability. One way to test this hypothesis with a small and fairly homogeneous group of dyslexics would be to subject them all to the procedure, but following baselines of different lengths. Hence the introduction of visual scanning training would be staggered, with each of four children starting the procedure at different times. If the training procedure is effective, each subject should improve, but only after the training in scanning is introduced for that subject. This particular design has been used in memory rehabilitation (Wilson and Moffat, 1984).

Variations on these designs are frequently made. See, for example, Wong and Liberman (1981) for a discussion of mixed single subject designs in clinical research, Singh, Beale, and Dawson (1981) for a description of an alternating treatments design, and Hersen and Barlow (1976) and Kratchowill (1978) for further explanation of the variations.

Although it would be accurate to state that up until now single case experimental designs have been used infrequently in the remediation of dyslexia, we hope we have, nevertheless, been able to show their potential usefulness in this area. In furtherance of this aim we include below a detailed description of the treatment given to a young woman with acquired dyslexia, when a multiple baseline across behaviours design was employed.

RELEARNING OF LETTERS OF THE ALPHABET IN A CASE OF ACQUIRED ALEXIA

At the age of 17 years, J.R. was involved in a horse-riding accident and sustained a severe head injury. She was unconscious for nearly 3 months. A CT scan at the time showed multiple contusions and haemorrhages. She began speaking two to three weeks after regaining consciousness. Slow progress was made for several months until she was admitted to Rivermead Rehabilitation Centre, nine months after her accident, by which time she was 18 years old. Prior to her accident she had been studying for public examinations at a standard which suggests at least an average level of intellectual functioning. One month after admission, i.e. ten months post-injury, she was assessed in the clinical psychology department. Her verbal IQ was in the borderline/low average range although she achieved a normal score on the vocabulary subtest of the Wechsler Adult Intelligence Scale (Wechsler, 1955). As she was unable to do most of the performance subtests, a performance IQ and a full-scale IQ were unobtainable. Her memory was severely impaired. She remembered very little of what happened to her, did not know what day it was, had difficulty learning new information and scored in the abnormal range on all memory tests administered. In addition there were severe and unusual recognition problems for all kinds of visual material—real objects, photographs, drawings, and written stimuli. For example she was unable to recognize an onion by sight or touch, but could provide the word when given a verbal description such as 'a highly flavoured vegetable that makes your eyes water when you peel it and smells when you fry it'.

Her recognition deficits could not be explained by impaired visual acuity as she could copy adequately and could describe the features of the stimuli in front of her. Neither could they be explained by dysphasia as she could usually supply the correct name of an object when its function was described to her. Furthermore, her language comprehension and expression were perfectly normal. Her agnosia is described elsewhere (Davidoff and Wilson, 1985).

Her reading difficulties were also severe. She failed to read any words on the Schonell graded word reading test (Schonell and Schonell, 1963) unless these were printed in large letters. Even then she read only two words correctly ('tree' and 'little'). She could also read her own name, her brother's name and 'horse', 'saddle', and 'stirrup' in large print. When asked to read individual letters of the alphabet, she correctly identified less than 25 per cent. She was much better at pointing to letters named by the tester, when she was correct for 23/26 letters. She was also able to write single letters to dictation, making only 3 errors out of 26. However, she only managed to write 4/12 words correctly (*tree*, *little*, *horse* and *bun*). Examples of her errors were: 'PlAine' for *playing*, 'BoorK' for *book* and 'darehrra' for *Barbara*. On the Vernon Spelling Test (Vernon, 1977), she scored 4/80.

Because her impaired reading of individual letters appeared to hamper her reading of words, it was decided to re-teach the letters of the alphabet before commencing a more ambitious reading programme. (She was at this time receiving physiotherapy and occupational therapy as well as help with her memory and agnostic difficulties from the clinical psychology department.) An investigation was carried out of her ability to read letters of different sizes. For each letter of the alphabet eight cards were made—four for upper case letters and four for lower case. Each of the four letters was a different size, the sizes being 7.0 mm, 5.0 mm, 3.0 mm and 2.0 mm. J.R. was given these 208 letters in random order and asked to identify them.

Mean overall performance of the function of size and case is shown in Figure 3, which suggests a tendency for upper case letters to be easier than lower case, and larger easier than small. Of the 26 letters, 11 showed an advantage for upper case and 4 for lower case ($0.05 < p < 0.1$, sign test). A simple indication of the size effect can be obtained by comparing performance on the largest and smallest example of the 26 upper case and 26 lower case letters. Of these comparisons, 32 showed equal performance for large and small letters, 18 showed an advantage to the largest size, and 2 to the smallest ($p < 0.01$, sign test).

Table 1 shows the confusion matrix for upper and lower case letters. Examination of common confusions offers a number of cues as to the nature of the underlying perceptual process. Some errors seem to occur because the letter presented and the response have a broadly similar shape, examples being D→O, Q→O, Q→G, and v→w. In other examples, common features seem to be present as for example with B→E, G→C, J→T, j→i, and l→I. Finally errors of orientation appear to occur including d→p, d→b, u→n and M→W. While it would obviously be unwise to draw strong conclusions from a small number of selected

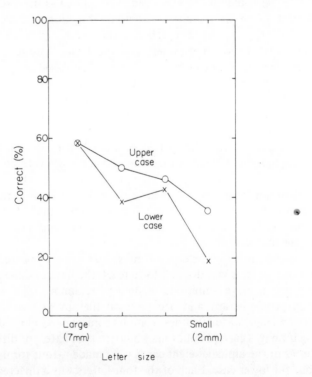

Figure 3. Mean overall performance (percentage) as a function of size and case.

Table 1. Confusion matrices for upper and lower case letters

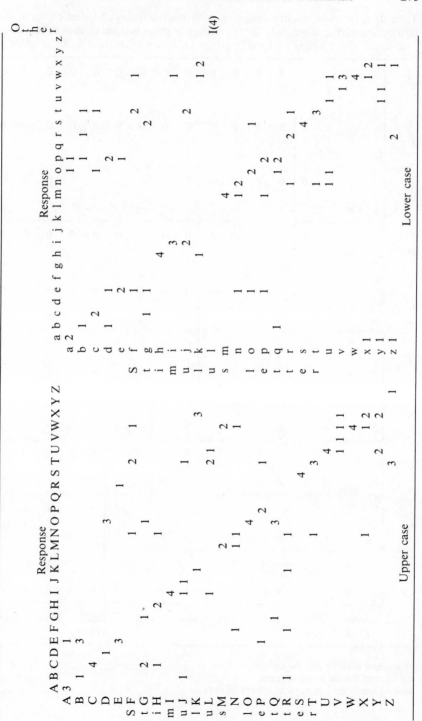

Table 2. A multiple baseline design to study the relearning of letters of the alphabet by a patient with acquired dyslexia. The reading of letters is tested on each of 18 successive sessions, with training on specific groups of letters introduced at different times

	Jun 1982		Jul/Aug		Sept		Oct		Nov		Dec		Jan 1983		Feb		March	
Y	×	×	×	×	0	0	0	0	0	0	0	0	0	0	0	0	0	0
J	×	×	0	0	0	0	0	0	0	0	0	0	0	0	0	0	0	0
R	×	×	0	0	0	0	0	0	0	0	0	0	0	0	0	0	0	0
D	×	×	×	×	0	0	0	0	0	0	0	0	0	0	0	0	0	0
L	×	×	×	×	×	×	0	0	0	0	0	0	0	0	0	0	0	0
V	×	×	×	×	×	×	×	×	0	0	0	0	×	0	0	×	0	0
K	×	×	×	×	×	×	×	×	×	×	×	×	0	×	×	0	×	0
B	×	×	×	×	×	×	×	×	×	0	0	0	0	0	0	0	0	0
Q	×	×	×	×	×	×	×	×	×	×	×	×	0	×	0	0	0	0
Z	×	×	×	×	×	×	×	×	×	×	×	×	×	×	0	0	×	×

× = errors made in test session.
0 = no errors made in test session.
Dashed line = next stage of treatment introduced.

errors, they do suggest the possibility of a breakdown in different components of the process of perceiving and identifying letters.

Although both size and case tended to influence performance, J. R. read certain letters consistently correctly regardless of size (e.g. S, C, m, and s). Other letters were always incorrect regardless of size (e.g. Q, Z, d, and y). The majority of letters, however, were correct some of the time but not consistently. We decided to select the ten most difficult letters and use a multiple baseline design to see whether or not it was possible for J.R. to relearn them. Baselines were taken and each letter introduced separately.

The actual teaching of the letters consisted of (a) practice, (b) feedback on whether or not she was correct, (c) description of the shape of the letter (e.g. J.R. was asked 'What does the letter look like?'—she replied 'An O with a tail'; she was then told 'An O with a tail is a Q'), (d) any other associations we could think of (e.g. when learning the letter Y we sang ' *Why* are we waiting' and chanted, ' *Why* can't I remember Y?', (e) rewards for 20 or 30 correct responses. Rewards consisted of a walk to the local fields to see the horses or being given a book on horses. The results may be seen in Table 2.

In July 1983 a post-treatment assessment revealed that she made only seven errors on all 208 letters, namely L→J, Z→K, q→b, z→x, and j→i (three times).

Having successfully taught most of the letters in the alphabet in several different sizes, the programme was extended to cover sound combinations, e.g. 'ir', 'wr', 'igh', etc. Baselines were taken in March 1983 and the ten sound combinations that J.R. always misread and misspelled were selected for treatment. It had been intended to do a multiple baseline approach as with the single letters. The first sound combination selected for treatment was 'oa'. Three

Table 3. Teaching sound combinations to a dyslexic girl

			TREATMENT			
Rule	Baseline 1 (March)	Baseline 2 (July)	Week 1	Week 2	Week 3	Week 4
oa	×	[a]√	√	√	√	√
ea	×	×	√	√	√	√
ur	×	×	×	×	×	√
ir	×	×	√	√	√	√
ai	×	×	√	√	√	√
aw	×	×	√	√	√	√
ie	×	×	×	×	√	×
igh	×	×	√	√	×	√
wr	×	×	√	√	×	√
Totals correct	0%	10%	80%	80%	70%	90%

[a] Taught following first baseline.

treatment sessions were spent practising this sound. Unexpectedly, however, J.R. was discharged home and the programme had to be abandoned. She returned for one month in July prior to her summer holiday and admission to a further education college for young handicapped adults. Given that a multiple baseline design would take longer than one month, it was decided to teach J.R. all ten sound combinations at once. A further baseline revealed that there had been no change in her ability to read or spell the ten sound combinations during the intervening 3-month break. Encouragingly, though, she still succeeded with the 'oa' combination, reading words like 'boat' and 'coat' successfully. Three times each week during that month all ten combinations were practised. Once a week the practice sessions were preceded by a test of her knowledge of the sound combinations. The testing consisted of asking J.R. to read a list of words containing the combinations. The results can be seen in Table 3.

J.R.'s ability to learn and retain information appeared to have improved considerably since the programme began with the introduction of the letter Y. That one letter took her 6 weeks to learn. It would have been possible to carry out a non-parametric statistical test on J.R.'s results. A Wilcoxon matched-pairs signed ranks test comparing pre- and post-treatment scores for the sound combinations would give a significant result. However, it is not necessary to employ statistics when the results are obvious. Statistics are less often employed in single case studies than in group designs. Some would argue that if statistics are needed in single case studies then it is unlikely that any real clinical significance has occurred. Others argue that on occasions statistics are important particularly when there is considerable variability in performance. Hersen and Barlow (1976), Yule and Hemsley (1977), Kratchowill (1978), and Edgington (1982) all provide further discussion of the arguments and the statistical techniques available in single case methodology.

In the case of J.R., we were using a single case design in order to evaluate a relatively complex treatment package. There was virtually no evidence to indicate that acquired agnosic dyslexia of this type was amenable to retraining so our first priority was to attempt to ascertain whether any form of rehabilitation was possible. Our results clearly suggest that it is, although progress is inevitably slow. We could equally well, however, have used the approach to study different methods of retraining which in themselves might have been selected to test different theoretical interpretations of the underlying process. The single case method is like any other scientific method, a way of answering a range of questions. However, since it can be applied to a single individual, it can be combined very effectively with the process of treating a child or patient with a reading or learning problem. As such it provides an important bridge between the theoretical concerns of the academic, and the more applied aims of the teacher or therapist.

REFERENCES

Baddeley, A. D., and Wilson, B. (1983), Differences among amnesias and between amnesics: the role of single case methodology in theoretical analysis and practical treatment. In: W. Hirst (Ed.), *Proceedings of the Princeton Amnesia Conference.* Hillsdale, NJ, Erlbaum.

Broca, P. (1861), Remarques sur le siège de la faculté du langage articule, suives d'une observation d'aphemie. *Bull. Soc. Anat.* **36**, 330–357.

Carr, S., and Wilson, B. (1983), Promotion of pressure relief exercising in a spinal injury patient: a multiple baseline across settings design. *Behavioural Psychotherapy* **11**, 329–336.

Davidoff, J., and Wilson, B. (1985), A case of associative visual agnosia showing a disorder of pre-semantic visual classification. *Cortex* **21**, 121–134.

DeRenzi, E., and Vignolo, L. A. (1962), The token test: a sensitive test to detect receptive disturbances in aphasics. *Brain* **85**, 665–678.

Dunn, L. M. (1965), *Expanded Manual for the Peabody Picture Vocabulary Test.* Circle Pines, Minn., American Guidance Service.

Edgington, E. S. (1982), Nonparametric tests for single-subject multiple schedule experiments. *Behavioural Assessment* **4**, 83–91.

Freud, S., and Breuer, J. (1974), *Studies on Hysteria.* Harmondsworth, Penguin.

Gianutsos, R., and Gianutsos, J. (1979), Rehabilitating the verbal recall of brain injured persons by mnemonic training: an experimental demonstration using single case methodology. *Journal of Clinical Neuropsychology* **1**, 117–135.

Hersen, M,. and Barlow, D. H. (1976). *Single Case Experimental Designs. Strategies for Studying Behavior Change.* New York, Pergamon Press.

Kratchowill, T. R. (Ed.) (1978), *Single Subject Research: Strategies for Evaluating Change.* New York, Academic Press.

Schonell, F. J., and Schonell, F. E. (1963), *Diagnostic Attainment Testing.* Edinburgh, Oliver & Boyd.

Shallice, T. (1979), Case study approach in neuropsychological research. *Journal of Clinical Neuropsychology* **1**, 183–211.

Singh, N. N., Beale, I. L., and Dawson, M. J. (1981), Duration of facial screening and suppression of self-injurious behaviour: analysis using an alternating treatments design. *Behavioural Assessment* **3**, 411–420.

Vernon, P. E. (1977), *The Graded Word Spelling Test.* London, Hodder & Stoughton.

Wechsler, D. (1955), *The Wechsler Adult Intelligence Scale.* New York, The Psychological Corporation.

Wilson, B. (1982), Success and failure in memory training following a cerebral vascular accident. *Cortex* **18**, 581–594.

Wilson, B., and Moffat, N. (1984), Rehabilitation of memory for everyday life. In: J. E. Harris and P. Morris (Eds.), *Everyday Memory, Actions and Absentmindedness.* London, Academic Press.

Wilson, B., White, S., and McGill, P. (1983), Remediation of acquired alexia following a gunshot wound. Paper presented at the Second World Congress on Dyslexia. Halkidiki, Greece.

Wong, S. E., and Liberman, R. P. (1981), Mixed single-subject designs in clinical research: variations of the multiple baseline. *Behavioural Assessment* **3**, 297–306.

Yule, W., and Hemsley, D. (1977), Single case method in medical psychology. In: S. Rachman (Ed.), *Contributions to Medical Psychology I.* Oxford, Pergamon Press.

Zlutnick, S., Mayville, W. J., and Moffat, S. (1975), Modification of seizure disorders: the interruptions of behavioural chains. *J. Appl. Beh. Anal.* **8**, 1–12.

CHAPTER 19

Computers and Reading Instruction: Lessons from the Past, Promise for the Future

JOSEPH K. TORGESEN and NANCY WOLF
Florida State University, USA

One of the most exciting and well-publicized developments in education in the last five years has been the introduction of computers to classrooms on a scale never before experienced. This explosion of computer availability is the direct result of huge reductions in both the start-up and ongoing costs of computer use that have accompanied the development of microcomputers. Educators have been ready to respond to the increased economic feasibility of using computers in the classroom because they have tremendous intuitive appeal as a device for aiding the instructional process. Computers can control the presentation of different kinds of stimuli very precisely, they can be programmed to respond in different ways to individual students, and they have an enormous capacity to measure responses and provide immediate and informative feedback. All of these characteristics suggest that computers have great promise as an educational tool. The challenge of the present is to find ways to use the unique capabilities of computers to aid in the solution of education's most important problems.

Certainly one of the most troublesome problems faced by educators today is teaching all children to read effectively. For example, there is good evidence from both short-term (Arter and Jenkins, 1979) and long-term (Horn, O'Donnell, and Vitulano, 1983) evaluations that techniques currently in use are not very effective in helping reading disabled, or dyslexic, children achieve advanced reading skills. While some children may have cognitive limitations that prevent the acquisition of fluent reading skills, many other children probably do not read well because of inadequate instruction or lack of opportunities for effective practice. This chapter is written to evaluate the possible uses that computers may have in helping to achieve more fluent and effective reading skills in children who do not learn to read well from regular classroom instruction.

279

The chapter will be organized around several issues. The first issue involves the general question of instructional effectiveness. What do we know for sure about the uses of computers to teach reading skills? The second issue concerns the setting of priorities for computer use with reading disabled children. Computers may come to be used in many different ways with dyslexic children, but we need to attack the most important problems first. The final section of the chapter will provide a selective discussion of some presently available software that will not only illustrate the present state of the art for microcomputers, but will also provide an indication of developments that are required in the future.

EFFECTIVENESS OF COMPUTER-ASSISTED INSTRUCTION (CAI) IN READING

In trying to understand what we know about the use of computers to teach reading skills, I will first provide a brief historical perspective on the use of computers in this area, and then will consider several recent evaluations of computer-assisted instruction in reading. Many educators who have only recently been introduced to computers through the wide availability of microsystems are unaware that attempts to use computers to provide instruction in reading have a 20-year history. In fact, the first systematic efforts to develop CAI in reading began in 1964 at the Institute for Mathematical Studies in the Social Sciences under the direction of Patrick Suppes (Suppes, Jerman, and Brian, 1968).

Extensive development efforts over several years led to the production of a tutorial program in beginning reading that was implemented using a central computer connected to 16 separate terminals. The terminals were quite elaborate, consisting of a television screen, a keyboard, a light pen, a film projector, and earphones. Students could view line drawings and letters on the television screen, see pictures via film projection, and listen to audio messages recorded on tape. The software designed for this system was conceptualized as being tutorial in that it provided instruction extending from the initial introduction of a concept to skill mastery. The program focused on both decoding and comprehension skills, but because it was designed for very young children, the primary emphasis was on decoding, or translating print to sound. Instruction in phonological correspondence rules and word analysis was provided along with exercises designed to strengthen sight word vocabularies. In one evaluation effort during the 1966–67 school year (Wilson and Atkinson, 1967), 100 children were exposed to the program for 20 minutes a day during about one-half of the school year. Standardized tests showed that children receiving the CAI tutorial in reading made significantly more progress in attaining basic word decoding skills than a comparable group of children who had been receiving CAI in math but not in reading.

Following their experience with the tutorial program, the Stanford group developed another reading program for young children that essentially provided drill and practice on skills that were initially introduced by the teacher. Not only was the tutorial system very expensive, but also it proved to be very difficult to anticipate all of the different instructional needs of children when they were first introduced to reading concepts. The drill and practice program again used a mainframe computer with separate terminals, but the terminals were much simpler than for the tutorial program. They consisted simply of a teletypewriter and earphones. The advantages of the new system were that it operated much faster, it used a digitized audio system that allowed rapid access (32 ms) to over 6000 messages, and it allowed elaborate computations to be made so that the drill and practice it provided to each student could be individualized, based on each child's response history. The program itself contained six 'instructional' strands that provided practice on different skills. The strands were letter identification, sight words, spelling patterns, phonics, word comprehension (vocabulary), and sentence comprehension. A formal evaluation of this program was reported in 1972 by Fletcher and Atkinson. First-graders who had been randomly assigned to 8–10 minutes a day of CAI scored roughly half a grade placement higher in reading skill than their counterparts who had not received CAI in reading. There were differences between groups in both decoding and paragraph reading skill, and it appeared that boys profited more from the CAI than girls.

In 1969, the Computer Curriculum Corporation was formed to provide a commercial outlet for the programs developed at Stanford. The program that has been most widely disseminated by this organization provides drill and practice in reading skills for children between the 2.5 and 6th grade. It uses a central computer controlling separate terminals, but these terminals are even simpler than those used by the previously developed experimental drill and practice program. They have no audio capability, but can simply send and receive typed messages. The largest use of this program has been in the Chicago public schools. The program was introduced in 1971 in seven schools, and by 1977 it was in use in 59 schools. It has been repeatedly evaluated, and appears to be one of the most cost-effective ways to provide the extra instruction that many inner-city children need in order to improve their reading skills (Hallworth and Brebner, 1980). This program has also been the subject of a large-scale evaluation in Los Angeles, and this evaluation will be reported in a later section.

At the same time that CAI in reading was being developed at Stanford, the PLATO project at the University of Illinois was developing its own early reading program called the Plato Early Reading Curriculum (PERC). This program was never subject to the same level of evaluation as the system developed at Stanford, but what evaluation data there were indicated that the program was not very effective (Swinton, Amarel, and Morgan, 1978; Yeager, 1977). However, the PLATO project has continued to develop CAI in reading, and now has an extensive variety of programs available that teach reading skills ranging from pre-primer (letter and sight word recognition) through evaluative comprehension. These programs are being used primarily in settings that service adult nonreaders. For example, a successful application of the PLATO Basic Skills Learning System was reported by Caldwell and Rizza (1979).

The reading curriculum in the Basic Skills Learning System provides instruction in five different areas, and each area has a tutorial section, a drill and practice section, a review-help sequence, an off-line activity (practice accomplished off the computer), and a mastery test. The types of reading skills covered are structural analysis (instruction on the structure of words), vocabulary development, literal comprehension, interpretive comprehension, and evaluative comprehension. Caldwell and Rizza (1979) found that adults who began the program with reading skills between the third and eighth grade made about 1.1 grade levels improvement in reading for each 15 hours of instruction. Unfortunately, the evaluation did not last very long, so there is no indication that initial rates of progress would be maintained with more extensive instruction.

From this brief treatment, it is clear that the history of CAI in reading did not begin with the popularization of microcomputers in the schools. Although there were other isolated attempts to develop CAI in reading prior to the advent of microsystems (e.g. Green, Henderson, and Richards, 1968; Golub, 1974), the contributions of the Stanford and Illinois projects are the ones that have had a major impact on the field. The Stanford curriculum has been used extensively in Texas and California, as well as Chicago. However, both the Stanford and PLATO systems are hampered by relatively high start-up and maintenance costs. Therefore, if computers are going to broadly affect the quality of reading instruction in schools, that impact will almost certainly come from software that is implemented on microcomputers.

Although the future of CAI in reading seems to lie with instructional programs implemented on microcomputers, almost all of the evaluative data on CAI in this area is derived from studies of instructional systems implemented on larger computers. The programs implemented on the larger systems are quite different in many ways from those currently available for microcomputers. So, most of the data currently available does not really answer questions about how effective the newer systems are going to be. In fact, there can be no general answer to questions about the effectiveness of CAI. The answer to this question depends on the specific hardware and software that is used, as well as the overall educational context in which it is applied. Perhaps a better question to consider is simply whether or not it is possible to program a computer to effectively aid children in the acquisition of basic skills in reading. When the question is phrased this way, the answer is affirmative.

For example, a recent meta-analysis (Roblyer and King, 1983) of 12 evaluation studies showed that groups exposed to CAI in reading achieved approximately two-thirds of a standard deviation above control groups on a variety of dependent measures. The analysis also indicated that CAI had been more effective in increasing decoding (average effect size = 1.03 s.d.) than comprehension (average effect size = 0.51 s.d.) skills. The studies considered in this analysis varied from one another in length of treatment (from 7 to 720 hours, median, 22.5 hours), sample size (from 22 to 629 subjects, median, 60), and age of subjects (elementary school to adults). Dependent measures included standardized tests of decoding and comprehension skills as well as special tests constructed to evaluate specific types of learning. All of these reading programs operated as supplements to teacher-administered instruction, and most of them employed a drill and practice format. Although these kinds of summary data do not provide much insight into the specific ways that computers can be used to teach reading, they are an impressive demonstration of the overall effectiveness of several different types of CAI programs.

The largest single formal evaluation of CAI in reading took place between 1976 and 1980 as a joint project between the Educational Testing Service and the Los Angeles Unified School District (Holland, 1980). The study actually evaluated CAI in reading, math, and language arts, but we will be concerned only with the evaluation of the reading curriculum. The subjects in the study were minority, or 'culturally disadvantaged' children primarily of Spanish-speaking origin. Over the three-year course of the study, approximately 2000 children from four different schools participated in the CAI curriculum. Although the study employed three different types of control groups against which the performance of students receiving CAI in reading was compared, we will consider only the comparison involving the 'within CAI' group. Within each grade level from fourth to sixth, children were randomly assigned to either a math or reading-language arts CAI curriculum. So, the control groups for children receiving the reading curriculum were other children from the same classes and schools who had approximately equal pre-test scores in reading, but who received CAI in math rather than reading.

The curriculum evaluated was Computer Curriculum Corporation's drill and practice program that requires children to be reading at least at the 2.5 grade level before they start. The four strands of the curriculum were word attack, vocabulary, literal comprehension, and work study skills. The CAI was delivered in 'computer labs' that contained up to 32 terminals served by one central minicomputer. Children in the reading curriculum received 10 minutes per day of reading instruction and ten minutes per day of instruction in language arts. Since the study lasted three years, it was possible to assess the effectiveness of the reading curriculum for periods ranging from one to three years.

The study employed two types of evaluation measures, a curriculum-specific test designed to measure improvement in the particular skills taught by the program, and the Comprehensive Test of Basic Skills, which is a nationally standardized measure of reading skill. On the curriculum specific test, a one-year exposure to CAI resulted in a difference of about 0.4 of a standard deviation in improvement in reading skills in favor of the children exposed to reading CAI. The comparable effect sizes for two-year and three-year exposure to the curriculum were 0.52 and 0.42, respectively. The evaluators concluded that the main effects of the reading curriculum, as measured by the curriculum-specific tests, took place in the first year of exposure to CAI, with no appreciable differential improvement in reading occurring after that.

As might be expected, the treatment effects were not as large when measured by the more general measure of reading skills, the CTBS. Although effects were still positive and significant for the reading vocabulary parts of the test (one-year effect size = 0.25 s.d., three-year = 0.58 s.d.), effects for reading comprehension were actually negative over three years (one-year effect size = 0.23 s.d., three-year = −0.24 s.d.). Thus, this specific curriculum appeared to be most effective in increasing the reading vocabulary skills of disadvantaged students, but did not address the need for training in reading comprehension.

The evaluators reported that both students and teachers were generally pleased with the CAI curriculum, and they also pointed out a number of specific characteristics of the program that may have helped to account for some of the positive results. First, the 'lab instructors' were highly trained teachers, who employed a number of different techniques such as oral praise, tokens, and contests, to keep the children motivated and involved in the instruction. In addition, the 'lab teachers' were readily available to help children if they experienced special difficulties with the curriculum. Although the curriculum in this study appeared to be administered in an efficient manner, a factor that may have seriously limited overall effectiveness was a general lack of coordination between the classroom and CAI reading curriculum. The CAI did not directly support classroom instruction, since it was adopted as a package with no attempt made to adapt it to the particular type of reading instruction being given in the different classrooms from which the children came.

One might argue that the study just reviewed tells us little about the potential applications of CAI with reading disabled children. After all, the children in the study were not formally classified as dyslexic, and the computer intervention (10 minutes a day) cannot be considered very intensive. However, the study does illustrate the potential impact of even small amounts of CAI in reading on minority group children who often have difficulty learning to read in the regular classroom. It is also consistent with other research (Fletcher and Atkinson, 1972; Jamison et al., 1975; Tait, Hartley, and Anderson, 1974) indicating that CAI often has its greatest impact on students who have difficulty with regular classroom instruction. Thus, although this large-scale study does not directly answer questions about the effects of CAI with dyslexic children, it does suggest that computers can be programmed to provide useful instructional support to at least one group of children who usually experience difficulty in learning to read.

In addition to subject population differences, of course, studies like those cited also used a different curriculum in a different context than is likely to be the case with dyslexic or learning disabled children. While instruction in the study cited occurred in computer laboratories under the supervision of highly trained teachers who focused exclusively on CAI, widespread use of computers with reading disabled children is likely to occur in resource rooms under the part-time supervision of the resource teacher. Also, the curriculum used in most early studies was both more elaborate, and in some ways more restricted, than that being offered for use on the newer microsystems. Finally, the CAI in many large-scale studies was not well coordinated with instruction being received from the teacher. If computers are used to reinforce instruction with reading disabled children, the skills practiced or taught on the computer will be closely allied to those being covered by regular classroom or remedial instructors.

Although almost all systematic evaluation of CAI in reading has focused on nonreading disabled populations, two recent studies have been reported that did use reading disabled children as subjects in evaluating CAI. One of the studies (Spring and Perry, in press) used a microcomputer to help fourth grade reading disabled children practice word decoding skills. Of course, the absence of good speech recognition capabilities in microcomputers makes it difficult to teach grapheme–phoneme correspondence and word analysis skills via computer. However, these investigators assured that their subjects accurately decoded nonsense words by requiring that one or more 'words' presented briefly on the screen be remembered for later re-entry into the computer. They assumed that children would only be able to meet the memory demands of the task if they were able to treat the nonsense words as units after accurately decoding them. Twelve reading disabled children were given practice on nonsense words composed of five different vowels and 17 different consonants. They practiced for 10 minutes a day over a period of two months. At the conclusion of training, the experimental group scored significantly better on a test requiring them to read both nonsense and real words than did a group of similar children who did not receive the training. The authors concluded that 'decoding ability, as measured by an accuracy criterion, was significantly improved by CAI training' (p. 18).

Another recent study (Rashotte and Torgesen, 1983) focused on increasing reading fluency in learning disabled children. This study used third through fifth grade children who were relatively accurate (above 90 per cent correctly read words) but slow (65 words per minute) readers of material at the second grade level. The basic training task involved repeatedly reading the same passages over and over. Each day, the child read the same passage over four times, and the next day a different passage was read repeatedly. The passages were presented on an Apple II microcomputer which also timed the reading and provided immediate feedback about reading speed. Although the study asked a number of different questions, the major result of interest here is that there was a generalized increase in fluency (across different passages) only when the passages had many words in common. There was no general improvement in fluency when passages on successive days did not share common words. Thus, the program was helpful primarily as a way of increasing individual word reading speed, rather than as a way of increasing general speed of processing text.

Both of these studies illustrate that computers can be used to enhance specific reading skills in reading disabled children. Of course, such data are no substitute for evaluation of more broadly based reading skills. We will not have convincing research evidence to support CAI with dyslexic children until we can show a socially significant impact on their overall reading skills in both short- and long-term evaluations. However, the absence of formal evaluation results for microcomputer systems will not, and should not, prevent special educators from beginning to use them in remedial work.

If computers are used in a way that is consistent with generally sound educational practice, children should benefit from interacting with them. After all, good CAI systems simply follow many of the procedures that good teachers follow. Computers can have a positive effect on the time children spend on academic tasks, they can be programmed for mastery-based learning, they employ direct instruction and practice, the instruction they deliver can be individualized, and they can offer timely and informative feedback. All of these instructional procedures have been shown to lead to higher achievement in the regular classroom, and they are also part of most modern recommendations for the education of children with special learning problems (Hallahan and Kauffman, 1976; Hammill and Bartel, 1975; Maxwell, 1980).

PRIORITIES FOR USE OF COMPUTERS
IN READING INSTRUCTION

While it is obvious that microcomputers currently have some important limitations in their capacity to support reading instruction (lack of high quality speech reproduction and recognition, limitations in memory capacity for elaborate branching programs), they also have some unique capabilities that may be particularly helpful in the instruction of reading disabled children. In setting priorities for the use of expensive computer resources in reading instruction, we should be guided both by a concern for the most basic educational needs of reading disabled children, and by an awareness of the unique capabilities of computers. As Fletcher and Suppes (1972) have pointed out, 'In designing computer-assisted instruction, the problem is not what teachers can do and what computers can do. The problem is to allocate to teachers and computers the tasks that each does best' (p. 45). In this discussion of priorities, I will first address some of the unique capabilities of computers, and then will suggest briefly how they might be focused on certain critical instructional areas with dyslexic children.

Computer capabilities may be divided roughly into two categories: those that have general instructional value for a variety of different content areas, and those that have specific instructional value for reading. In the general category, four characteristics suggest themselves as fairly obvious advantages of computer-assisted instruction. First, computers have clear motivational value (Lepper, 1982). Part of the motivational impact of computers at present is derived from their novelty, but they also may be programmed to provide inherently interesting and varied activities that can increase the time children are willing to spend practicing important academic skills. Lesgold (1982) has suggested that one of the major uses of computers in reading instruction may be to provide 'practice games' that will induce children with learning difficulties to spend the large amounts of time that may be required for them to learn important component skills in reading. A second obvious advantage of CAI over many traditional forms of instruction is the capacity to deliver immediate and informative feedback during instruction or practice. Although educators generally recognize the importance of timely feedback as an aid to learning, immediate feedback may be more beneficial for some types of learning than others (Kulhavey, 1977). Methods of delivering performance feedback is clearly an area that needs close research scrutiny in the further development of CAI.

Computers also have a strong capability to individualize instruction. Senf (1983) has suggested that computers can individualize instruction in either or both of two different ways. They can vary the amount of instruction or practice in a given area based on student performance, or they can provide different kinds of instruction based on student needs. The former type of individualization is essentially quantitative, while the latter implies qualitative variation in instruction. Historically, computers have excelled at providing quantitative individualization based on student learning rates, but qualitative variation in instruction has been much more rare. The latter type of instruction is difficult to provide because it requires a well-developed theory specifying the important ways that children differ from one another in their instructional needs.

A final characteristic of computers that is generally useful for instruction is their capacity to collect large amounts of precise response data. The computer's specific capability to measure response rates may be helpful in establishing more appropriate criteria for the mastery of component skills in children with learning disabilities. Both general theory in reading (LaBerge and Samuels, 1974), and specific discussions of the needs of learning disabled children (Lesgold, 1983; Sternberg and Wagner, 1982) indicate the potential utility of instructional activities that monitor both speed and accuracy of children's responses. Many reading programs now allow advancement to higher levels of instruction based only on an accuracy criterion (Lesgold and Resnick, 1982). Since rapid responding is also important in mastery of component skills, many children may have difficulties in reading because they are required to move to higher level tasks before they have really mastered basic ones.

Wilkenson (1983) has identified three capabilities of computers that may make unique contributions specifically to instruction in reading. The first of these is the control that computers make possible over the framing of text. Textual material may be presented as pages, paragraphs, lines, words, or even single letters. In a later discussion of some of the currently available software in reading, we will examine one program that makes use of the framing capabilities of microcomputers to address a problem that may be experienced by some poor readers. A second capability of computers that may be of specific aid to reading instruction is the ability to vary the pace of presentation of text. This capability, of course, might be used to address problems involving either too fast, too variable, or too slow processing of various kinds of text. The final capability that computers introduce to reading instruction involves allocation of control over both framing and pacing. In traditional reading situations, students have complete control over the way they process the text. They can re-read, or skip ahead as they like. However, for some instructional purposes, it may be appropriate to reserve some of the control over which portions of text are available for processing.

Some of the capabilities described above may have more immediate application to reading instruction than others. A few of the capabilities of modern computers are so new that they may actually lead to the development of new instructional goals. However, the point of this discussion is that there is a set of computer capabilities that do have immediate application to reading instruction, and our task is to identify ways that they may be employed most effectively. One aspect of instructional efficiency is to focus on the most important problems first. A number of authors (Lesgold, 1983; Torgesen and Young, 1983; Wilkenson, 1983) have suggested that the first use of computers should be to provide the extensive practice that learning disabled children require for the attainment of rapid and efficiently executed component skills in reading.

There is now a great deal of information about individual differences in reading supporting the idea that the primary locus of difficulty for most poor readers is at the individual word rather than discourse level of processing (Stanovich, 1982a, 1982b). Children with severe reading disabilities have problems both applying phonetically based word analysis procedures to new words and with rapidly recognizing words that they can pronounce accurately if given sufficient time. Given that teachers frequently find it difficult to provide the kind of closely monitored practice (involving both a speed and accuracy criterion) that children with reading disabilities may require to master word processing skills (Berliner and Rosenshine, 1977), computer applications in this area provide an opportunity to focus some of the unique capabilities of computers on a problem of first importance.

Many of the capabilities of computers discussed earlier make them particularly able to provide the practice that may be required to build rapid and efficient word reading skills in disabled children. Wilkenson (1983) has discussed a program called READINTIME that uses the framing and pacing capabilities of computers to help children become more acquainted with the structure of words. Lesgold (1983, 1982) has also indicated how the dynamic gaming capabilities of computers can be used to support practice in word recognition skills.

The use of computers to enhance word reading skills in disabled readers implies that computers be used primarily in a 'drill and practice' format at present. Because of limitations in speech recognition and production capacity, microcomputers are not able to provide initial tutoring in phonetically based word analysis skills. However, as Spring and Perry (in press) have shown, computers can be programmed to provide practice in these skills. Lesgold (1983) has also suggested that we have much better knowledge of the elements required for effective practice than we do about the exact ways to deliver good initial instruction in reading. This makes it likely that we will be able to do a better job programming practice activities than developing complex tutorials for new concepts. A final point in favor of an initial focus on using computers to provide practice that is supplemental to teacher-administered instruction is that the memory capabilities of currently available microcomputers cannot support the rapid and complex branching activities of good tutorial programs. One of the reasons the initial PLATO program in reading failed was that it simply operated too slowly (Yeager, 1977). Extremely complex programs on micros also must operate slowly because of the necessity of retrieving extra program steps from disk or tape storage.

Although most of the reading comprehension difficulties of disabled readers can be accounted for in terms of their inefficiency in decoding text, they also may have general comprehension problems related to lack of knowledge about complex syntax (Vogel, 1974), lack of background knowledge, or failure to use effective comprehension strategies while reading or listening (Bransford, Stein, and Vye, 1982; Paris, 1981). Computers will probably have important applications in enhancing abilities in a variety of these areas, although these problems are less well understood, and may be more difficult to program instruction for, than inefficient decoding skills.

CURRENTLY AVAILABLE SOFTWARE IN READING

The discussion of reading programs in this section is, of course, not comprehensive. There are at least several hundred individual computer programs now available that purport to teach a variety of skills important in reading. Instructional programs were selected for discussion here because they serve as examples of the best software available. Each of them also represents a particular approach to reading instruction and focuses on different skill areas.

Probably the most comprehensive reading instruction program currently available for microcomputers is the Micro-Read program published by American Educational Computer, Inc. This program employs excellent graphics and high quality audio output from digitially recorded speech to provide practice in reading skills ranging from simple grapheme–phoneme correspondence to advanced comprehension and study skills. Although it is a visually more attractive and interesting program than the earlier curriculum developed for larger computers, it lacks the latter program's sophisticated record-keeping capabilities and also has only a limited set of practice activities in each strand.

Limitation in the number of practice exercises that have an audio component are the result of the large storage requirements for digitally recorded speech. For example, although 74 floppy disk sides are required to store the 261 separate lessons covering skills from grade levels one through eight, 54 of the disk sides are used to store lessons in the first three levels. These levels, of course, focus more on phonics than comprehension skills, and more of their lessons require digital speech. Therefore, the limited memory capacity of currently available microsystems makes it difficult to program large amounts of reading practice that requires high quality audio output. This limitation in the number of practice activities for individual skills may make Micro-Read more appropriate as a back-up reading activity for children who learn normally than as a device for providing the extensive practice needed by dyslexic children.

A further limitation of the Micro-Read program is that it does not push children to a mastery criteria involving both speed and accuracy of response, but simply measures accuracy. It is to be hoped that programs such as Micro-Read can be further developed to provide both more individualized practice with larger numbers of exercises and emphasis on speed and accuracy in the execution of component skills in reading.

At the opposite extreme from the Micro-Read program in terms of compre-hensiveness are the Hint and Hunt programs (Hint and Hunt I, and Hint and Hunt II) offered by DLM Teaching Resources. Although these latter programs focus on a very limited range of reading skills, they offer the kind of intensive skill-building activities that appear particularly suited to children with moderate to severe reading problems.

The Hint and Hunt program was designed by researchers at the Learning Research and Development Center of the University of Pittsburgh to provide extensive practice recognizing and analysing words varying in medial vowels and vowel combinations. Hint and Hunt I provides practice on five short vowels and four vowel digraphs and diphthongs contained in simple words. Level II of the program practices the same vowels in more complex word environments and also teaches three new digraphs and diphthongs. Two aspects of the program make it attractive for use with reading disabled children. First, it focuses on a skill (recognizing the often variable sounds associated with medial vowels and vowel combinations) that is extremely difficult for poor readers. Second, it provides extensive practice activities in word analysis and recognition that emphasize both speed and accuracy of response.

There are two basic instructional activities to each Hint and Hunt program. First, the vowel sounds are introduced and practiced in an 'instructional mode' that employs a simple response format and does not emphasize speed. High quality digitized speech (similar to that used for the Micro-Read program) is used to present the sounds associated with the different vowels. The second activity employs a game format to provide extensive speed-oriented practice in recognizing words and nonsense syllables that contain the vowel sounds introduced in the instructional phase of the program. As in other programs currently available, the record-keeping and program control functions of the Hint and Hunt programs are primitive in comparison to the older, mainframe programs. Children must record their own scores for each activity, so that efficient use of the program may require a significant amount of teacher monitoring. However, the programs do focus on an area of special importance to disabled readers, and the use of exciting graphics and speed-based practice exemplifies the current state of the art in microcomputer-based programs to teach basic reading skills.

The 'Fundamental Word Focus' package offered by Random House also seeks to provide extensive practice on word-recognition skills, and some of these practice activities require children to respond rapidly. 'Fundamental Word Focus' is essentially a group of ten different games that provide different kinds of practice at reading and manipulating individual words. It is designed for children with fourth through ninth grade reading skills, so that it is not appropriate for children who are having problems mastering basic grapheme–phoneme translations. Rather, it is supposed to help students develop fluency and efficiency in word recognition once they have progressed beyond a basic instructional level.

A number of the games are modeled after traditional teaching or workbook activities, such as word search puzzles or alphabetization activities. Although these activities may be interesting to children, they do not fully utilize computer capabilities, nor do they provide the kind of direct practice in speeded word recognition that appears vital for dyslexic children. However, a number of other activities in the set do provide direct practice in word-recognition skills using a dynamic, game-like format that more fully utilizes computer capabilities. For example, one game called 'syllable attack' presents an initial consonant cluster in a box in the middle of the screen. At each side of the box, columns of word elements (vowel–consonant) descend at varying speed to smash 'cities' at the bottom of the screen. The child's task is to indicate which word elements form acceptable words with the consonant cluster in the box before the columns can reach the bottom of the screen. This program demands rapid processing and integration of word elements for successful performance.

Although the graphics and record keeping capabilities of 'Fundamental Word Focus' are primitive in comparison to both other programs for micros and the comprehensive programs for larger computers, the general focus of the programs may prove helpful in improving the word-processing fluency of disabled readers. One important feature of this program is the attempt that the program developers have made to show how activities on the computer can be integrated with off-line instructional activities by the teacher. If computers are to be used effectively as supplemental reading activities, then interactions with teacher-directed activities must be clearly articulated. Although there is a need for further development in this area, 'Fundamental Word Focus' does provide an example of beginning efforts in the right direction.

A program that was specifically developed to meet a particular instructional need of dyslexic children is the 'Compensatory Reading Program' developed by Fisher (in press) and available from Instructional/Communications Technology, Inc. Fisher's program is derived from a theory of reading disability (Fisher, 1979) that suggests the two primary problems of dyslexic children are: (1) difficulties learning to make translations between graphemic and phonemic information; and, (2) inability to use information available in the visual periphery while processing text. This theory is in agreement with the point made earlier that dyslexic children experience their most severe difficulties in the area of decoding, or individual word reading. However, it goes on to suggest that dyslexic children also have a problem utilizing cues available in the visual periphery to aid the processing of horizontally arranged text. Thus, Fisher suggests that dyslexic children may be trained to recognize individual words well, but may still be inefficient readers because they do not use peripheral information, such as word shape and spacing, to help them process connected text efficiently.

Fisher is careful to point out that his program is not sufficient to teach children to read. Rather, it is designed to improve reading fluency after basic word reading skills have been mastered. The program was designed for children in the fourth grade and above who have large sight vocabularies for words read individually, but who still follow a slow, word-by-word reading strategy when processing text. The basic operation of the program is simple. It uses the framing capabilities of the computer to present story text in a variety of visual formats. The child reads stories, or parts of stories, over and over in increasingly complex formats. The first time through a selection, there is only one word per line. The second time, two well spaced words are presented per line, and by the fifth reading of the entire story, the child is reading normally spaced text. The emphasis is for the child to read the stories orally as rapidly as possible, and a teacher or aide must be present to correct any word-reading errors that occur. The program is designed to be used for 15–20 minutes a day over a period of approximately five to eight weeks.

As Fisher (in press) presents them, the specific goals of the program are to: (1) help children become more rapid word recognizers; (2) make them better word sequencers; and, (3) help them become 'reacquainted' with left-to-right word attack sequencing skills. The initial word spacing is thought to reduce 'competition' between information available to foveal and peripheral vision, and to establish a habit of large, purposeful left–right eye movements while reading. The hope is that the particular sequence of training activities in the program will help dyslexic children learn to use information available in the visual periphery to more efficiently process horizontally arranged text.

The most important question about the 'Compensatory Reading Program' is whether it is more effective in increasing reading skills than other forms of extensive practice in processing text. For example, many of the goals and methods of a new technique called 'repeated reading' are similar to those outlined by Fisher for his program (Moyer, 1982). Although 'repeated reading' does not require the same modifications of text as are used in the Compensatory Reading Program, its proponents claim many of the same effects (increased fluency in processing text) as are claimed for the newer computer program. Clearly, we need much more careful, analytic research to determine if the method used by the Compensatory Reading Program is the best way to help reading disabled children develop the skills needed to process text rapidly and efficiently.

Although, as I mentioned before, we know very little about how to directly instruct comprehension skills, there are a number of programs available that have been designed to help increase reading comprehension in poor or beginning readers. As with most efforts to build comprehension skills, these programs do not explicitly teach special techniques to improve comprehension such as those being investigated in recent research on comprehension processes (Brown, Campione, and Day, 1981; Brown and Palincsar, 1982), but rather, they provide practice in responding to many different kinds of comprehension questions.

Two examples of comprehension programs that can both be used with children who have second grade reading skills and above are the Cloze-Plus program offered by Milliken, and Diascriptive Reading offered by Educational Activities, Inc. The strengths of the Cloze-Plus program include a well-developed record-keeping system that allows the teacher to pre-prescribe several different aspects of each child's assignment, such as starting point, length, and criteria for mastery. The program also has the capability to underline relevant portions of the text if a student has difficulty with a question and requests assistance.

The Diascriptive Reading Program (Level I) is simpler to operate than the Cloze-Plus, but it also provides broadly based practice in extracting a variety of different kinds of information from text or other printed material. The different lesson areas are called Details, Inference, Main Idea, Sequence, and Vocabulary, and each lesson draws attention to different kinds of information contained in text. The program uses an attractive format with large, easy-to-read letters, and attractive graphic reinforcers for correct responding. The program's developers have attempted to provide informative feedback for wrong answers that can help children learn to focus on critical features of text.

The main advantage of both of these programs over printed materials is that they provide immediate feedback about right and wrong answers. The format of the questions is multiple choice (although the Cloze-Plus does have some open-ended questions), and the actual exercises themselves are very similar to those available in cheaper printed materials. Both programs also provide good records of student performance, so they may save some teacher time in evaluating responses from paper-and-pencil tasks. Overall, the unique capabilities of computers currently appear to be less fully utilized in the area of comprehension practice than they are in programs designed to enhance speed and efficiency of decoding skills.

CONCLUDING COMMENTS

Microcomputers are currently being assimilated into classrooms largely on the basis of their intuitive appeal as instructional devices. Evaluation studies using large computer systems have shown that computers can help children learn to read better. However, both the hardware capabilities and the software used in the early studies are different from those currently available with microsystems. Thus, although we know in general that computers can be useful instructional devices in reading, we do not know if the instructional activities available on microcomputers can substantially alter children's reading skills.

For individuals concerned with the education of reading disabled children, the microcomputer provides many instructional capabilities not previously available. A central point of this chapter is that computers are most appropriately used at present in a supplemental role in resource rooms. It is clear that they cannot do some things as well as teachers (i.e. present new concepts in reading), but they may be capable of doing other things better, or at least for longer periods of time. For example, they may prove particularly helpful in providing the extensive practice (closely monitored for both speed and accuracy of response) that reading disabled children may require to master component skills in reading. A conclusion from this chapter is that the component skills most in need of CAI in dyslexic children are those involved in rapid word recognition and decoding.

Finally, although there are some promising beginnings in the production of software for microcomputers, an enormous amount of development work remains to be done. A lot of the software currently available merely mimics activities that can be accomplished with other, less expensive, media. The challenge is to develop software that will make maximum use of the unique capabilities offered by computers. From my vantage point, it seems that research efforts to develop the microcomputer as a useful tool in reading instruction will be one of the most exciting and productive areas of educational research over the next several years.

REFERENCES

Arter, J. A., and Jenkins, J. R. (1979), Differential diagnosis–prescriptive teaching: a critical appraisal. *Review of Educational Research* **49**, 517–555.

Berliner, D. C., and Rosenshine, B. (1977), The acquisition of knowledge in the classroom. In: Anderson, R. C., Spiro, R. J., and Montague, W. E. (Eds.), *Schooling and the Acquisition of Knowledge*. Hillsdale, NJ, Lawrence Erlbaum Associates.

Bransford, J. D., Stein, B. S., and Vye, N. J. (1982), Helping students learn how to learn from written texts. In: M. Singer (Ed.), *Competent Reader, Disabled Reader: Research and Application*. Hillsdale, NJ, Lawrence Erlbaum Associates.

Brown, A. L., Campione, J., and Day, J. D. (1981), Learning to learn: on training students to learn from texts. *Educational Researcher* 10, 2, 14–21.

Brown, A. L., and Palincsar, A. S. (1982), Inducing strategic learning from texts by means of informed, self-control training. *Topics in Learning and Learning Disabilities* 2, 1, 1–17.

Caldwell, R. M., and Rizza, P. A. A computer-based system of reading instruction for adult non-readers. *AEDS Journal* 12, 4, 155–162.

Fisher, D. F. (1979), Dysfunction in reading disability: there's more than meets the eye. In: L. Resnick and P. Weaver (Eds.), *Theory and Practice of Early Reading*, Vol. 1. Hillsdale, NJ, Lawrence Erlbaum.

Fisher, Dennis (1981), Compensatory training for disabled readers: implementing and refining. *Journal of Learning Disabilities* 14, 451–454.

Fisher, D. F. (in press), *Teacher's Guide: Compensatory Reading Program*. Huntington Station, NY, Instructional/Communication Technology, Inc.

Fletcher, J. D., and Atkinson, R. C. (1972), Evaluation of the standard CAI program in initial reading. *Journal of Educational Psychology* 63, 6, 597–602.

Fletcher, J. D., and Suppes, P. (1972), Computer assisted instruction in reading: grades 4–6. *Educational Technology* August, 45–49.

Golub, L. S. (1974), A computer-assisted literacy development program. *Journal of Reading* 17, 4, 279–284.

Green, D. R., Henderson, R. L., and Richards, H. C. (1968), Learning to recognize words and letters on a CAI terminal. ED 027 177, Arlington, Va., ERIC Document Reproduction Service.

Hallahan, D. P., and Kauffman, J. M. (1976), *Introduction to Learning Disabilities: A Psycho-behavioural Approach*. Englewood Cliffs, NJ, Prentice-Hall.

Hallworth, H. J., and Brebner, A. (1980), CAI for the developmentally handicapped: nine years of progress. Paper presented at the Association for the Development of Computer-Based Instructional Systems, Washington, DC, April, 1980. (ERIC Document Reproduction Service No. 198–792.)

Hammill, . and Bartel, N. R. (1975), *Teaching Children with Learning and Behavior Problems*. Boston, Allyn & Bacon.

Holland, P. W. (1980), Computer-assisted instruction: a longitudinal study panel presentation at the AERA Annual Conference, April, 1980.

Horn, W. F., O'Donnell, J. P., and Vitulano, L. A. (1983), Long-term follow-up studies of learning-disabled persons. *Journal of Learning Disabilities* 16, 542–555.

Jamison, D., Fletcher, J. D., Suppes, P., and Atkinson, R. C. (1975), Cost and performance of computer assisted instruction for compensatory education. In: R. R. Radner, and J. Froomkin (Eds.), *Education as an Industry*. New York, Columbia University Press.

Kulhavey, R. W. (1977), Feedback in written instruction. *Review of Educational Research* 47, 211–232.

LaBerge, D., and Samuels, S. J. (1974), Toward a theory of automatic information processing in reading. *Cognitive Psychology* 6, 293–323.

Lepper, M. R. (1982), Microcomputers in education: motivational and social issues. Paper presented at the annual meeting of the American Psychological Association, Washington, DC, August, 1982.

296   DYSLEXIA: ITS NEUROPSYCHOLOGY AND TREATMENT

Lesgold, A. M. (1982), Computer games for the teaching of reading. *Behavior Research Methods and Instrumentation* **14**, 224-226.

Lesgold, A. M. (1983), A rationale for computer-based reading instruction. In: A. C. Willienson (Ed.), *Classroom Computers and Cognitive Science*. New York, Academic Press.

Lesgold, A. M., and Resnick, L. B. (1982), How reading difficulties develop: perspectives from a longitudinal study. In: J. P. Das, R. F. Mulcaky, and A. E. Wall (Eds.), *Theory and Research in Learning Disabilities*. New York, Plenum Press.

Maxwell, M. (1980), *Improving Student Learning Skills*. San Francisco, Jossey-Bass.

Moyer, S. B. (1982), Repeated reading. *Journal of Learning Disabilities* **45**, 619-623.

Paris, S. G. (1981), Comprehension monitoring memory, and study strategies of good and poor readers. *Journal of Reading Behavior* **13**, 5-22.

Rashotte, C. A., and Torgesen, J. K. (1983), Repeated reading and reading fluency in learning disabled children. Unpublished manuscript, Florida State University.

Raynor, K., and McConkie, G. W. (1976), What guides a reader's eye movements? *Vision Research* **16**, 829-837.

Roblyer, M. D., and King, F. J. (1983), Reasonable expectations for computer-based instruction in basic reading skills. Paper presented at a meeting of the Association for Educational Communications and Technology, January, 1983.

Senf, G. M. (1983), Learning disabilities challenge coursework. *The Computing Teacher* **110**, 18-20.

Spring, C., and Perry, L. (in press), Computer-assisted instruction in work decoding for educationally-handicapped children. *Journal of Educational Technology Systems*.

Stanovich, K. E. (1982a) Individual differences in the cognitive processes of reading, I: Word decoding. *Journal of Learning Disabilities* **15**, 485-493.

Stanovich, K. E. (1982b) Individual differences in the cognitive processes of reading, II: Text-level processes. *Journal of Learning Disabilities* **15**, 549-554.

Sternberg, R. J., and Wagner, R. K. (1982), Automatization failure in learning disabilities. *Topics in learning and learning disabilities* **2**, 12-23.

Suppes, P., Jerman, M., and Brian, D. (1968), *Computer-assisted instruction: Standord's 1965-1966 Arithmetic Program*. New York, Academic Press.

Swinton, S., Amarel, M., and Morgan, J. (1978), The PLATO elementary demonstration education outcome evaluation. ED 106 020. Arlington, Va., ERIC Document Reproduction Service.

Tait, K., Hartley, J., and Anderson, R. C. (1974), Feedback procedures in computer-assisted arithmetic instruction. *British Journal of Educational Psychology* **43**, 2, 161-171.

Torgesen, J. K., and Young, K. (1983), Priorities for the use of micro-computers with learning disabled children. *Journal of Learning Disabilities* **16**, 234-237.

Vogel, S. A. (1974), Syntactic abilities in normal and dyslexic children. *Journal of Learning Disabilities* **7**, 103-109.

Wilkenson, A. C. (1983), Learning to read in real time. In A. C. Wilkenson, (Ed.), *Classroom computers and cognitive science*. N.Y.: Academic Press.

Wilson, H. A., and Atkinson, R. C. (1967), *Computer-based instruction in initial reading: A progress report on the Stanford Project*, Technical Report No. 119. Stanford University, Institute for Mathematical Studies in the Social Sciences.

Yeager, R. F. (1977), Lessons in the PLATO Elementary Reading Curriculum Project. ED 139 966. Arlington, Va.: ERIC Document Reproduction Service.

Author Index

297

Subject Index

304

Laterality, 45, 46, 59, 60, 172, 173
asymmetries, 173
bilateral anomalies, 45
of language, 52
quotient, 56
unilateral anomalies, 45
Lateralization, 45, 46, 173
Lateralized brain development, 47
Learned helplessness, 218, 219, 227
Learning, 35
pictographs, 35
symbols, 35
Learning disabilities, x, xi, 6, 9, 10, 11,
12, 13, 19, 20, 23, 24, 35, 55, 58,
59, 60, 61, 62, 73, 139, 145, 176,
204, 207, 212, 215, 216, 220, 222,
223, 224, 226, 227, 231, 232, 233,
234, 235, 236, 237, 238, 239, 240,
241, 242, 243, 244, 249, 250, 252,
290, 292, 293
assessment techniques, 12
attentional, 12
causes, 9
characteristics, xi, 24, 35
control group, 24
defined, xi, 9, 11, 250
developmental lag, 24
diagnosis, 11, 12, 238
educational opportunities, 35
emotional, 12
etiology, xi, 20, 35
exclusionary criteria, 12
experience factor, 24
inclusionary criteria, 12
learning, 12
linguistic status, 12
markers, 9, 20
neurological, 12
neurophysiological dysfunction, xi
perceptual-motor, 12
problems, 10
problems in mathematics, 9, 16, 17
processing breakdown, 24
proficiency factor, 24
referral conditions, 10
research, 10, 11, 12, 13, 20, 24, 34,
249
sampling, 9, 10, 11, 18, 20
selecting criteria for, 12
subtypes, xi, 20
symptomatology, 35

symptoms, 9, 10, 12, 20
teacher training, 249
treatments, 20
Learning disorders, 58, 59, 60, 206,
243
Left-handedness, xiv, 44, 52, 53, 54,
55, 56, 57, 58, 59, 60, 61, 71, 72,
74, 75, 77, 78, 80, 170, 171, 172
allergies, 59
autism, 54
dyslexia, 54
immune disorders, 44, 46, 47
immune system, 54
learning disabilities, 44
left–right confusion, 74
males, 61
migraine, 54, 59
migraine headaches, 44
myasthenia gravis, 59
rheumatoid arthritis, 59
stuttering, 54, 59
Lesion, 39, 44, 51, 53
Letters, 210, 211
Lexical ambiguity, 136, 139, 140, 141,
144
Lexical encoding, 160
Lexical levels, 144, 146
Lexical system, 160
Linguistic ability, 24, 33, 35
Linguistic awareness, 253, 259
Linguistic competence, 51
Linguistic context, 145
Linguistic deficits, 24
Linguistic factors, 166
Linguistic rules, 253
Linguistic skills, 34, 253, 254
accuracy on, 24
Linguistic structure, 32
Linguistic systems, 134
pictographic sentence construction,
32
Locus of control, 218

Magnetic resonance imaging, xiv 70,
78, 79, 84, 171
inversion recovery images, 78
spin echo, 78
Males, 14, 25, 53, 61
Manual dominance, 55
Marker system, 17, 18, 20
background, 18